HETEROSTRUCTURE LASERS

PART B ☐ **MATERIALS AND OPERATING CHARACTERISTICS**

QUANTUM ELECTRONICS — PRINCIPLES AND APPLICATIONS

A Series of Monographs

EDITED BY

YOH-HAN PAO
Case Western Reserve University
Cleveland, Ohio

PAUL KELLEY
Lincoln Laboratory
Massachusetts Institute of Technology
Lexington, Massachusetts

N. S. Kapany and J. J. Burke. OPTICAL WAVEGUIDES, 1972

Dietrich Marcuse. THEORY OF DIELECTRIC OPTICAL WAVEGUIDES, 1974

Benjamin Chu. LASER LIGHT SCATTERING, 1974

Bruno Crosignani, Paolo Di Porto, and Mario Bertolotti. STATISTICAL PROPERTIES OF SCATTERED LIGHT, 1975

John D. Anderson, Jr. GASDYNAMIC LASERS: AN INTRODUCTION, 1976

W. W. Duley. CO_2 LASERS: EFFECTS AND APPLICATIONS, 1976

Henry Kressel and J. K. Butler. SEMICONDUCTOR LASERS AND HETEROJUNCTION LEDs, 1977

H. C. Casey and M. B. Panish. HETEROSTRUCTURE LASERS: PART A, FUNDAMENTAL PRINCIPLES; PART B, MATERIALS AND OPERATING CHARACTERISTICS, 1978

In preparation

Robert K. Erf (Ed.). SPECKLE METROLOGY

HETEROSTRUCTURE LASERS

H. C. Casey, Jr.

Bell Laboratories
Murray Hill, New Jersey

M. B. Panish

Bell Laboratories
Murray Hill, New Jersey

PART B

Materials and Operating Characteristics

ACADEMIC PRESS   New York   San Francisco   London   1978

A Subsidiary of Harcourt Brace Jovanovich, Publishers

ACADEMIC PRESS, INC.
111 Fifth Avenue, New York, New York 10003

United Kingdom Edition published by
ACADEMIC PRESS, INC. (LONDON) LTD.
24/28 Oval Road, London NW1 7DX

Library of Congress Cataloging in Publication Data

Casey, Horace Craig, Date
     Heterostructure lasers.

     (Quantum electronics series)
     Includes bibliographical references and index.
     1. Semiconductor lasers. I. Panish, M. B., joint
author. II. Title. III. Series.
TA1700.C37   621.36'61   77–11211
ISBN 0–12–163102–8 (pt. B)

PRINTED IN THE UNITED STATES OF AMERICA

To Jean Anne and Evelyn

CONTENTS

CHAPTER 8 □ DEGRADATION

The evolution of early GaAs homostructure lasers into a variety of heterostructure lasers and the present commercial implementation of these devices have required the collaboration of scientists and engineers from several areas of the physical sciences. Many diverse skills had to be brought together to achieve an understanding of the fundamental principles, the preparation, and the operating characteristics of these devices. Future work, which will extend the research to other materials and structures, will continue to require an interdisciplinary understanding of this field. This book is a tutorial research monograph with emphasis on the interdisciplinary nature of the subject. It should be noted that we have included only those topics that are sufficiently well understood to be suitable in a tutorial work. Applications are not considered.

Each major topic is introduced along with the basic laws that govern the observed phenomena. The expressions relevant to heterostructure lasers are derived from the basic laws, and realistic numerical examples are given. For example, a crystal grower may not have studied the propagation of electromagnetic radiation or gain in a laser, while a physicist interested in those subjects may not have dealt previously with phase equilibria and crystal growth. The derivations, therefore, contain definitions and considerable detail to permit the reader to study an unfamiliar subject.

Both rigorous and approximate solutions are derived. In most cases, the resulting expressions may readily be evaluated with a hand calculator or simple computer programs. The availability of a minicomputer with a hard copy graphic output permitted us to easily illustrate numerical results in graphic form. Therefore, the reader can either follow the detailed derivations or simply obtain a brief overview from the numerous illustrations. The numerical examples are based on the GaAs–$Al_xGa_{1-x}As$ heterostructure. At the present time, the $Al_xGa_{1-x}As$ system provides the only heterostructures for which there are sufficient data to evaluate numerically the derived expressions.

There are several unique difficulties encountered in the preparation of a book on a rapidly evolving interdisciplinary subject. One is the notation in which the same symbols have been used to represent different quantities. Rather than defy convention, we have attempted, where possible, to use different fonts and other minor modifications. For example, the usual symbol for electron concentration and refractive index has been n, and these two cases are distinguished by adding a bar for refractive index $\bar{n}$. To distinguish x, y, and z as spatial coordinates, script x, y, and z have been used for solid-solution compositions. In other cases, the usage should identify the symbol. The second problem is the almost daily publication of papers on hetero-structure lasers. Not only do these papers provide additional data, but they often modify the interpretation of a particular concept. Chapter 4 had to be modified when the correct Γ, L, and X conduction band ordering in GaAs was established. We have attempted to be sufficiently fundamental so that continuing publications in the field will build on the principles presented here. Additional work will surely modify some of our present ideas. The third problem is the large number of publications on semiconductor lasers. Rather than attempt to include all papers, enough representative references are given to permit the interested reader to start a library search on a particular topic. Finally, the absence of students in an industrial laboratory environment prevented us from having an audience on which to try out the various presentations. However, Bell Laboratories provided access to a broad range of experts on many diverse subjects. As a result, the interdisci-plinary nature of the presentation was enhanced, and topics were included that otherwise would have been omitted.

ACKNOWLEDGMENTS

We wish to thank numerous colleagues both at Bell Laboratories and elsewhere that greatly aided the organization and preparation of this book. In Chapter 2, the approach used in the beam divergence derivation was suggested by L. Lewin. Discussions with J. L. Merz were helpful in the initial stages of the wave propagation derivations. W. T. Tsang provided insight into several of the derivations and made useful suggestions for the distributed-feedback presentation. In Chapter 3, F. Stern provided extensive guidance in the optical matrix element derivation as well as calculated (unpublished) gain coefficient spectra. Discussions with W. B. Joyce were useful in the description of blackbody radiation, and discussions with J. R. Brews were helpful in the screening length derivation. M. Lax provided useful suggestions on the proper use of Fermi's "Golden Rule." In the preparation of Chapter 4, discussions with W. B. Joyce were helpful in the presentation of the Fermi-level assignment. We want to thank R. Dingle for making his unpublished data on the composition dependence of the energy gap of $Al_xGa_{1-x}As$ available to us, and D. E. Aspnes for numerous discussions on the band structure of GaAs and $Al_xGa_{1-x}As$. In Chapter 6, comments by M. Ilegems were very helpful in deriving the thermodynamic relationships for the liquidus equation. Discussions with C. D. Thurmond aided the presentation of the phase equilibria. Discussions with A. Y. Cho contributed to the description of molecular-beam epitaxy. In Chapter 7, numerous discussions with W. B. Joyce and T. L. Paoli helped clarify many concepts and analyses. W. T. Tsang suggested the approximation used in combining the current spreading and lateral diffusion in stripe-geometry lasers. In Chapter 8, numerous discussions with B. C. De Loach, Jr., R. W. Dixon, R. L. Hartman, T. L. Paoli, C. H. Henry, P. M. Petroff, and D. V. Lang aided the presentation of degradation. M. Urbano made useful suggestions throughout the manuscript.

We would especially like to thank Miss Carol Eigenbrod and Mrs. Sylvia Lipton for typing the numerous drafts of this book in addition to their usual duties.

CONTENTS OF PART A

FUNDAMENTAL PRINCIPLES

5.1 INTRODUCTION

The semiconductor materials that have been used most extensively to fabricate heterostructure injection lasers are combinations of III–V compounds. Combinations of IV–VI compounds are also used in order to obtain much longer wavelength emission. Heterostructure lasers with low threshold current density and long operating life at room temperature have been made with GaAs–$Al_xGa_{1-x}As$ heterojunctions which were used as the illustrative case in Chapters 1–4. However, there are important wavelength regions that are not attainable by varying x in the active layers of $Al_xGa_{1-x}As$–$Al_yGa_{1-y}As$ DH lasers. There is considerable interest in the wavelength region between 1.0 and 1.4 μm because optical fibers have the lowest loss[1] and material dispersion[2] in this wavelength region. The variation of loss and material dispersion with wavelength for multimode fibers is illustrated in Fig. 5.1-1. In Fig. 5.1-1a, it is shown that the loss in state-of-the-art fibers with a germania-doped-silica (GeO_2–SiO_2) core and a borosilicate (B_2O_3–SiO_2) cladding is presently very close to the fundamental limits resulting from scattering and from absorption by the Si–O bond. Scattering loss is due to refractive index fluctuations within the fiber. Low-loss fibers are also obtained with phosphosilicate (P_2O_5–SiO_2) cores.[3] The material dispersion plot of Fig. 5.1-1b is for a GeO_2–SiO_2 core and B_2O_3–SiO_2 cladding fiber and shows that the material dispersion for this fiber goes through zero near 1.25 μm. Cohen and Lin[2] also consider the dependence on doping of the wavelength for the zero material dispersion. The waveguide dispersion of a mode due to the frequency dependence of the propagation constant of the individual modes is believed to be negligible, and intermodal dispersion due to transit time differences between modes can be very small in graded-index multimode fibers.[2] Because low-loss fibers are expected to be available routinely, considerable effort has been concentrated on materials that emit in the 1.0–1.4 μm wavelength region. That effort has resulted in cw room-temperature operation at about 1.1 μm with $GaAs_{0.88}Sb_{0.12}$–$Al_{0.4}Ga_{0.6}As_{0.88}Sb_{0.12}$ (Ref. 4), InP–$Ga_{0.12}In_{0.88}$-$P_{0.77}As_{0.23}$ (Ref. 5), and $Ga_xIn_{1-x}As$–$Ga_yIn_{1-y}P$ (Ref. 6) DH lasers. In addition to these systems, other combinations of binary, ternary, or quaternary III–V compounds are expected to be studied in order to match various optical fiber transmission properties, to obtain visible laser emission, and to satisfy various application requirements. In the IV–VI system, hetero-

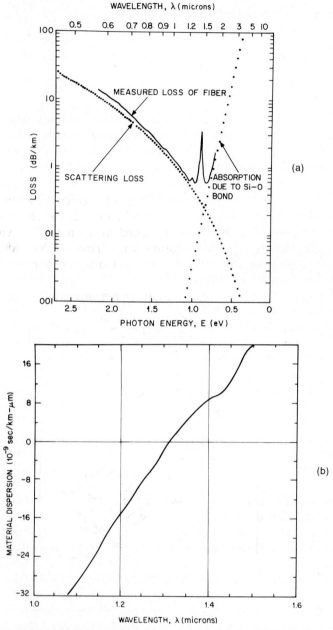

FIG. 5.1-1   Transmission properties of state-of-the-art GeO$_2$–SiO$_2$ core and B$_2$O$_3$–SiO$_2$ cladding optical fibers. (a) Transmission loss for a 0.23 numerical aperature (NA) and a 60-μm-diameter core fiber (Ref. 1). (b) Material dispersion for a 0.26 NA and a 50-μm-diameter core fiber (Ref. 2).

structure lasers have been made primarily with PbTe–Pb$_{1-x}$Sn$_x$Te hetero-junctions.

With III–V heterostructure lasers, the performance of the device appears to depend not only upon the energy gap E_g and refractive index disconti-nuities at the heterojunctions that provide carrier and optical confinement, but also upon the structural quality of the heterojunction interface and the epitaxial layers. A particular problem is the formation of lattice defects due to lattice mismatch between the semiconductors that comprise the hetero-junctions. These defects, particularly dislocations, may reduce the efficiency of radiative recombination and, as described in Chapter 8, reduce the operating life of the device. In III–V systems, the ability to achieve a hetero-junction of sufficiently high quality to yield useful heterostructure lasers appears to be strongly dependent upon the achievement of a close lattice match between the heterojunction materials. In fact, the ability to grow high-quality heteroepitaxial layers is dependent upon a reasonably close lattice match at the growth temperature. This chapter is devoted to a dis-cussion of the various binary, ternary, and quaternary systems that may be useful for heterostructure lasers.

Examples of such III–V solid solutions are given in Figs. 5.1-2 and

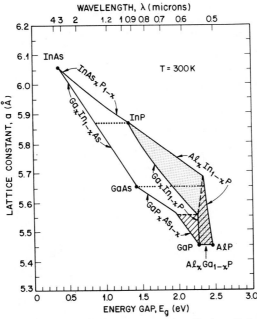

FIG. 5.1-2 Energy gap and lattice constant for Ga$_x$In$_{1-x}$P$_y$As$_{1-y}$ (clear) and (Al$_x$Ga$_{1-x}$)$_y$In$_{1-y}$P (shaded). Dashed lines separate direct- and indirect-energy-gap re-gions, and the cross hatch designates the indirect-energy-gap regions. Dotted lines show lattice match to binary compounds.

5.1-3. These figures show the variation of the energy gap (emission wavelength) with lattice constant for several ternary and quaternary solid solution systems that are discussed in this chapter. Note that for conversion between photon energy E and wavelength λ,

$$E \text{ (eV)} = 1.2398/\lambda \text{ (μm)}. \tag{5.1-1}$$

The boundaries joining the binary compounds give the ternary energy gap and lattice constant. The cross-hatch indicates indirect-energy-gap material. Note that both direct- and indirect-energy-gap material may be useful for heterostructure lasers. The active region requires an energy gap that is direct, while the surrounding wider energy-gap material may be direct or indirect. Regions where there is a lattice match to a binary are of particular interest. The dotted lines in these figures give the lattice match to the indicated binary.

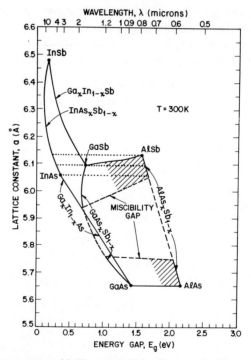

FIG. 5.1-3 Energy gap and lattice constant for $Ga_xIn_{1-x}As_ySb_{1-y}$ and $Al_xGa_{1-x}As_y$-Sb_{1-y}. The dashed lines show the edge of a miscibility gap of uncertain extent in the $Al_xGa_{1-x}As_ySb_{1-y}$ system. The miscibility gap along $GaAs_xSb_{1-x}$ must extend into the $Ga_xIn_{1-x}As_ySb_{1-y}$ system, but is not shown in the figure because of its uncertain extent. Cross hatch designates indirect-energy-gap regions. Dotted lines show lattice match to binary compounds.

Figure 5.1-2 shows the $Ga_xIn_{1-x}P_yAs_{1-y}$ and $(Al_xGa_{1-x})_yIn_{1-y}P$ quaternary solid solutions as the clear and shaded regions, respectively. The dotted lines indicate solid solutions that lattice match GaAs or InP. As shown by this figure, solid solutions that are lattice matched to InP can have emission energies (wavelengths) from about 0.85 eV (1.46 μm) to 1.2 eV (1.03 μm), while solid solutions lattice matched to GaAs have emission energies from about 1.4 eV (0.89 μm) to 2.1 eV (0.59 μm). Similarly, Fig. 5.1-3 shows the $Al_xGa_{1-x}As_ySb_{1-y}$ and $Ga_xIn_{1-x}As_ySb_{1-y}$ systems. The dotted lines indicate solid solutions that lattice match to AlSb, GaSb, and InAs. Also, GaAs and $Al_xGa_{1-x}As$ lattice match along the GaAs–AlAs boundary. These lattice matched systems permit laser emission from about 0.4 eV (3.0 μm) to 1.1 eV (1.1 μm). In Fig. 5.1-3, a region of compositions that may not exist due to a miscibility gap is also illustrated. The various sections of this chapter are devoted to a detailed description of these solid solutions as well as other III–V and IV–VI systems. Figure 5.1-4 summarizes the presently or potentially available wavelengths for many of the laser materials discussed in this chapter.

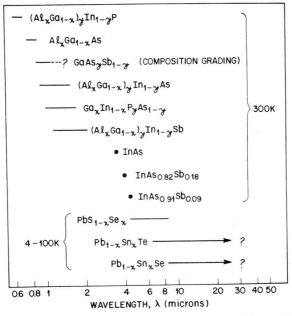

FIG. 5.1-4 Emission wavelengths either presently or potentially available with III–V and IV–VI heterostructure lasers. Except for $GaAs_ySb_{1-y}$ and $Ga_xIn_{1-x}As$, where low threshold lasers have been obtained with composition grading, all the III–V systems listed are for the active regions of lattice-matched heterostructure lasers. Binary and ternary active regions are included here in some cases as the end points of ternary and quaternary composition ranges.

The properties of the binary III–V compounds that are relevant to heterostructure lasers are given in Section 5.2. As shown in Figs. 5.1-2 and 5.1-3, the binary compounds are required as bulk crystal substrates for subsequent epitaxial growth of heterostructure layers. The extension of the binary III–V compounds to the III–V ternary solid solutions is presented in Section 5.3 with emphasis on the compositional dependence of the energy gap. A discussion of the various III–V binary and ternary lattice-matching systems for heterostructure lasers is given in Section 5.4. The lattice-matched DH of GaAs–$Ga_{0.51}In_{0.49}P$ is discussed in considerable detail to illustrate carrier confinement when ΔE_c is zero. Additional lattice-matched hetero-structure lasers are possible with III–V binary and quarternary systems discussed in Section 5.5. A successful example is InP–$Ga_{0.12}In_{0.88}P_{0.77}As_{0.23}$. Other heterostructure lasers are made possible by growing compositionally graded layers on a substrate so that the ternary or quaternary active layer and adjacent layers have the same lattice constant. A discussion of dislocation generation in compositionally graded epitaxial layers and heterostructure lasers prepared on these layers is presented in Section 5.6. Although reasonably complete examples are given in each section, not all of the properties necessary for a quantitative description of heterostructure lasers are well known for many of the III–V crystalline solid solutions.

The properties of the binary IV–VI compounds and their extension as crystalline ternary solid solutions for heterostructure lasers are given in Section 5.7. These materials are in an earlier stage of development than the III–V compounds. The calculated energy gaps and experimental data for $Pb_{1-x}Sn_xTe$ and $Pb_{1-x}Sn_xSe$ show that the energy gap decreases as x increases from zero and as x decreases from unity, so that it passes through zero within the ternary composition range. This unusual feature permits heterostructure lasers capable of emitting far into the infrared. Another unusual feature is the variation of E_g with temperature which is opposite to the behavior observed in III–V compounds. Unlike the III–V hetero-structures, lattice mismatch does not appear to be a serious problem either for epitaxial growth or for nonradiative recombination center formation. The relaxation of one set of difficulties has, however, been offset by the acquisition of another problem. The lattice vacancies that are at equilibrium during growth persist when the crystal is cooled and influence the crystal conductivity at the IV–VI laser operating temperature.

5.2 III–V BINARY COMPOUNDS

Crystal Structure and Lattice Constants

The III–V compounds of interest here are those between Al, Ga, and In (group III) and P, As, and Sb (group V). They crystallize in the zinc-blende

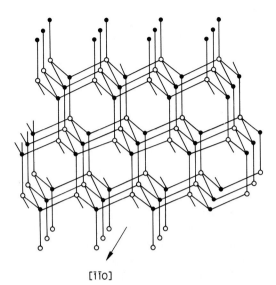

[$\bar{1}\bar{1}0$]

FIG. 5.2-1   The zinc-blende structure.

structure. That structure consists of two interpenetrating face-centered cubic lattices with the atoms tetrahedrally coordinated as shown in Fig. 5.2-1. A unit cell for this structure is shown in Fig. 5.2-2. The symbol { } represents a family of planes and the symbol ( ) generally represents a specific plane. The six faces of the cube in Fig. 5.2-2 with lattice constant a representing

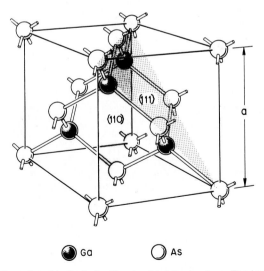

● Ga   ○ As

FIG. 5.2-2   The unit cell in GaAs for the zinc-blende structure. The lattice constant is a. The six faces of the cube are the six equivalent {100} planes.

the unit cell are the six equivalent {100} planes. The diagonal plane that includes both Ga and As atoms is one of the four {110} planes which are the natural cleavage planes in III–V compounds. The triangular cut through As atoms in the unit cell represents one of the eight {111} crystal planes. Equivalent sets of {100} and {111} planes can be drawn through Ga atoms when the equivalent unit cell with Ga atoms in the corners is used. Frequently the orientation is described in terms of the direction in the crystal. For zinc-blende crystals, the crystal directions are normal to the crystal planes and in the general case are represented in angled brackets $\langle\ \rangle$. Thus in Fig. 5.2-1, one arrow represents the specific $[1\bar{1}0]$ direction, and the general designation is $\langle 110\rangle$ for all $\langle 110\rangle$ directions.

The lattice constants of the III–V binary compounds are summarized in Table 5.2-1. The nominal stoichiometry of the III–V compounds is obviously one group III atom per group V atom. Deviations from this stoichiometry which result from the presence of vacancy and interstitial atoms are influenced by the crystal growth conditions.[7] Annealing results for GaAs[8] suggest that the variations of the lattice constant with stoichiome-

TABLE 5.2-1   Lattice Constants of the Binary III–V Compounds

Compound	Lattice constant, a(Å)	$T°C$	Reference
AlP	5.451	—	a
AlAs	5.6605	0	b
AlSb	6.1355	18	c
GaP	5.45117	25	d
GaAs	5.65325	27	e
GaSb	6.09593	—	f
InP	5.86875	18	c
InAs	6.0584	18	c
InSb	6.47937	25	f

a A. Addamiano, *J. Am. Chem. Soc.* **82**, 1537 (1960).

b M. Ettenberg and R. J. Paff, *J. Appl. Phys.* **41**, 3926 (1970).

c G. Giesecke and H. Pfister, *Acta Crystallogr.* **11**, 369 (1958).

d R. L. Barns, Private communication. This value represents the average for vapor-grown (5.45114 Å) and solution-grown (5.45120 Å) samples.

e C. M. H. Driscoll, A. F. W. Willoughby, J. B. Mullin, and B. W. Straughan, "Gallium Arsenide and Related Compounds, 1974," p. 275. Inst. of Phys., London, 1975.

f M. E. Straumanis and C. D. Kim, *J. Appl. Phys.* **36**, 3822 (1965).

try will be less than $\sim 10^{-3}$ Å and for the purposes of this chapter can be ignored. The effects of impurities on the lattice constant are smaller.[9]

Energy Gaps

The band structures of most of the binary III–V compounds are well known and are generally rather similar. The band structure of GaAs was illustrated in Fig. 4.2-1. The energy gaps E_g for the III–V compounds of interest are summarized in Table 5.2-2. As mentioned in Section 3.8, it is

TABLE 5.2-2   Energy Gaps of the Binary III–V Compounds

Compound	Type of energy gap	Experimental energy gap, E_g (eV)				Temperature dependence of energy gap, $E_g(T)$ (eV)	Ref.
		0°K	Ref.	300°K	Ref.		
AlP	indirect	2.52	a	2.45	a	$2.52 - 3.18 \times 10^{-4} T^2/(T + 588)^r$	n
AlAs	indirect	2.239	b	2.163	b	$2.239 - 6.0 \times 10^{-4} T^2/(T + 408)^r$	b
AlSb	indirect	1.687	c	1.58	d	$1.687 - 4.97 \times 10^{-4} T^2/(T + 213)^r$	c
GaP	indirect	2.338	e	2.261	e	$2.338 - 5.771 \times 10^{-4} T^2/(T + 372)$	o
GaAs	direct	1.519	f	1.424	g	$1.519 - 5.405 \times 10^{-4} T^2/(T + 204)$	o
GaSb	direct	0.810	h	0.726	i	$0.810 - 3.78 \times 10^{-4} T^2/(T + 94)^r$	p
InP	direct	1.421	j	1.351	j	$1.421 - 3.63 \times 10^{-4} T^2/(T + 162)^r$	j
InAs	direct	0.420	k	0.360	l	$0.420 - 2.50 \times 10^{-4} T^2/(T + 75)^r$	q
InSb	direct	0.236	m	0.172	i	$0.236 - 2.99 \times 10^{-4} T^2/(T + 140)^r$	p

^{a} M. R. Lorenz, R. Chicotka, G. D. Pettit, and P. J. Dean, *Solid State Commun.* **8**, 693 (1970).

^{b} B. Monemar, *Phys. Rev.* **B8**, 5711 (1973). This value in Table 5.2-2 includes an exciton binding energy of 0.010 eV.

^{c} N. N. Sirota and A. I. Lukomskii, *Sov. Phys.-Semicond.* **7**, 140 (1973) [*Translated from.: Fiz. Tekh. Poluprov.* **7**, 196 (1973)].

^{d} K.-Y. Cheng, Stanford Electron. Lab., Tech. Rep. No. 5111-5 (August 1975).

^{e} M. R. Lorenz, G. D. Pettit, and R. C. Taylor, *Phys. Rev.* **171**, 876 (1968).

^{f} D. D. Sell, S. E. Stokowski, R. Dingle, and J. V. DiLorenzo, *Phys. Rev.* **B7**, 4568 (1973).

^{g} D. D. Sell and H. C. Casey, Jr., *J. Appl. Phys.* **45**, 800 (1974).

^{h} E. J. Johnson. I. Filinski, and H. Y. Fan, *Proc. Int. Conf. Phys. Semiconduct., Exeter,* 1962 p. 375. Inst. of Phys. and Phys. Soc., London, 1962.

^{i} D. Auvergne, J. Camassel, H. Mathieu, and A. Joullie, *J. Phys. Chem. Solids* **35**, 133 (1974).

^{j} W. J. Turner and W. E. Reese, "Radiative Recombination in Semiconductors, Paris, 1964," p. 59. Dunod, Paris, 1965.

^{k} C. R. Pidgeon, D. L. Mitchell, and R. N. Brown, *Phys. Rev.* **154**, 737 (1967).

^{l} S. Zwerdling, B. Lax, and L. M. Roth, *Phys. Rev.* **108**, 1402 (1957).

^{m} S. Zwerdling, W. H. Kleiner, and J. P. Theriault, *J. Appl. Phys.* **32**, 2118 (1961).

^{n} B. Monemar, *Solid State Commun.* **8**, 1295 (1970). The technique used to assign E_g in this paper will give a value less than E_g. Therefore, $0.030 + 4 \times 10^{-5} T$ has been added to the values in this paper to agree with the values in Lorenz *et al.*^{a}

^{o} C. D. Thurmond, *J. Electrochem. Soc.* **122**, 1133 (1975).

^{p} J. Camassel and D. Auvergene, *Phys. Rev.* **B12**, 3258 (1975).

^{q} J. R. Dixon and J. M. Ellis. *Phys. Rev.* **123**, 1560 (1961).

^{r} The parameters α and θ were assigned from the experiment data by C. D. Thurmond, private communication.

necessary to have a direct-energy-gap material in order to obtain net stimulated emission; however, the confining wider energy-gap layers may be direct or indirect. In Section 4.2, the temperature dependence of the direct-energy gap was given by Eq. (4.2-1). This equation has the general form of[10]

$$E_g(T) = E_g(0) - \alpha T^2/(T + \theta), \tag{5.2-1}$$

where $E_g(0)$ is the energy gap at $0°K$, α an empirical parameter of $\sim 5 \times 10^{-4}$ eV/°K, and θ an empirical parameter often near the Debye temperature. Expressions of the form of Eq. (5.2-1) are also given in Table 5.2-2. The temperature dependence of E_g is useful because it represents approximately the variation of the laser emission photon energy with temperature. The energy gap as a function of temperature also occurs in the expression for the intrinsic carrier concentration that was given by Eq. (4.3-43).

Properties Relevant to Heterojunctions

Numerous properties of the III–V binary compounds have been reported. A useful summary was given by Neuberger.[11] The properties summarized in Table 5.2-3 have been limited to those useful in consideration of heterostructure lasers.

Equation (4.3-1) gave the step in the conduction band ΔE_c as the electron affinity χ_1 of the narrow-energy-gap semiconductor minus the electron affinity χ_2 of the wide-energy-gap semiconductor. Thus, for a positive ΔE_c, χ_1 must be larger than χ_2. Unfortunately, it is not clear how well the available values represent the actual electron affinities, and the applicability of χ to assignment of ΔE_c has not been demonstrated. As discussed in Chapter 4, measured values of ΔE_c have been given only for $Al_xGa_{1-x}As$. Therefore, estimates of ΔE_c for other cases must be based on the electron affinity data available at the present time. The values of χ in Table 5.2-3 have been revised from the original references to account for the more recent values of E_g. Note that the electron affinity of III–V binary compounds increases with atomic weight of the group III element.

As summarized in Table 4.3-3, the heterojunction built-in potential requires evaluation of the Fermi levels. The Fermi level is influenced by the effective mass through the effective density of states. Therefore, the next two columns in Table 5.2-3 summarize the density of states electron effective mass m_n and hole effective mass m_p. The division of the potential between the sides of the heterojunction depends on the fully ionized impurity concentration and the dielectric constant. The dielectric constants are given next in Table 5.2-3.

In Section 2.4, it was shown by Eq. (2.4-44) that for guided modes the refractive index $\bar{n}$ of the active layer must be larger than $\bar{n}$ of the bounding layers. The room-temperature refractive indices at the photon energy of the energy gap are given in Table 5.2-3. As illustrated in Fig. 5.2-3, the variation of $\bar{n}$ with photon energy E is different near E_g for the direct-energy-gap semiconductor GaAs in Fig. 5.2-3a[12] and for the indirect-energy-gap semiconductor AlAs in Fig. 5.2-3b.[13] The variation of $\bar{n}$ with carrier concentration for GaAs was given in Figs. 2.5-2 and 2.5-3. The refractive index also has a temperature dependence, and a good example of this dependence for GaAs has been given by Marple.[14] An extensive summary of $\bar{n}$ over a large range in photon energy for the various III–V binary compounds has been given by Seraphin and Bennett.[15]

The last column of Table 5.2-3 gives the thermal conductivities which are important for the determination of heat flow at high excitation. These values have been taken mostly from the critical assessment by Maycock.[16] Further details may be found in Ref. 16. The thermal conductivity depends also on temperature and impurity content of the crystal.[16] A discussion of the heat flow problem for stripe-geometry GaAs–Al$_x$Ga$_{1-x}$As DH lasers is given in Section 7.8.

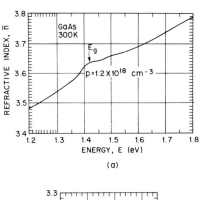

(a)

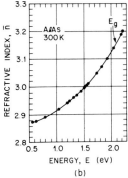

(b)

FIG. 5.2-3   Refractive index as a function of photon energy. (a) GaAs (Ref. 12). (b) AlAs (Ref. 13).

TABLE 5.2-3 Selected Properties of III–V Binary Compounds

Compound	Electron affinity χ(eV)	Ref.	Conduction band effective mass m_n	Ref.	Valence band effective mass m_p	Ref.	Dielectric constant ε	Ref.	Refractive index at E_g, $\bar{n}$	Ref.	Thermal conductivity σ (W/cm-deg)	Ref.
AlP	—	—	—	—	$0.70m_0$	f	—	—	3.027	y	0.9	ff
AlAs	—	—	$0.15m_0$	g	$0.79m_0$	f	$10.1\varepsilon_0$	q	3.178	q	0.91	gg
AlSb	3.64	a	$0.12m_0$	h	$0.98m_0$	f	$14.4\varepsilon_0$	r	>3.4	z	0.57	ff
GaP	4.0^{est}	b	$0.82m_0$	i	$0.60m_0$	j	$11.1\varepsilon_0$	s	3.452	aa	0.77	ff
GaAs	4.05	c	$0.067m_0$	k	$0.48m_0$	k	$13.1\varepsilon_0$	t	3.655	bb	0.44	ff
GaSb	4.03	c	$0.042m_0$	h	$0.44m_0$	l	$15.7\varepsilon_0$	u	3.82	cc	0.33	ff
InP	4.4	d	$0.077m_0$	m	$0.64m_0$	n	$12.4\varepsilon_0$	v	3.450	dd	0.68	ff
InAs	4.54	e	$0.023m_0$	m	$0.40m_0$	o	$14.6\varepsilon_0$	w	~3.52	w	0.27	ff
InSb	4.59	c	$0.0145m_0$	p	$0.40m_0$	p	$17.7\varepsilon_0$	x	~4.0	ee	0.17	ff

[a] T. E. Fischer, *Phys. Rev.* **139**, A1228 (1965).
[b] A. M. Cowley and S. M. Sze, *J. Appl. Phys.* **36**, 3212 (1965).
[c] G. W. Gobeli and F. G. Allen, *Phys. Rev.* **137**, A245 (1965).
[d] T. E. Fischer, *Phys. Rev.* **142**, 519 (1966).
[e] T. E. Fischer, F. G. Allen, and G. W. Gobeli, *Phys. Rev.* **163**, 703 (1967).
[f] P. Lawaetz, *Phys. Rev. B* **4**, 3460 (1971).
[g] D. J. Stukel and R. N. Euwema, *Phys. Rev.* **188**, 1193 (1969).
[h] H. Mathieu, D. Auvergne, P. Merle, and K. C. Rustagi, *Phys. Rev. B* **12**, 5846 (1975).
[i] A. Onton, *Phys. Rev.* **186**, 786 (1969) has given $m_t = 0.191m_0$ and $m_l = 1.7m_0$. For three equivalent minima, $m_n = 3^{2/3}(m_l m_t^2)^{1/3} = 0.82m_0$.

[j] C. C. Bradley, P. E. Simmonds, J. R. Stockton, and R. A. Stradling, *Solid State Commun.* **12**, 413 (1973).

[k] Q. H. F. Vrehen, *J. Phys. Chem. Solids* **29**, 129 (1968).

[l] D. Auvergne, J. Camassel, H. Mathieu, and A. Joullie, *J. Phys. Chem. Solids* **35**, 133 (1974).

[m] E. D. Palik and R. F. Wallis, *Phys. Rev.* **123**, 131 (1961).

[n] J. Leotin, R. Barbaste, S. Askenzy, M. S. Skolnick, R. A. Stradling, and J. Tuchendler, *Solid State Commun.* **15**, 693 (1974).

[o] C. R. Pidgeon, D. L. Mitchell, and R. N. Brown, *Phys. Rev.* **154**, 737 (1967).

[p] C. R. Pidgeon and R. N. Brown, *Phys. Rev.* **146**, 575 (1966).

[q] R. E. Fern and A. Onton, *J. Appl. Phys.* **42**, 3499 (1971).

[r] D. Shaw and H. D. McKell, *Brit. J. Appl. Phys.* **14**, 295 (1963).

[s] A. S. Barker, Jr., *Phys. Rev.* **165**, 917 (1968).

[t] I. Strzalkowski, S. Joshi, and C. R. Crowell, *Appl. Phys. Lett.* **28**, 350 (1976).

[u] M. Hass and B. W. Henvis, *Phys. Chem. Solids* **23**, 1099 (1962).

[v] C. Hilsum, S. Fray, and C. Smith, *Solid State Commun.* **7**, 1057 (1969).

[w] O. G. Lorimor and W. G. Spitzer, *J. Appl. Phys.* **36**, 1841 (1965).

[x] R. B. Sanderson, *J. Phys. Chem. Solids* **26**, 803 (1965).

[y] B. Monemar, *Solid State Commun.* **8**, 1295 (1970).

[z] B. O. Seraphin and H. E. Bennett, "Semiconductors and Semimetals, Vol. 3" (R. K. Willardson and A. C. Beer, eds.), p. 499. Academic Press, New York, 1967.

[aa] D. F. Nelson and E. H. Turner, *J. Appl. Phys.* **39**, 3337 (1968).

[bb] D. D. Sell, H. C. Casey, Jr., and K. W. Wecht, *J. Appl. Phys.* **45**, 2650 (1974).

[cc] D. F. Edwards and G. S. Haynes, *J. Opt. Soc. Am.* **49**, 414 (1959).

[dd] G. D. Pettit and W. J. Turner, *J. Appl. Phys.* **36**, 2081 (1965).

[ee] T. S. Moss, S. D. Smith, and T. D. F. Hawkins, *Proc. Phys. Soc. London* **B70**, 776 (1957).

[ff] P. D. Maycock, *Solid State Electron.* **10**, 161 (1967).

[gg] M. A. Afromowitz, *J. Appl. Phys.* **44**, 1292 (1973).

5.3 III–V TERNARY SOLID SOLUTIONS

Crystalline Solid Solutions

When compounds are formed that have more than one group III element distributed randomly on group III lattice sites or more than one group V element distributed randomly on group V lattice sites, those compounds are crystalline solid solutions. As described in Chapter 1, the notation most frequently used, and used throughout this book, is $A_x B_{1-x} C_y D_{1-y}$ with A and B for the group III elements and with C and D for the group V elements. If A, B, and C are group III elements and D is a group V element, the notation $(A_x B_{1-x})_y C_{1-y} D$ is convenient. A similar notation is used for the solid solution with three group V elements and one group III element. If solid solutions with all values of x or y between 0 and 1 can exist, the system is said to consist of a complete series of solid solutions. This is a condition that occurs for a number of III–V systems. Phase and thermodynamic studies suggest that the tendency towards unmixing, i.e., a limiting of the possible range of x and y to less than 0 to 1, increases with increasing difference in the covalent radii of the different atoms occupying the same set of lattice sites.

In ternary III–V solid solutions, the lattice constant of the crystal generally scales linearly with composition (Vegard's law), and this behavior can be reasonably assumed to occur also for the quaternary solid solutions. Linear variation with composition does not, in general, occur for the other properties. However, when detailed data are unavailable, it is often necessary to use linear interpolation.

The variation of E_g with composition is the primary property of interest when considering heterojunctions. As illustrated in Chapter 4, not only is the energy difference from the valence band to the lowest lying conduction band important, but the energy separating the various conduction band minima can influence heterostructure laser performance. Therefore, it is useful to know the compositional dependence of the Γ, L, and X conduction-band minima. There are 18 conceivable ternary systems among the group III and group V elements of interest, and experimental data are available for more than half of these. For most of the rest, it is likely that extensive solid solutions do not exist. The energy-gap compositional dependence often can be represented by

$$E_g = a + bx + cx^2 \qquad (5.3\text{-}1)$$

for the ternary solid solution $A_x B_{1-x} C$ or $AC_y D_{1-y}$. The bowing parameter c has been treated theoretically by Van Vechten and Bergstresser.[17] Their theory may be used to estimate c when experimental data are unavailable.

The available experimental compositional dependence of E_g in the ternary solid solutions is summarized in this section.

Because no data are available for the ternaries, properties such as electron affinity and dielectric constant that were given in Table 5.2-3 for III–V binaries are taken to have a linear compositional dependence. The effective mass, however, can have a quadratic dependence on composition.[18] Depending on the system, the bowing parameter can be small so that the more convenient linear dependence may be used.

The compositional dependence of the refractive index has been determined for only a few of these ternary systems. The refractive index for $Al_xGa_{1-x}As$ has been measured over the composition range of interest for heterostructure lasers[19] and was summarized in Figs. 2.5-4 and 2.5-5. Data has also been obtained for GaP_xAs_{1-x}.[20,21] Afromowitz[22] used a modification of the semi-empirical single-effective-oscillator model[23] to include an approximation of the absorption spectrum and evaluated $\bar{n}$ as a function of x for photon energies less than E_g for $Al_xGa_{1-x}As$, GaP_xAs_{1-x}, and $Ga_xIn_{1-x}P$. These models in Refs. 22 and 23 can be useful for the calculation of $\bar{n}$ as a function of E for systems where no experimental data are available.

The thermal conductivity in the ternary solid solution is generally a minimum near $x = 0.50$.[16,24] For $Al_xGa_{1-x}As$, the thermal conductivity decreases from the binary values by a factor of four when x is between 0.4 and 0.6.[24] This behavior means that the thermal resistance is more of a problem in the ternaries than in the binary compounds. Additional properties of the III–V ternary solid solutions may be found in the compilation by Neuberger.[25] The next part of this section presents many of the available E_g versus x diagrams for the III–V ternary solid solutions. An earlier compilation was given by Onton.[26]

$Al_xIn_{1-x}P$

The room temperature compositional dependence of the Γ direct-energy gap and the X indirect-energy gap have been measured by cathodoluminescence.[27,28] The composition was determined by x-ray microprobe analysis. The results of Onton and Chicotka[27] are shown in Fig. 5.3-1. This system has the direct–indirect transition at $x = 0.44$ with $E_g = 2.33$ eV. The linear variation of the direct-energy gap shown in Fig. 5.3-1 is represented by the expression given in Table 5.3-1.

$Al_xGa_{1-x}As$

The most intensively studied III–V ternary solid solution for heterostructure lasers is $Al_xGa_{1-x}As$. Many of the properties of this system have

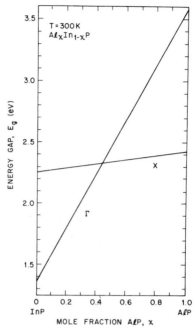

FIG. 5.3-1 Compositional dependence of the direct-energy gap Γ and the indirect-energy gap X for $Al_xIn_{1-x}P$ (Ref. 27).

TABLE 5.3-1 Compositional Dependence of the Energy Gap in the III–V Ternary Solid Solutions at 300°K[a]

Compound	Direct energy gap E_g (eV)	Indirect energy gap, E_g (eV)	
		X minima	L minima
$Al_xIn_{1-x}P$	$1.351 + 2.23x$	—	—
$Al_xGa_{1-x}As$	$\begin{cases} [b]1.424 + 1.247x \\ [c]1.424 + 1.247x + 1.147 \\ \quad \times (x - 0.45)^2 \end{cases}$	$1.900 + 0.125x + 0.143x^2$	$1.708 + 0.642x$
$Al_xIn_{1-x}As$	$0.360 + 2.012x + 0.698x^2$		
$Al_xGa_{1-x}Sb$	$0.726 + 1.129x + 0.368x^2$	$1.020 + 0.492x + 0.077x^2$	$0.799 + 0.746x + 0.334x^2$
$Al_xIn_{1-x}Sb$	$0.172 + 1.621x + 0.43x^2$	—	—
$Ga_xIn_{1-x}P$	$1.351 + 0.643x + 0.786x^2$	—	—
$Ga_xIn_{1-x}As$	$0.36 + 1.064x$	—	—
$Ga_xIn_{1-x}Sb$	$0.172 + 0.139x + 0.415x^2$	—	—
GaP_xAs_{1-x}	$1.424 + 1.150x + 0.176x^2$	—	—
$GaAs_xSb_{1-x}$	$0.726 - 0.502x + 1.2x^2$	—	—
InP_xAs_{1-x}	$0.360 + 0.891x + 0.101x^2$	—	—
$InAs_xSb_{1-x}$	$0.18 - 0.41x + 0.58x^2$	—	—

[a] See text for references.   [b] $(0 < x < 0.45)$.   [c] $(0.45 < x < 1.0)$.

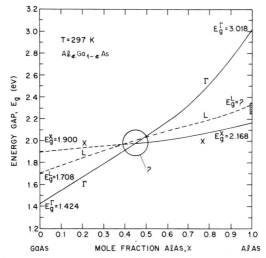

FIG. 5.3-2   Compositional dependence of the direct-energy gap Γ and the indirect-energy gaps X and L for Al$_x$Ga$_{1-x}$As (see Section 4.2 for references and assignment of the energy gap values).

been presented in Chapters 2–4. The importance of this system is based on the close lattice match to GaAs. To consolidate all the E_g versus x ternary diagrams in one place, Fig. 4.2-2 has been repeated here as Fig. 5.3-2. In Chapter 2, $\bar{n}$ as a function of photon energy for various values of x was given in Fig. 2.5-4, and $\bar{n}$ versus x at a fixed photon energy was given in Fig. 2.5-5. Numerous properties were given in Chapter 4. The variation of the donor and acceptor ionization energy were given in Fig. 4.3-3. Numerical expressions for the compositional dependence of the energy gaps and effective masses were summarized in Table 4.2-1, and the E_g dependence is given here in Table 5.3-1. The compositional dependence of the thermal conductivity was given by Afromowitz.[24] The temperature dependence of the direct-energy gap for selected values of x up to $x = 0.4$ has been given by Vorobkalo et al.[29]

Al$_x$In$_{1-x}$As

The compositional dependence of the Γ direct-energy gap and X indirect-energy gap were assigned from cathodoluminescence measurements.[28] The E_g versus x behavior is summarized in Fig. 5.3-3 and Table 5.3-1. The composition was determined by x-ray microprobe analysis. The energy gap was given as direct up to $x = 0.68$ with $E_g = 2.05$ eV.

Al$_x$Ga$_{1-x}$Sb

Very complete data are available for this system.[30–32] Cheng et al.[32] determined the energy gaps by a variety of optical techniques including a

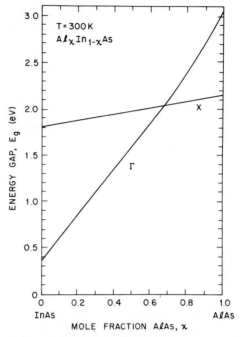

FIG. 5.3-3 Compositional dependence of the direct-energy gap Γ and the indirect-energy gap X for $Al_x In_{1-x} As$ (Ref. 28).

differential technique called wavelength modulated absorption spectra. The composition was determined by x-ray microprobe analysis. The compositional dependence from Ref. 32 of the direct energy gap and the X and L indirect energy gaps are summarized in Fig. 5.3-4 and Table 5.3-1. The direct–indirect transition occurs at $x = 0.2$ where $E_g = 0.96$ eV. Compositional dependence of the electron effective mass and heavy-hole effective mass were given by Mathieu et al.[30] It should be noted that the separation between the L indirect-conduction band and the Γ direct-conduction band for GaSb at $x = 1$ is only ~ 0.08 eV. Thus heterostructure lasers with GaSb or $Al_x Ga_{1-x} Sb$ active layers can be expected to have a significant fraction of the conduction electrons in the indirect-conduction band (see Section 4.6), which would result in a high J_{th} at room temperature.

$Al_x In_{1-x} Sb$

The compositional dependence of the direct energy gap was determined by electroreflectance by Isomura et al.[33] The composition was assigned by lattice constant measurements. No information is available on the direct–indirect transition and the estimated X indirect band has been drawn in Fig. 5.3-5 on the basis of the X band in AlSb. The quadratic dependence of E_g in Table 5.3-1 is from Ref. 33.

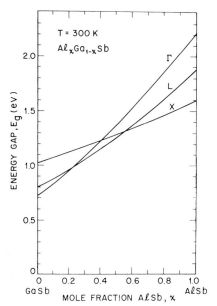

FIG. 5.3-4   Compositional dependence of the direct-energy gap Γ and the indirect-energy gaps X and L for Al$_x$Ga$_{1-x}$Sb (Ref. 32).

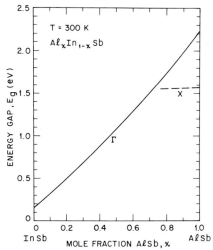

FIG. 5.3-5   Compositional dependence of the direct-energy gap Γ for Al$_x$In$_{1-x}$Sb (Ref. 33).

Ga$_x$In$_{1-x}$P

Considerable controversy has been involved in the position of the direct–indirect transition x_c. One value is $x_c = 0.74$, while the other is $x_c = 0.63$. Numerous references to both designations have been given by Lee *et al.*[34] The careful work of Nelson and Holonyak gives $x_c = 0.73$. The energy gap was obtained by Nelson and Holonyak by observation of the exciton absorption. Composition was determined by x-ray microprobe analysis. The compositional dependence shown in Fig. 5.3-6 is from Ref. 35 and gives $x_c = 0.73$ with $E_g = 2.239$ eV. Similar data with $x_c = 0.73$ were obtained by Onton *et al.*[36] by simultaneous cathodoluminescence and x-ray microprobe analysis.

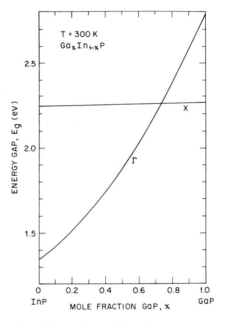

FIG. 5.3-6 Compositional dependence of the direct-energy gap Γ and the indirect-energy gap X for Ga$_x$In$_{1-x}$P (Ref. 35).

Ga$_x$In$_{1-x}$As

The early data for E_g versus x in this system exhibited considerable bowing. The more recent data of Baliga *et al.*[37] suggest a linear dependence. In that work, the energy gap was assigned from the photoresponse of an electrolyte–semiconductor junction. The composition was determined by using x-ray dispersive analysis in a scanning electron microscope. Their results cover x between 0.5 and 1.0. Similar results were obtained by Nahory *et al.*[38] over a smaller range in x by photoluminescence and photoreflectance. The compositional dependence of E_g from Ref. 37 is summarized in Fig. 5.3-7 and Table 5.3-1. Earlier references that give results with bowing are summarized in Ref. 37.

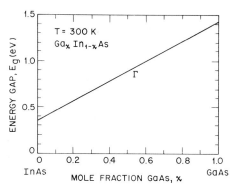

FIG. 5.3-7   Compositional dependence of the direct-energy gap Γ for $Ga_x In_{1-x} As$ (Ref. 37).

$Ga_x In_{1-x} Sb$

The compositional dependence of the direct energy gap between 77°K and 300°K was determined by Auvergne *et al.*[39] by piezoreflectance measurements. Composition was determined by x-ray microprobe analysis. Their results are summarized in Fig. 5.3-8 and Table 5.3-1. Compositional dependence of the effective masses is also given in Ref. 39.

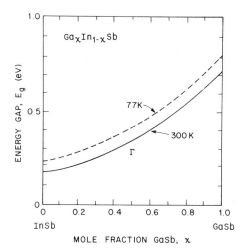

FIG. 5.3-8   Compositional dependence of the direct-energy gap Γ for $Ga_x In_{1-x} Sb$ (Ref. 39).

GaP$_x$As$_{1-x}$

This III–V ternary has been used extensively for visible-light-emitting diodes. The compositional dependence has been determined by electro-reflectance by Thompson et $al.$[40] The direct–indirect transition of $x_c = 0.45$ was obtained by pressure measurements[41] which gives $E_g = 1.977$ eV. The energy-gap dependence versus x is summarized in Fig. 5.3-9 and Table 5.3-1.

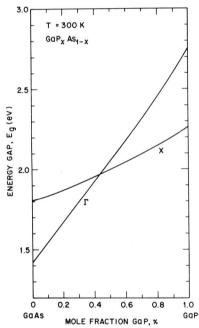

FIG. 5.3-9   Compositional dependence of the direct-energy gap Γ and indirect-energy gap X for GaP$_x$As$_{1-x}$ (Ref. 40).

GaAs$_x$Sb$_{1-x}$

This ternary is of interest because it has an energy gap in the wavelength region near 1 μm where the optical fiber transmission losses and dispersion are at a minimum. Double-heterostructure (DH) lasers with GaAs$_{0.88}$Sb$_{0.12}$ active layers were used by Nahory et $al.$[4] to obtain cw room-temperature operation. Since this composition does not lattice match any binary substrate, intermediate step-graded layers were used between the GaAs substrate and the heterostructure. This DH laser is considered in further detail in Section 5.6. This system has a miscibility gap, but its exact width is not known. Energy-gap data are available for $0 < x < 0.38$ and $0.75 < x < 1.0$.[42–44]

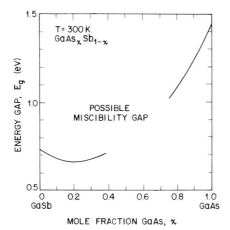

FIG. 5.3-10   Compositional dependence of the direct-energy gap Γ for GaAs$_x$Sb$_{1-x}$ (Ref. 43).

The energy gap as a function of x from Ref. 43 is summarized in Fig. 5.3-10 and Table 5.3-1.

InP$_x$As$_{1-x}$

The compositional dependence of E_g for this system was assigned from photoluminescent measurements by Antypas and Yep.[45] The composition was determined by measurement of the lattice constant. Their value of E_g at $x = 0$ has been increased by 0.01 eV to agree with the value for InAs in Table 5.2-2. The resulting room temperature expression is given in Table 5.3-1 and is plotted in Fig. 5.3-11.

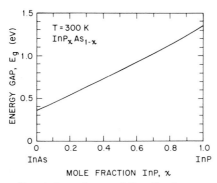

FIG. 5.3-11   Compositional dependence of the direct-energy gap Γ for InP$_x$As$_{1-x}$ (Ref. 45).

InAs$_x$Sb$_{1-x}$

The room temperature absorption data of Woolley and Warner[46] were used by Thompson and Woolley[47] to give the quadratic expression given in Table 5.3-1. The values at $x = 0$ and $x = 1$ are slightly different than the E_g given for the binary compounds in Table 5.2-2. This expression is plotted in Fig. 5.3-12.

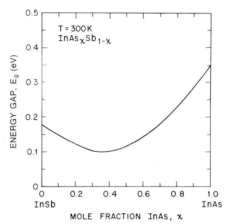

FIG. 5.3-12 Compositional dependence of the direct-energy gap Γ for InAs$_x$Sb$_{1-x}$ (Ref. 47).

5.4 III–V BINARY AND TERNARY LATTICE-MATCHING SYSTEMS FOR HETEROSTRUCTURE LASERS

General Considerations

In this section, a number of lattice-matching III–V binary and ternary heterojunctions and the potential use of these semiconductors for heterostructure lasers is discussed. A detailed description of each case would require information as extensive as that presented for GaAs–Al$_x$Ga$_{1-x}$As in Chapters 2–4. Such information is not available. Even the distribution of ΔE_g between ΔE_c and ΔE_v is only known from the electron affinities of the binary compounds as given in Table 5.2-3. These values of χ are subject to errors in excess of 0.1 eV and interpolation for ternary or quaternary solid solutions is perilous. Even with this limited amount of information, it is useful to survey the possible heterojunction combinations. Only the case of GaAs–Ga$_{0.51}$In$_{0.49}$P will be considered in some detail.

The binary lattice constants given in Table 5.2-1 are plotted in Fig. 5.4-1 together with ternary lattice constants that have been taken to scale linearly

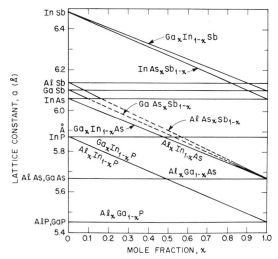

FIG. 5.4-1 Lattice constant as a function of composition for ternary III–V crystalline solid solutions in which the end components differ by less than 0.5 Å. Vegard's law is assumed to be obeyed in all cases. The dashed lines show regions where miscibility gaps are expected.

with composition. Ternary systems in which the lattice constants of the end components differ by more than ~0.5 Å are expected to have large miscibility gaps that will greatly limit the range of compositions at which they can exist. These ternaries have been omitted from Fig. 5.4-1. Lattice-matching combinations for binary to ternary III–V compounds are readily seen from an inspection of Fig. 5.4-1. These combinations occur where the plot of the ternary compound lattice constant crosses the horizontal line for a binary compound. In most cases, that occurs at only one composition, but GaAs and $Al_xGa_{1-x}As$, and GaP and $Al_xGa_{1-x}P$ are closely matched for all values of x. Heterojunctions of GaP–$Al_xGa_{1-x}P$ are not considered further, however, because $Al_xGa_{1-x}P$ has an indirect energy gap over the entire composition range. Each of the possible binary–ternary lattice-matched combinations are briefly considered as potential heterostructure lasers. The systems discussed in the remainder of this section are summarized in Table 5.4-1.

AlSb–$Ga_{0.9}In_{0.1}Sb$

The only Al binary III–V compound that appears to have been prepared as a bulk single crystal is AlSb.[48] Since AlSb surfaces oxidize quite rapidly in air, epitaxial growth techniques will be required that permit *in situ* removal

TABLE 5.4-1 Binary to Ternary III–V Lattice-Matched Systems for Heterostructure Lasers

System	Laser emission			Comments
	Energy, E (eV)	Wavelength, λ (μm)	Temperature (°K)	
AlSb–Ga$_{0.9}$In$_{0.1}$Sb[a]	$\begin{cases}0.63\\0.71\end{cases}$	2.0 1.75	300 0	Problems with AlSb surface oxidation
AlSb–InAs$_{0.82}$Sb$_{0.18}$[a]	0.38	3.26	0	Problems with AlSb surface oxidation
GaAs[a]–Al$_x$Ga$_{1-x}$As	1.42	0.87	300	Extensively used
GaAs[b]–Al$_x$Ga$_{1-x}$As– Al$_y$Ga$_{1-y}$As[a] $y < x$ }	1.42–1.61	0.87–0.773	300	Extensively used
GaAs[a]–Ga$_{0.51}$In$_{0.49}$P	1.42	0.87	300	Preparation by chemical-vapor deposition. No apparent advantages over other GaAs cases.
GaP–Al$_x$Ga$_{1-x}$P	Indirect E_g	—	—	—
GaSb[a]–AlAs$_{0.08}$Sb$_{0.92}$	0.72	1.72	300	A possible system for λ near 2 μm. J_{th}(300°K) may be high.
GaSb–InAs$_{0.91}$Sb$_{0.09}$[a]	0.347	3.57	0	Long wavelength at low temperature
InP–Ga$_{0.47}$In$_{0.53}$As[a]	0.86	1.44	300	A possible system for λ near 1.5 μm
InP[a]–Al$_{0.47}$In$_{0.53}$As	1.35	0.92	300	Must compete with successful GaAs lasers
InAs[a]–AlAs$_{0.16}$Sb$_{0.84}$	0.42	3.0	0	Long wavelength at low temperature
InAs[a]–GaAs$_{0.08}$Sb$_{0.92}$	0.42	3.0	0	Long wavelength at low temperature

[a] Active layer.
[b] Substrate.

of the oxide and subsequent protection of the AlSb surfaces. The compositional dependence of the energy gap was given in Fig. 5.3-8, and the expression in Table 5.3-1 gives $E_g = 0.633$ eV at 300°K for $x = 0.9$. From Table 5.2-2, E_g for GaSb is ~ 0.08 eV greater at 0°K than at 300°K. This increase is added to the ternary value at 300°K to give $E_g \approx 0.71$ eV at 0°K for $Ga_{0.9}In_{0.1}Sb$. Examination of E_g, χ, and $\bar{n}$ in Tables 5.2-2 and 5.2-3 indicates that carrier and optical confinement can be expected. Double heterostructures of

$$N–AlSb|n– \text{ or } p–Ga_{0.9}In_{0.1}Sb|P–AlSb$$

would have emission energies from ~ 0.63 eV (~ 2.0 μm) at 300°K to ~ 0.71 eV (~ 1.75 μm) at 0°K. Heterostructure lasers in this system have not been reported.

AlSb–InAs$_{0.82}$Sb$_{0.18}$

Work with this system will engender the same difficulties as with the preceding system because of the AlSb oxidation. The compositional dependence of the energy gap was illustrated in Fig. 5.3-12, and the expression in Table 5.3-1 gives $E_g = 0.23$ eV at 300°K for $x = 0.82$. From Table 5.2-2, E_g for InAs at 0°K is greater by ~ 0.060 eV than at 300°K, so that $E_g \approx 0.29$ eV at 0°K for $InAs_{0.82}Sb_{0.18}$. Examination of E_g, χ, and $\bar{n}$ in Tables 5.2-2 and 5.2-3 indicates that carrier and optical confinement can be expected. However, the small conduction-band effective mass means that the quasi-Fermi level would be high above the conduction band edge at high excitation. Double heterostructures of

$$N–AlSb|n– \text{ or } p–InAs_{0.82}Sb_{0.18}|P–AlSb$$

would have emission energies from ~ 0.23 eV (5.39 μm) at 300°K to ~ 0.29 eV (4.28 μm) at 0°K. The narrow energy gap of the active region would restrict operation of this laser to low temperatures. Heterostructure lasers in this system have not been reported.

GaAs–Al$_x$Ga$_{1-x}$As or Al$_x$Ga$_{1-x}$As–Al$_y$Ga$_{1-y}$As

The lattice constants of GaAs and AlAs differ by less than 0.2% at 300°K and are the same near 1200°K. They form a complete series of solid solutions with lattice constants following Vegard's law. Partly because of the close lattice match, heteroepitaxy of $Al_xGa_{1-x}As$ multilayers with differing values of x has been relatively simple, and the resulting heterojunctions do not contain significant concentrations of interface recombination centers.[48a] The utilization of the nearly lattice-matched heterojunctions and the relatively simple liquid-phase epitaxial (LPE) techniques described in Chapter 6 has led to the evolution of the various types of heterostructure lasers described in Chapter 7.

Waveguiding in GaAs–Al$_x$Ga$_{1-x}$As symmetric and asymmetric DH infinite-slab waveguides was described in Chapter 2. This description included discussion of the far-field emission patterns from the DH, distributed feedback, and waveguiding in various four- and five-layered heterostructures. The theory for stimulated emission and the expressions for threshold current density were derived for GaAs active layers in Chapter 3. The energy-band diagrams for various GaAs–Al$_x$Ga$_{1-x}$As heterojunctions were illustrated in Chapter 4. In Chapter 7, the experimental behavior of GaAs–Al$_x$Ga$_{1-x}$As heterostructure lasers is summarized.

The most widely studied lasers in this system have been with the DH

$$N\text{–}Al_xGa_{1-x}As|n\text{–} \text{ or } p\text{–}GaAs|P\text{–}Al_xGa_{1-x}As.$$

The emission wavelength can be decreased by the use of Al$_y$Ga$_{1-y}$As in the active layer with $y < x$. In this manner, Miller et al.[49] first achieved cw lasers operating in the visible with laser emission as high as 1.61 eV (0.7730 μm). The lasing threshold remained relatively unchanged in the range $y = 0$ to 0.21. As shown in Fig. 4.6-4, the fraction of electrons in the Al$_x$Ga$_{1-x}$As direct conduction band begins to decrease rapidly for $x > 0.20$. Alferov et al.[50] and Kressel and Hawrylo[51] have also studied DH lasers with Al$_x$Ga$_{1-x}$As active layers. Further description of the experimental properties of GaAs–Al$_x$Ga$_{1-x}$As and Al$_x$Ga$_{1-x}$As–Al$_y$Ga$_{1-y}$As heterostructure lasers is given in Chapter 7.

GaAs–Ga$_{0.51}$In$_{0.49}$P

Figure 5.4-1 shows that a lattice-matched DH laser can be made with the structure

$$N\text{–}Ga_{0.51}In_{0.49}P|n\text{–} \text{ or } p\text{–}GaAs|P\text{–}Ga_{0.51}In_{0.49}P.$$

Since $\bar{n}$ for GaP at 1.424 eV is less than 3.2,[52] there will be waveguiding. From the expression in Table 5.3-1, E_g for Ga$_{0.51}$In$_{0.49}$P is 1.883 eV. However, if the electron affinity is taken as the average of the InP and GaP values given in Table 5.2-3, a value of 4.2 eV is obtained. From Eq. (4.3-1), ΔE_c is $\chi(\text{GaAs}) - \chi(\text{Ga}_{0.51}\text{In}_{0.49}\text{P})$, and a value of -0.15 eV for ΔE_c is obtained for this heterojunction. Since there is considerable uncertainty in this value, ΔE_c will be taken here as zero and ΔE_v taken as ΔE_g. The energy-band diagram will be drawn to illustrate carrier confinement in such a case. The achievement of cw room-temperature operation[53] with this structure demonstrates that there is adequate carrier confinement within the active layer.

The energy-band diagram for the GaAs–Ga$_{0.51}$In$_{0.49}$P p–P heterojunction has been drawn in Fig. 5.4-2. This figure serves to illustrate that in the absence of a positive value for ΔE_c, the electron barrier in the conduction

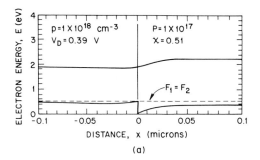

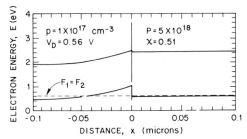

FIG. 5.4-2 Energy-band diagram for GaAs–Ga$_{0.51}$In$_{0.49}$P p–P heterojunction at 297°K. (a) $(N_{A_1}^- - N_{D_1}^+) = 1.1 \times 10^{18}$ cm^{-3} and $F_1 - E_{v_1} = 0.054$ eV on the p-side, and $(N_{A_2}^- - N_{D_2}^+) = 2 \times 10^{17}$ cm^{-3} and $F_2 - E_{v_2} = 0.120$ eV on the P-side. (b) $(N_{A_1}^- - N_{D_1}^+) = 1.1 \times 10^{17}$ cm^{-3} and $F_1 - E_{v_1} = 0.113$ eV on the p-side, and $(N_{A_2}^- - N_{D_2}^+) = 7 \times 10^{18}$ cm^{-3} and $F_2 - E_{v_2} = 0.016$ eV on the P-side.

band may be appreciably influenced by the impurity concentrations. The built-in potential for the p–P heterojunction was given in Chapter 4 as

$$V_D \text{(volts)} = [(F_1 - E_{v_1}) + \Delta E_v - (F_2 - E_{v_2})]/q. \qquad (4.3\text{-}122)$$

This equation shows that for large V_D it is desirable to make the Fermi level $(F_2 - E_{v_2})$ small, which means large hole concentrations in the P-Ga$_{0.51}$In$_{0.49}$P layer. A large value of the Fermi level $(F_1 - E_{v_1})$ requires small hole concentrations in the GaAs layer. This behavior is illustrated by the two cases shown in Figs. 5.4-2a, b. The nominal values of $m_n = 0.1 m_0$ and $m_p = 0.60 m_0$ were assigned to Ga$_{0.51}$In$_{0.49}$P in order to obtain the Fermi levels for these examples. The expressions necessary to calculate the energy-band diagrams were given in the isotype heterojunction part of Section 4.3.

The DH is illustrated in Fig. 5.4-3a for zero bias. In this heterostructure, the bias necessary to give $n = 2 \times 10^{18}$ cm^{-3} $(F_c - E_c = 0.079$ eV) in the GaAs active layer requires V_a across the N–p heterojunction to exceed V_D [see Eq. (4.6-2)]. For an applied bias of 1.55 V in Fig. 5.4-3b, 1.47 V is across

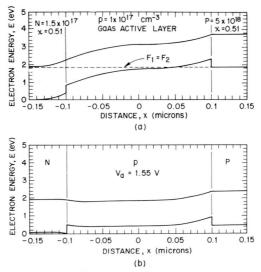

FIG. 5.4-3   Energy-band diagram for GaAs–Ga$_{0.51}$In$_{0.49}$P N–p–P double heterostructure at 297°K. The N–p heterojunction is for Ga$_{0.51}$In$_{0.49}$P with $(N_D{}^+ - N_A{}^-) = 3 \times 10^{17}$ cm^{-3} and $(E_c - F) = 0.042$ eV. The p–P heterojunction is from Fig. 5.4-2b. (a) Zero bias. (b) Forward bias of 1.55 V.

the N–p heterojunction. The built-in potential that remains at the p–P heterojunction is 0.48 V and provides electron confinement. A lower value of P would result in sufficient carrier confinement, and the value of 5×10^{18} cm^{-3} was selected only to illustrate the effect. The interesting result of this example is that carrier confinement can be achieved in heterojunctions without a positive ΔE_c.

It should also be pointed out that lasers with this heterostructure have been prepared by chemical-vapor deposition (CVD).[53-55] These devices had room-temperature threshold current densities as low as 1.14×10^3 A/cm^2 and differential quantum efficiencies of 30 to 45%.[53] Because Ga$_{0.51}$In$_{0.49}$As also is lattice matched to Al$_x$Ga$_{1-x}$As, double heterostructures of

$$Al_xGa_{1-x}As | Ga_{0.51}In_{0.49}P | Al_xGa_{1-x}As$$

with $x \gtrsim 0.6$ have been prepared by LPE.[56] Only optically pumped devices at low temperature were reported. At 77°K, Schul and Mischel[57] have operated Ga$_{0.51}$In$_{0.49}$P–Ga$_{0.32}$Al$_{0.68}$As SH lasers that were grown on GaAs substrates.

GaAs–Al$_{0.51}$In$_{0.49}$P

The ternary compound Al$_{0.51}$In$_{0.49}$P lattice matches to GaAs. As shown in Fig. 5.3-1, the energy gap E_g at $x = 0.51$ will be indirect with a value of about 2.3 eV. Heterostructure lasers in this system with GaAs active layers are possible, but would have no obvious advantages over the other lasers with GaAs active regions.

GaSb–AlAs$_{0.08}$Sb$_{0.92}$

As indicated in Fig. 5.4-1, this ternary is expected to have a miscibility gap. However, double heterostructures of

$$N–AlAs_{0.08}Sb_{0.92}|n– \text{ or } p–GaSb|P–AlAs_{0.08}Sb_{0.92}$$

are possible. The energy gap of AlSb is indirect and about twice the value of E_g for GaSb. The laser emission energy would be 0.72 eV (1.72 μm) at 300°K. No studies have been reported for this heterostructure. However, closely related DH lasers with Al$_x$Ga$_{1-x}$As$_y$Sb$_{1-y}$ are discussed in Section 5.5.

GaSb–InAs$_{0.91}$Sb$_{0.09}$

The compositional dependence of the energy gap of InAs$_x$Sb$_{1-x}$ was given in Fig. 5.3-12, and the expression in Table 5.3-1 gives $E_g = 0.287$ eV at 300°K for $x = 0.91$. From Table 5.2-2, E_g for InAs is 0.060 eV greater at 0°K than at 300°K. When this increase is added to the value at 300°K, $E_g = 0.347$ eV for InAs$_{0.91}$Sb$_{0.09}$ at 0°K. Double heterostructures of

$$N–GaSb|n– \text{ or } p–InAs_{0.91}Sb_{0.09}|P–GaSb$$

would have an emission energy of ~ 0.347 eV (3.57 μm) at 0°K. Values of $\bar{n}$ in this wavelength region for GaSb indicate that waveguiding can be expected. Heterostructure lasers in this system have not been reported.

InP–Ga$_{0.47}$In$_{0.53}$As

The compositional dependence of the energy gap of Ga$_x$In$_{1-x}$As was illustrated in Fig. 5.3-7, and the expression in Table 5.3-1 gives $E_g = 0.860$ eV at 300°K for $x = 0.47$. Double heterostructures of

$$N–InP|n– \text{ or } p–Ga_{0.47}In_{0.53}As|P–InP$$

have been prepared by chemical-vapor deposition on InP substrates by Nuese et al.[58] Room-temperature threshold current densities of 6×10^3 A/cm^2 were obtained for an emission wavelength of 1.7 μm.

InP–Al$_{0.47}$In$_{0.53}$As

The compositional dependence of the energy gap was illustrated in Fig. 5.3-3, and the expression in Table 5.3-1 gives $E_g = 1.460$ eV at 300°K for $x = 0.47$. Double heterostructures of

$$N–Al_{0.47}In_{0.53}As|n– \text{ or } p–InP|P–Al_{0.47}In_{0.53}As$$

would have an emission energy of 1.351 eV (0.92 μm) at room temperature and should have waveguiding. Because the GaAs DH lasers emit near 1.4 eV, DH lasers with InP active layers offer no obvious advantages. Heterostructures have not been prepared with this heterojunction.

InAs–AlAs$_{0.16}$Sb$_{0.84}$

As indicated in Fig. 5.4-1, the ternary is expected to have a miscibility gap. However, double heterostructures of

$$N\text{–}AlAs_{0.16}Sb_{0.84}|n\text{– or } p\text{–}InAs|P\text{–}AlAs_{0.16}Sb_{0.84}$$

may be possible. Because the energy gap of InAs is 0.360 eV at room temperature, this heterostructure laser would be for low-temperature operation and would have an emission energy of 0.420 eV ($\sim$ 3.0 μm) at 0°K. No heterostructures have been prepared with this system.

InAs–GaAs$_{0.08}$Sb$_{0.92}$

As indicated in Fig. 5.4-1, this ternary is also expected to have a miscibility gap. However, double heterostructures of

$$N\text{–}GaAs_{0.08}Sb_{0.92}|n\text{– or } p\text{–}InAs|P\text{–}GaAs_{0.08}Sb_{0.92}$$

may be possible. The active layer is InAs and would have the same emission properties as the preceeding system and no heterostructures have been prepared.

5.5 III–V BINARY AND QUATERNARY LATTICE-MATCHING SYSTEMS FOR HETEROSTRUCTURE LASERS

Introductory Comments

An added degree of freedom in lattice matched III–V heterostructures may be obtained with quaternary crystalline solid solutions. The InP–Ga$_x$In$_{1-x}$P$_y$As$_{1-y}$ heterojunction serves as a successful example of a binary–quaternary lattice-matching system. The work by Hsieh et al.[5] has resulted in cw room-temperature DH lasers with emission wavelengths in the 1.0–1.1 μm range. Yamamoto et al.[59] have prepared DH lasers with this heterojunction to give cw operation for wavelengths from 1.22 to 1.34 μm. As shown in Fig. 5.1-1, the transmission loss and material dispersion are lowest in this wavelength region.

In this section, the reduction of stress in Al$_x$Ga$_{1-x}$As layers grown on GaAs substrates is illustrated by the introduction of small amounts of P to give the quaternary Al$_x$Ga$_{1-x}$P$_y$As$_{1-y}$. Then the possible binary–quaternary lattice-matched heterojunction combinations are briefly considered for application to heterostructure lasers. The systems discussed in the remainder of this section are summarized in Table 5.5-1.

TABLE 5.5-1 Binary to Quaternary III–V Lattice-Matched Systems for Heterostructure Lasers

Quaternary	Lattice matching binary	Comments
Al$_x$Ga$_{1-x}$P$_y$As$_{1-y}$	GaAs	No binary lattice match except at low y (≈ 0.01). Used to adjust Al$_x$Ga$_{1-x}$As lattice constant.
Al$_x$Ga$_{1-x}$P$_y$Sb$_{1-y}$	GaAs, InP, InAs	Mostly indirect-energy gap and probable miscibility gaps.
Al$_x$Ga$_{1-x}$As$_y$Sb$_{1-y}$	InP, InAs, GaSb	Regions of probable miscibility gaps at compositions where lattice matched to InP. Step-graded DH lasers grown on GaAs for 1-μm emission. Lattice match to InAs for emission at ~ 3 μm at low temperature. Lattice match to GaSb for 1.7 μm emission at 300°K, possible high J_{th}.
Al$_x$In$_{1-x}$P$_y$As$_{1-y}$	InP	InP active region not at an interesting emission wavelength.
Al$_x$In$_{1-x}$P$_y$Sb$_{1-y}$	GaAs, InAs, AlSb, GaSb	Probable miscibility gaps.
Al$_x$In$_{1-x}$As$_y$Sb$_{1-y}$	InP, GaSb, AlSb	Very similar in lattice constant variation with composition to Ga$_x$In$_{1-x}$As$_y$Sb$_{1-y}$. Less interest than that system because of greater growth problems and indirect-energy-gap regions.
Ga$_x$In$_{1-x}$P$_y$As$_{1-y}$	InP, GaAs	For laser emission in the 1–1.5-μm region with lattice match to InP. Low threshold cw lasers have been prepared.
Ga$_x$In$_{1-x}$P$_y$Sb$_{1-y}$	GaAs, InP, InAs, AlSb	Probable extensive miscibility gaps.
Ga$_x$In$_{1-x}$As$_y$Sb$_{1-y}$	InP, GaSb, AlSb	For low-temperature DH lasers at wavelengths greater than ~ 2 μm. Miscibility gap over part of the InP lattice match region.
(Al$_x$Ga$_{1-x}$)$_y$In$_{1-y}$P	GaAs, Al$_x$Ga$_{1-x}$As	Heterostructure lasers with visible emission to 2.15 eV.
(Al$_x$Ga$_{1-x}$)$_y$In$_{1-y}$As	InP	Heterostructure lasers with emission between 0.8 and 1.5 μm.
(Al$_x$Ga$_{1-x}$)$_y$In$_{1-y}$Sb	AlSb	Heterostructure lasers with emission between 1.1 and 2.1 μm. Problems with AlSb surface oxidation.
Al(P$_x$As$_{1-x}$)$_y$Sb$_{1-y}$	InP	All indirect energy gap, probable miscibility gap.
Ga(P$_x$As$_{1-x}$)$_y$Sb$_{1-y}$	InP	Probable miscibility gap in desired composition range.
In(P$_x$As$_{1-x}$)$_y$Sb$_{1-y}$	AlSb, GaSb, InAs	Heterostructure lasers with emission between ~ 2–4 μm. Expected difficulties with miscibility gaps over part of the desired composition ranges.

$Al_xGa_{1-x}P_yAs_{1-y}$

This quaternary system is a special case. Data are available at low P composition where an exact room-temperature lattice match to GaAs may be obtained. At higher P compositions there is no lattice match to a binary III–V compound. Only the low P composition range will be considered here. As previously discussed in Section 5.4, the GaAs–$Al_xGa_{1-x}As$ system is closely lattice matched. The temperature dependence of the GaAs[60] and AlAs[61] lattice constants are shown in Fig. 5.5-1. An assumed behavior of $Al_{0.3}Ga_{0.7}As$ is also shown. Even though an almost perfect lattice match is achieved at the ~800°C growth temperature, considerable stress is introduced into GaAs–$Al_xGa_{1-x}As$ heteroepitaxial layers upon cooling. The stress results from the slight difference in thermal expansion coefficients of the two materials. By using an x-ray topographic camera which is also equipped to plot substrate lattice curvature, Rozgonyi et al.[62,63] determined

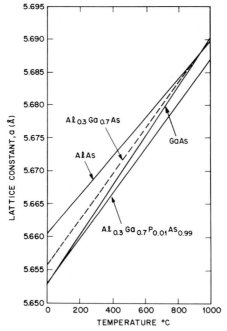

FIG. 5.5-1 Lattice constants of GaAs, AlAs, $Al_{0.3}Ga_{0.7}As$, and $Al_{0.3}Ga_{0.7}P_{0.01}As_{0.99}$ as a function of temperature. The lines for AlAs and GaAs were drawn through the data of Refs. 60 and 61, respectively. The line for $Al_{0.3}Ga_{0.7}As$ was drawn from the measured lattice constant at room temperature and the intersection of the binary compounds at high temperature. The line for $Al_{0.3}Ga_{0.7}P_{0.01}As_{0.99}$ was drawn from the measured lattice constant at room temperature and the assumption of the same thermal expansion coefficient as the ternary.

the average stress of $Al_xGa_{1-x}As$ layers on GaAs substrates as a function of AlAs mole fraction. Their results are shown in Fig. 5.5-2. Since stress is possibly detrimental to the life of heterostructure lasers,[64] the possibility of stress compensation by the addition of small amounts of P to the wide energy gap layers was investigated by Rozgonyi et al.[65,66] Phosphorus is an excellent candidate for such stress compensation because it is isoelectronic with As, and the covalent radius of P is much smaller than for As. A very small amount of P in As sites has no significant effect on either the electrical or optical properties.

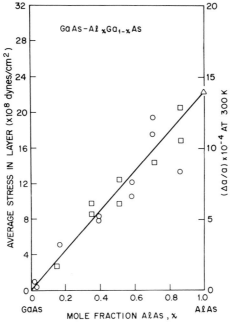

FIG. 5.5-2   Average layer stress as a function of composition for $Al_xGa_{1-x}As$ (Ref. 62). The circles and squares represent data from two different LPE systems. The data point for $x = 1$ is from Ref. 60.

The addition of P to the ternary to almost exactly stress compensate GaAs–$Al_{0.3}Ga_{0.7}As$ at room temperature translates the $Al_{0.3}Ga_{0.7}As$ curve of Fig. 5.5-1 to the $Al_{0.3}Ga_{0.7}P_{0.01}As_{0.99}$ curve. The slopes of the $Al_{0.3}Ga_{0.7}As$ and $Al_{0.3}Ga_{0.7}P_{0.01}As_{0.99}$ curves are assumed identical, since the amount of P in the quaternary to lattice match GaAs at room temperature is $y < 0.02$. Experimental verification of the reduction in stress by the use of the quaternary was obtained by LPE growth of single layers of $Al_xGa_{1-x}As$ and $Al_xGa_{1-x}P_yAs_{1-y}$ on GaAs substrates. The results of

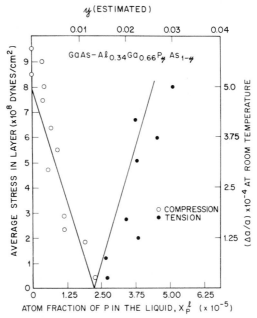

FIG. 5.5-3   Stress compensation as a function of the atom fraction of P in the growth liquid and the estimated P content of $Al_{0.34}Ga_{0.66}P_yAs_{1-y}$ layers grown on GaAs. The value of y is estimated from the change in stress as compared to $Al_{0.34}Ga_{0.66}As$ grown on GaAs. The stress is converted to a lattice-constant difference Δa between the quaternary and the binary substrate, and Δa with Vegard's law yields y (Ref. 62).

these studies are given in Fig. 5.5-3. For that work, the solution composition range investigated was estimated from the thermodynamic calculations for quaternary solutions described in Section 6.2. It should be noted that the extent to which stress can be eliminated by this technique is dependent upon the uniformity of the layers. Layer uniformity is influenced by P and Al depletion from the melt during growth. The amount of depletion is dependent upon the quaternary phase equilibria, the LPE growth system, and the growth conditions. Afromowitz and Rode[67] have shown that a stress reduction by a factor of ten may be obtained for 2-μm-thick layers by adding P to the appropriate solutions in the heterostructure laser growth apparatus. Presumably the growth procedure and apparatus would have to be modified for further improvement.

It may be seen in Fig. 5.5-1 that the addition of P to $Al_xGa_{1-x}As$ to achieve a lattice match to GaAs at room temperature results in lattice mismatch at the growth temperature. When sufficiently great, this mismatch can lead to the formation of edge and inclined dislocations as will be described in Section 5.6. Some evidence suggests that P addition may result in longer operating life for properly fabricated injection lasers.[68] This improvement may be related to stress reduction, but has been difficult to demonstrate conclusively. It was also observed by Dyment *et al.*[69] that the addition of P results in DH lasers with somewhat lower threshold current densities. The reasons for the lower threshold are not understood.

$Al_xGa_{1-x}As_ySb_{1-y}$

In this quaternary, Al and Ga have very similar covalent radii so that the major change in lattic constant is achieved by varying y. The variation of the energy gap and lattice constant with composition is illustrated in Fig. 5.5-4. The iso-energy gap lines were drawn with the aid of experimental data from Nahory *et al.*[69a] Since the ratio of the total number of group III atoms to the total number of group V atoms is unity, the composition of

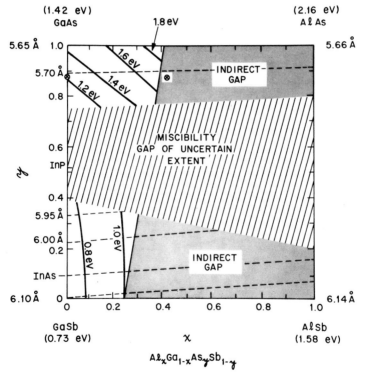

FIG. 5.5-4 The x–y compositional plane for $Al_xGa_{1-x}As_ySb_{1-y}$ at 300°K. The x–y coordinate of any point in the plane gives the composition. The solid lines are constant direct-energy-gap values interpolated from experimental data of Nahory *et al.*[69a] The dashed lines are constant lattice constants. The compositions used by Nahory *et al.*[4] are indicated by ⊗.

the quaternary is uniquely represented by the two parameters x and y. The composition of this solid solution is represented by a square in the x–y plane with the four binary compounds at the corners. The schematic energy gap–lattice parameter–composition diagram for this class of compounds was given in Fig. 1.5-1. In Fig. 5.5-4, constant values of the energy gap and the lattice constant are projected onto the x–y plane.

Three of the four ternary energy gap–composition diagrams that describe the ternary sides of Fig. 5.5-4 were given in Figs. 5.3-2, 5.3-4, and 5.3-10. Data are not available for the $AlAs_xSb_{1-x}$ system. The diagram of Fig. 5.5-4 shows that there are potential lattice-matching compositions to InP, InAs, and GaSb. The lattice match to InP is in a composition range that is not achievable because of the extensive miscibility gap in this system.[70,71] For lattice matching to InAs, the binary would be the active region. No DH lasers of $InAs–Al_xGa_{1-x}As_ySb_{1-y}$ have been reported. As can be seen in Fig. 5.5-4, DH lasers with both quaternary and GaSb active regions are possible when the compositions lattice match to GaSb. Dolginov et al.[72] prepared DH lasers of $GaSb–Al_xGa_{1-x}As_ySb_{1-y}$ at apparently a lattice-matching composition. Emission wavelengths from 1.5 to 1.8 μm were obtained between 77° and 300°K with a room-temperature threshold current density of 6.2×10^3 A/cm^2. As noted in the section on $Al_xGa_{1-x}Sb$, a portion of the conduction band electrons in the GaSb active layer would be expected to be in the L indirect-conduction band at room temperature and give a high $J_{th}(300°K)$.

Step-graded DH lasers that utilize $Al_{0.4}Ga_{0.6}As_{0.88}Sb_{0.12}$ cladding layers and a $GaAs_{0.88}Sb_{0.12}$ active layer emit near 1 μm and have operated cw at room temperature.[4] Discussion of this step-graded DH is given in the next section on compositionally graded heterostructures.

$Ga_xIn_{1-x}P_yAs_{1-y}$

The three-dimensional compositional dependence of the energy gap for the $Ga_xIn_{1-x}P_yAs_{1-y}$ system has been drawn in Fig. 5.5-5. The bounding ternary diagrams were given in Figs. 5.3-6, 5.3-7, 5.3-9, and 5.3-11. There are some experimental data reported[73,74] for the compositional dependence of the energy gap in the quaternary system at 300°K. Moon et al.[75] have used those data to show that the assumption of little additional bowing due to quaternary interactions is reasonable. The direct- and indirect-energy-gap surfaces are shown in Fig. 5.5-5 and their intersection demonstrates that most of this system is in the direct-energy-gap region. The lattice match to GaAs is not very interesting because the energy-gap range is from 1.42 eV to approximately 1.75 eV. This energy-gap range is the same as for $Al_xGa_{1-x}As$. However, the compositions that lattice match to InP are of considerable interest because this range of $Ga_xIn_{1-x}P_yAs_{1-y}$ has an

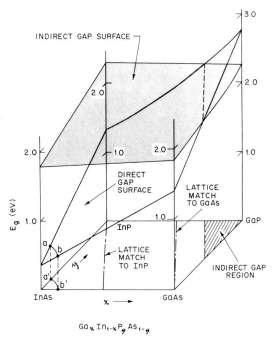

$$Ga_x In_{1-x} P_y As_{1-y}$$

FIG. 5.5-5 Three-dimensional representation of the compositional dependence of the direct- and indirect-energy-gap surfaces in $Ga_x In_{1-x} P_y As_{1-y}$ at 300°K. The square base gives the composition in terms of x and y.

energy gap that varies from 0.74 to 1.35 eV (1.7–0.9 μm). Since InP with an energy gap of 1.351 eV is the widest-energy-gap material in the lattice-matching range, DH lasers with the structure

$$P\text{–}InP\,|\,n\text{– or }p\text{–}Ga_x In_{1-x} P_y As_{1-y}\,|\,N\text{–}InP$$

may be prepared for laser emission in the wavelength region where optical-fiber transmission losses and dispersion are a minimum.

Moon *et al.*[75] constructed the energy gap–lattice constant–composition diagram that is a projection of Fig. 5.5-5 onto the x–y plane. This diagram is given in Fig. 5.5-6. There is a small difference in the compositional dependence for E_g of $Ga_x In_{1-x} As$ in Figs. 5.3-7 and 5.5-6. This difference represents the uncertainty in the assignment of E_g with x at the present time. Constant E_g values are shown by solid lines and the energy-gap value is given in steps of 0.1 eV. Constant lattice constants are shown by the broken lines. The broken line from the upper left-hand corner represents the lattice-match compositions to InP, while the broken line from the lower right-hand corner represents the lattice-match compositions to GaAs. From Fig. 5.5-6, it may

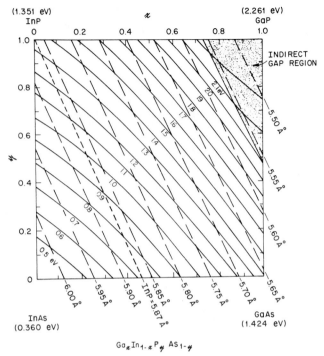

FIG. 5.5-6 The $x-y$ compositional plane for $Ga_xIn_{1-x}P_yAs_{1-y}$ at 300°K. The $x-y$ coordinate of any point in the plane gives the composition. The solid lines are constant direct-energy-gap values that were obtained by projection from the direct-energy-gap surface in Fig. 5.5-5. The broken lines are constant lattice constants. The lattice constant of InP is shown to illustrate the range of x and y that lattice match InP (Ref. 75).

readily be seen that $Ga_xIn_{1-x}P_yAs_{1-y}$ active layers which are lattice matched to InP can give DH lasers with emission energies (wavelengths) from 1.25 eV (0.99 μm) to 0.73 eV (1.7 μm).

Bogatov et al.[76] and Hsieh[77] prepared InP–$Ga_xIn_{1-x}P_yAs_{1-y}$DH lasers that operated with pulse excitation and gave emission wavelengths of 1.0–1.1 μm. As previously discussed, Hsieh et al.[5] obtained cw operation at an emission wavelength of 1.1 μm, and Yamamoto et al.[59] extended the emission wavelength to 1.34 μm. The DH lasers prepared by Hsieh et al.[77] have operated cw at room temperature for 5000 hr without significant degradation.[78] For the active layers in the DH lasers reported by Hsieh[5,77] the energy gap of the $Ga_{0.12}In_{0.88}P_{0.77}As_{0.23}$ is approximately 1.13 eV. These values are in reasonable agreement with Fig. 5.5-6. With this value of E_g, the heterojunction ΔE_g is 0.22 eV which is 2/3 of the ΔE_g for the usual choices of x in GaAs–$Al_xGa_{1-x}As$. Therefore, the use of high impurity concentrations in the InP cladding layers, as described in Section 5.4 for GaAs–$Ga_{0.51}In_{0.49}P$, may be helpful in providing carrier confinement in this DH laser. Efficient light-emitting diodes (LED's) have also been prepared with $Ga_xIn_{1-x}P_yAs_{1-y}$.[79] Considerable further effort can be expected to be devoted to producing heterostructure lasers and LED's that take advantage of the lattice match of InP–$Ga_xIn_{1-x}P_yAs_{1-y}$ for the low loss and dispersion of the optical fibers near 1.1–1.3 μm. Double heterostructures with red emission near 1.70 eV with the structure

$$N–Ga_{0.51}In_{0.49}P|p–Ga_{0.57}In_{0.43}P_{0.8}As_{0.2}|P–Ga_{0.51}In_{0.49}P$$

were prepared by Alferov *et al.*[80] The value of $J_{th}(300°K)$ was 2×10^4 A/cm².

$Ga_xIn_{1-x}As_ySb_{1-y}$

This system has a direct-energy gap at all compositions. The lattice constant has been taken as linear with composition. The lattice-matching compositions to AlSb, GaSb, and InP together with the 0°K constant energy-gap values in the $x–y$ compositional plane are shown in Fig. 5.5-7. The ternary compositional dependence of E_g was given for these systems

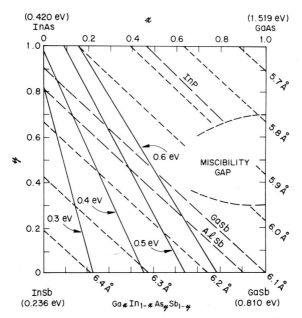

FIG. 5.5-7 The $x–y$ compositional plane for $Ga_xIn_{1-x}As_ySb_{1-y}$ at 0°K. The solid lines are constant direct-energy-gap values and the broken lines are constant lattice constants. The lattice constants of AlSb, GaSb, and InP are shown to illustrate the range of x and y for binary–quaternary lattice match.

in Fig. 5.3-7, 5.3-8, 5.3-10, and 5.3-12. These room-temperature values of E_g were translated to 0°K with the aid of the binary values in Table 5.2-2. The exact width of the miscibility gap in the ternary and the extent to which it penetrates into the quaternary is not known. Therefore, lattice-matching compositions to InP may not be useful. The systems that lattice match to AlSb and GaSb result in emission wave lengths $\gtrsim 2$ μm. The oxidation problems previously mentioned for AlSb may prevent its use.

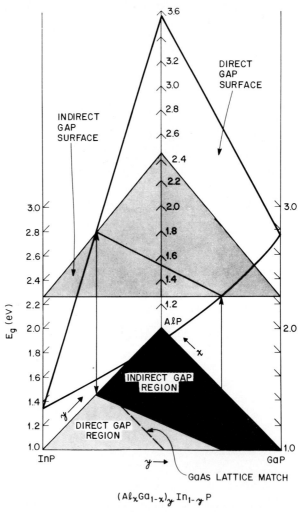

FIG. 5.5-8   Three-dimensional representation of the compositional dependence of the direct- and indirect-energy-gap surfaces in $(Al_xGa_{1-x})_yIn_{1-y}P$ at 300°K. The triangular base gives the composition in terms of x and y.

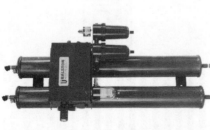

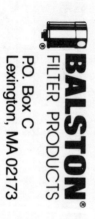

$(Al_xGa_{1-x})_yIn_{1-y}P$

This quaternary is the first system of the form $(A_xB_{1-x})_yC_{1-y}D$ to be considered and will be discussed more extensively than the others that follow. This system was represented schematically in Fig. 1.5-2. Both GaAs and $Al_xGa_{1-x}As$ lattice match $(Al_xGa_{1-x})_yIn_{1-y}P$ at all values of x for which $y = 0.51$. The three-dimensional compositional dependence of the energy gaps for this system has been drawn in Fig. 5.5-8. Two of the bounding ternary diagrams were given in Figs. 5.3-1 and 5.3-6. The compositional dependence of E_g for $Al_xGa_{1-x}P$ was not given because it is indirect at all compositions and experimental data are not available. A linear compositional dependence is assumed for both the direct and indirect-energy gaps. Because some additional bowing is expected in the quaternary, the intersection of the two surfaces is not really a straight line as shown. However, the bowing effects are expected to be small and have been neglected.

The base compositional plane is now a triangle rather than the previous square. The designation of the composition is illustrated in Fig. 5.5-9. An arbitrary system $(A_xB_{1-x})_yC_{1-y}D$ is shown. In order to permit x and y to be read directly from the edges of the triangular diagram, a procedure slightly different from that usually used for ternary triangular composition diagrams is employed. On the perimeter of the triangle, y along CD to BD is for $x = 0$,

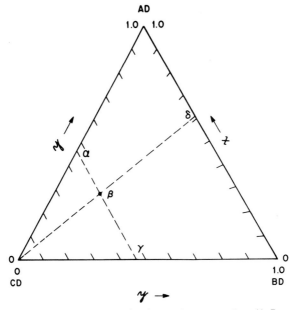

FIG. 5.5-9 Compositional diagram for the quaternary system $(A_xB_{1-x})_yC_{1-y}D$. See text for further description.

while y along CD to AD is for $x = 1.0$. To find the composition of an arbitrary point β, the line CD–β–δ is drawn from $y = 0$ to the x scale, and the line α–β–γ is drawn through β parallel to the x scale. The value of x is the value at δ, i.e., (BD to δ)/(BD to AD), while the value of y is the value at α or γ since α–β–γ will be a constant y line.

In the same manner as for $Ga_xIn_{1-x}P_yAs_{1-y}$, lines of constant energy gap and lattice constant are superimposed on the x–y compositional plane as shown in Fig. 5.5-10. The direct-to-indirect energy-gap crossover for a composition lattice matched to GaAs occurs at $x = 0.66$ and $y = 0.51$ at $E_g \approx 2.3$ eV. In principle, it is possible to prepare heterostructure lasers that are lattice matched to GaAs of the type

$$N-(Al_{x'}Ga_{1-x'})_{0.51}In_{0.49}P|n- \text{ or } p-(Al_xGa_{1-x})_{0.51}In_{0.49}P|$$
$$P-(Al_{x'}Ga_{1-x'})_{0.51}In_{0.49}P$$

with $x' > x$ and $x \lesssim 0.4$. For the condition of $x \lesssim 0.4$, it has been assumed that the direct energy gap in the active layer should be less than the indirect gap by ~ 0.15–0.20 eV to prevent transfer of injected electrons from the direct to indirect conduction band as considered in Section 4.6. This struc-

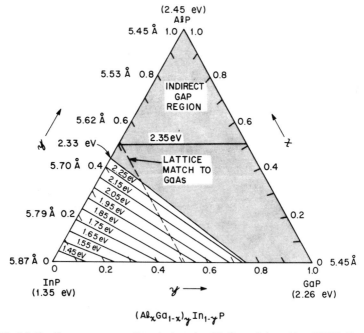

$$(Al_xGa_{1-x})_yIn_{1-y}P$$

FIG. 5.5-10 The x–y compositional plane for $(Al_xGa_{1-x})_yIn_{1-y}P$ at 300°K. The solid lines are constant direct-energy-gap values obtained by projection from the direct-energy-gap surface in Fig. 5.5-8. The broken line represents the GaAs lattice constant and is shown to illustrate lattice match to GaAs for $y = 0.51$ and $x = 0$ to 1.0.

ture with an energy gap of ~2.15 eV (0.58 μm) potentially has the highest energy emission at room temperature of any III–V heterostructure with complete lattice matching. It is doubtful that any substantial increase in emission energy can be achieved with graded systems. However, the thermodynamic arguments presented in Section 6.2 suggest that the controlled, simultaneous incorporation of Al and In in a III–V system that contains P will be very difficult.

(Al$_x$Ga$_{1-x}$)$_y$In$_{1-y}$As

In the same manner as for the previous quaternary, lines of constant energy gap and lattice constant are superimposed on the x–y compositional plane as shown in Fig. 5.5-11. The compositional dependence of the ternary energy gaps were given in Figs. 5.3-2, 5.3-3, and 5.3-7. Again, additional bowing in the quaternary has been neglected. All compositions with $y = 0.47$ lattice match to InP and are expected to have direct energy gaps. The smallest direct energy gap along $y = 0.47$ occurs at $x = 0$ and is approximately 0.80 eV at 300°K. The energy gap increases with x along the $y = 0.47$ composition line and is 1.5 eV at $x = 1.0$. Two possible heterostructures utilizing

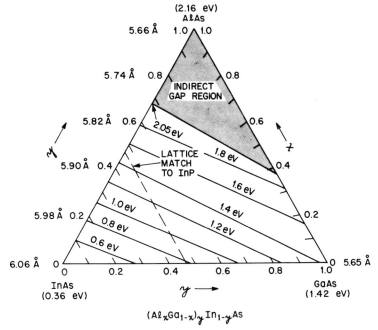

FIG. 5.5-11   The x–y compositional plane for (Al$_x$Ga$_{1-x}$)$_y$In$_{1-y}$As at 300°K. The solid lines are constant direct-energy-gap values obtained by a linear extrapolation of E_g from Al$_y$In$_{1-y}$As and Ga$_y$In$_{1-y}$As. The dashed line represents the InP lattice constant.

the $y = 0.47$ quaternary are of particular interest. The simplest is

$$N\text{–}InP\big|n\text{– or } p\text{–}(Al_xGa_{1-x})_{0.47}In_{0.53}As\big|P\text{–}InP,$$

which with $0 < x < 0.54$ would give laser emission from about 0.8 eV (1.6 μm) to about 1.2 eV (1.03 μm). The upper limit on x would be determined by the ΔE_g between InP and $(Al_xGa_{1-x})_{0.47}In_{0.53}As$ necessary for carrier confinement. A more complex structure on an InP substrate of

$$N\text{–}(Al_{x'}Ga_{1-x'})_{0.47}In_{0.53}As\big|n\text{– or } p\text{–}(Al_xGa_{1-x})_{0.47}In_{0.53}As\big|$$
$$P\text{–}(Al_{x'}Ga_{1-x'})_{0.47}In_{0.53}As$$

with $x' > x$ would give laser emission from 0.8 eV (1.6 μm) to 1.35 eV (0.92 μm) for x up to $\sim$0.8. The possibility of obtaining laser emission in the 1.2–1.3 μm range is an interesting possibility for this system. However, as described in Section 6.2, the large distribution coefficient of Al in this system will make the growth of layers by conventional epitaxy techniques difficult.

$(Al_xGa_{1-x})_yIn_{1-y}Sb$

Lines of constant energy gap and the AlSb lattice constant are super-imposed on the x–y compositional plane as shown in Fig. 5.5-12. The com-

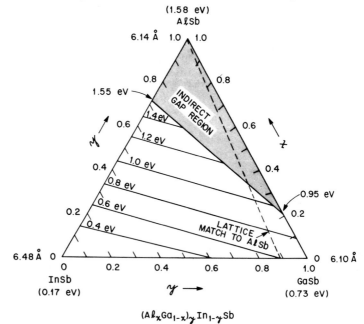

FIG. 5.5-12   The x–y compositional plane for $(Al_xGa_{1-x})_yIn_{1-y}Sb$ at 300°K. The solid lines are constant energy-gap values obtained by linear extrapolation of E_g from the terna-ries. The dashed line represents the AlSb lattice match.

positional dependence of the ternary energy gaps were given in Figs. 5.3-4, 5.3-5, and 5.3-8. The direct-to-indirect crossover was estimated in Fig. 5.3-5 for $Al_xIn_{1-x}Sb$. Although quaternary lattice matching occurs for AlSb, this system is of limited interest because of the anticipated growth problems due to the AlSb oxidation. If the growth problems could be overcome, hetero-structures of the form

$$N\text{–}AlSb|n\text{– or }p\text{–}(Al_xGa_{1-x})_yIn_{1-y}Sb|P\text{–}AlSb$$

would give laser emission from 1.0 eV (1.24 μm) to 0.6 eV (2.07 μm). The compositions for lattice matching to AlSb may be taken from Fig. 5.5-12.

$In(P_xAs_{1-x})_ySb_{1-y}$

Lines of constant energy gap and the lattice constant of AlSb, GaSb, and InAs are superimposed on the x–y compositional plane as shown in Fig. 5.5-13. The compositional dependence of the InP_xAs_{1-x} energy gap was given in Fig. 5.3-11. The compositional dependence of E_g for InP_xSb_{1-x}

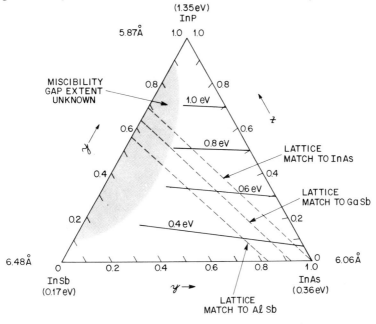

FIG. 5.5-13 The x–y compositional plane for $In(P_xAs_{1-x})_ySb_{1-y}$ at 300°K. The solid lines are estimated constant energy-gap values. The dashed lines represent the compositions for lattice matching to AlSb, GaSb, and InAs. The corresponding 0°K curves are obtained by adding 0.06 eV.

was not given because of the expected extensive miscibility gap. The compositional dependence of E_g for $InAs_xSb_{1-x}$ was given in Fig. 5.3-12. To draw approximate values for E_g in the quaternary, a linear composition dependence has been assumed for the energy gap of InP_ySb_{1-y} even though the miscibility gap prevents the existence of the solid solution. This diagram in Fig. 5.5-13 shows that lattice-matched quaternaries are possible for laser emission from about 0.6 eV (2.07 μm) to 0.3 eV (4.1 μm). Designation of the extent of the miscibility gap is necessary before the possible heterostructure lasers in this system can be considered.

5.6 COMPOSITIONAL GRADING FOR HETEROSTRUCTURE LASERS

Introductory Comments

Additional heterostructure combinations are possible when compositionally graded epitaxial layers are used with binary to ternary substrates in order to change the lattice constant. The composition is graded in an intermediate layer between the substrate and the heterostructure so that the active layer and adjacent layers have the same lattice constant at the active layer–heterojunction interface. There has been substantial experience in the growth of compositionally graded III–V ternary compounds by chemical-vapor deposition (CVD). This experience has been achieved primarily with the growth of GaP_xAs_{1-x} on GaAs for the production of red-light emitting diodes. The CVD process is described in Section 6.7. Compositional grading has also been used for other III–V solid solutions. The first example of composition grading to produce low threshold injection lasers was by Nahory et al.[4] They used liquid-phase epitaxy to prepare an intermediate step-graded $GaAs_xSb_{1-x}$ layer on a GaAs substrate for cw room-temperature DH lasers that emit at about 1 μm. The DH consisted of $Al_xGa_{1-x}As_ySb_{1-y}$ wide-energy-gap layers which are lattice matched to a $GaAs_ySb_{1-y}$ active layer. These DH lasers will be discussed in greater detail later in this section.

In this section, problems unique to compositionally graded layers will be considered. When an epitaxial layer is grown onto a substrate crystal which has a different lattice constant, the bond lengths of the material on each side of the heterojunction may be modified slightly from their normal values. This difference in lattice constant is taken up as strain, or if the mismatch is too great, misfit dislocations may be formed. In order to establish the terminology and concepts relevant to dislocations in III-V solid solutions, a qualitative description of dislocations is given in the next part of this section. Detailed texts on dislocations,[81,82] including a review article pertaining particularly to diamond-like semiconductors,[83] are available.

Dislocations in Crystals

Dislocations in crystalline solids are usually either "grown-in" or process induced. The process induced dislocations are usually the result of plastic flow which is caused by strain. They may be pure edge or pure screw dislocations, or they may be a mixture of both pure types. In a crystal consisting of only one kind of atom, an edge dislocation results from the presence of an extra plane of atoms as illustrated in Fig. 5.6-1. This extra plane may be the result of deformation of the crystal in the direction of the slip vector illustrated in the figure. The dislocation core is the edge of the extra plane. The plane along which atoms have had to move to create the dislocation is the slip plane, and the pure edge dislocation is perpendicular to the slip vector. The edge dislocation may also be the result of lattice mismatch at a heterojunction interface as illustrated in Fig. 5.6-2 for elemental cubic crystals, or it may result from strain induced by composition variation in a

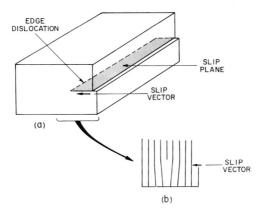

(a)

(b)

FIG. 5.6-1   Schematic representation of an edge dislocation Part (a) shows macroscopic view. Part (b) shows the extra plane of atoms resulting from slip, along the slip plane and in the direction of the slip vector.

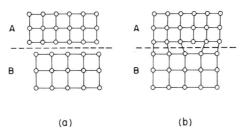

(a)   (b)

FIG. 5.6-2   Schematic representation of an edge dislocation that results from the epitaxial joining of crystal A to crystal B. The lattice constant of crystal A is smaller than for crystal B. (a) Before joining crystals A and B. (b) After epitaxial joining with the formation of an edge dislocation in crystal A.

compositionally graded layer. The screw dislocation, like the edge dislocation, may be created by slip. In this case, as illustrated in Fig. 5.6-3a, part
of the crystal slips parallel to the slip vector and part does not. The result is
a dislocation parallel to the slip vector as shown in Fig. 5.6-3b. The crystal
plane normal to the slip vector is a single plane in the form of a spiral ramp
with the dislocation at its axis. Thus, the name screw dislocation. The region
of the crystal in the immediate vicinity of both edge and screw dislocations
is distorted and therefore strained.

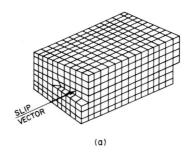

(a)

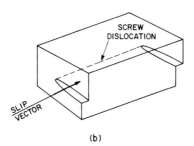

(b)

FIG. 5.6-3   Schematic representation of a screw dislocation. (a) Macroscopic view.
(b) Illustration that the slip vector is parallel to the dislocation.

It is useful at this point to mention the use[81] of the Burgers vector to
describe a dislocation. A Burgers vector is the representation of the closure
failure of a circuit in the crystal lattice consisting of atom to atom steps
along translation vectors in material that is perfect except for elastic strain.
The circuit, called a Burgers circuit, is such that it must close when it encircles
perfect material, and the Burgers vector is the vector joining the incomplete
ends of the circuit when it encircles a dislocation. For example, in Fig. 5.6-2
a Burgers circuit for the dislocation normal to the plane of the paper can
start at the upper left-hand corner. A path may have four atom steps down-
ward, four to the right, four upward and then four to the left. If the crystal
were perfect, the circuit would now be complete. Actually, the path described

requires one additional step to the left to be completed. This is the Burgers vector b that describes the enclosed dislocation.

The discussion given here is primarily concerned with III-V crystals. They consist of two different kinds of atoms, each on its own sublattice as was illustrated in Fig. 5.2-1 and 5.2-2. The group III and group V atoms are arranged so that the nearest-neighbor atoms are from the other group. In this case, the slip to form an edge or screw dislocation must traverse pairs of planes. Each pair must consist of one plane from each sublattice for the crystal to remain perfect beyond the distorted region.

Real dislocations often are mixtures with both screw and edge components. They are not constrained to be straight line features, as are pure screw and edge dislocations. A very common mixed dislocation in III–V compounds is the one illustrated in Fig. 5.6-4 (Ref. 84) for the perfect zinc-blende structure of Fig. 5.2-1. Figure 5.6-4 permits illustration of some significant features of the behavior of these dislocations. The dislocation shown in Fig. 5.6-4 is parallel to a $\langle 110 \rangle$ direction at D. The removal of a $\{112\}$ plane[82,83] at E, which consists of two sublattice planes, or the insertion of the same two sublattice planes at F would eliminate it. The Burgers vector is at $60°$ to the dislocation and the dislocation is thus designated as a $60°$ dislocation. Its Burgers vector joins two adjacent parallel $\langle 110 \rangle$ planes. The usual matrix notation for the Burgers vector of the $60°$ dislocation is $b = (a/2)\langle 110 \rangle$. Although the dislocation consists of the entire distorted region, it is interesting to note that two distinctly different $60°$ dislocations are possible. The two possibilities depend on whether group III or group V

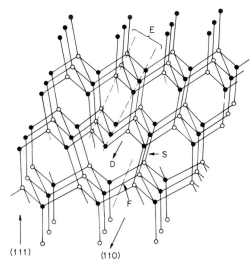

FIG. 5.6-4 The zinc-blende lattice with a $60°$ dislocation (Ref. 84).

atoms constitute the unbounded row. If the bonds at S move to the open bonds at D (as may occur with strain), the dislocation will move parallel to the {111} slip plane with no change in the total number of atoms involved. Such motion, with no change in the number of atoms in the extra plane, is called glide. If, however, there is any component of the motion of the dislocation out of any possible slip plane, part of each of a pair of {112} sublattice planes must be added or removed. Such dislocation motion, where there is atom transport to or away from the dislocation, is referred to as dislocation climb. This second type of dislocation motion has important implications for laser degradation, and the discussion is extended in Chapter 8. In this section, the primary concern is with dislocations that result from strain induced by compositional inhomogeneity or lattice mismatch at a heterojunction.

Dislocations in Compositionally Graded Layers

If all of the lattice mismatch at a heterojunction were taken up by edge dislocations, as illustrated in Fig. 5.6-2, then mismatched substrates would probably not be a serious problem for heterostructure lasers. The edge dislocations are parallel to the plane of the growing surface and would be completely overgrown after growth of a thin epitaxial layer with dislocation free material above the initial interface. Then the epitaxial material could serve as the new substrate surface for the lattice matched heterostructures such as those described in Sections 5.4 and 5.5.

Unfortunately, when mismatched III–V epitaxial layers are grown by either CVD[85–88] or LPE, it is experimentally observed that in addition to edge dislocations there are high concentrations of dislocations that penetrate through the grown structure. These penetrating dislocations may consist of mixed and screw dislocations, and it is convenient to refer to them as inclined dislocations. As described in Chapter 8, these dislocations may be very detrimental to laser operating life. Furthermore, semiconductor layers with dislocations that result from lattice mismatch have reduced luminescent efficiency in the region of the dislocation.[89]

Compositional grading during growth of the layer, in order to gradually change the substrate lattice constant to that of the desired solid solution composition, does not prevent the formation of dislocations because the lattice mismatch must be accommodated. Only edge dislocations or the edge component of mixed dislocations help accommodate strain. Dislocations that contribute to strain accommodation are referred to as misfit dislocations. Defects, such as dislocations and stacking faults may be observed by transmission-electron microscopy (TEM). The distorted region of the crystal at the defect diffracts electrons differently from the bulk lattice and because of that an image of the defect can be obtained. Abrahams et al.[85] observed by TEM that the density of inclined dislocations remains constant in graded layers with a constant gradation. In ungraded layers grown subsequently, the inclined dislocation density was dependent on the composition gradient in the graded region. According to their model, and also the model of Matthews *et al.*,[87,88] the strain introduced by the increased lattice change as the graded layer grows is accommodated by motion of portions of the underlying inclined dislocations. This motion increases the component of the dislocation that is parallel to the growing surface. The result of this mechanism is a dislocation network with portions or a component of each dislocation parallel to the interfacial plane. This type of dislocation is illustrated schematically in Fig. 5.6-5, where it is seen traversing several atomic planes in the crystal. At some planes, it simply passes through, but at others it becomes a mixed dislocation and is then parallel to the set of planes as shown in the figure. An example for GaP_xAs_{1-x} is shown in the transmission electron micrograph of Fig. 5.6-6. (Ref. 85) Portions of the dislocation network are not observed because they do not satisfy the diffraction conditions for imaging in the TEM. A transmission electron micrograph of a step-graded $In_xGa_{1-x}P$ layer is shown in Fig. 5.6-7, where the three distinct dislocation regions correspond to the three composition steps.

Both the dislocations frequently found in substrate crystals and the dislocations that form the networks illustrated in Figs. 5.6-5–5.6-7 are

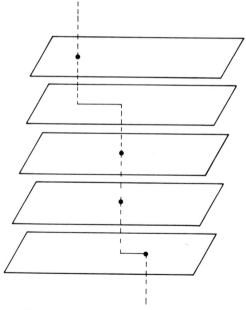

FIG. 5.6-5   Schematic representation of misfit dislocations to illustrate how they have edge dislocation portions parallel to the growing surface and inclined portions that penetrate up through the growing layer.

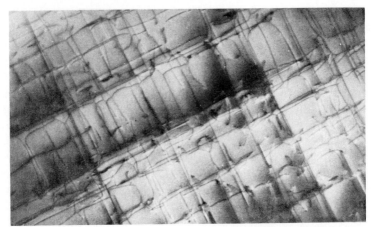

FIG. 5.6-6 Transmission electron micrograph of a dislocation network in a compositionally graded CVD layer of GaP_xAs_{1-x} grown on a GaAs substrate. The junction plane is parallel to the surface (Ref. 85).

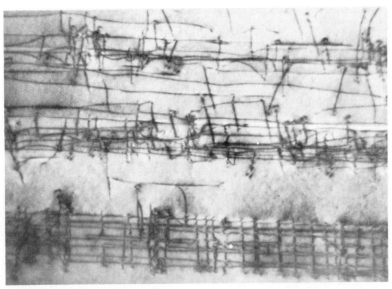

FIG. 5.6-7 Cross-sectional transmission electron micrograph of a step-graded $In_xGa_{1-x}P$ layer grown on GaP. The substrate–layer interface is at the bottom, and there are three steps where three distinct regions of dislocations are observed (Ref. 86).

commonly referred to as threading dislocations. The density of the inclined portions of the threading dislocations in a plane parallel to the growth direction is usually $10^5 - 10^6$ cm^{-2} for III–V epitaxial compositionally graded layers grown by CVD. This density may be too high for injection lasers or even high radiance light-emitting diodes (LED's) in which long operating life is required (Chapter 8). There is, however, some evidence that the inclined dislocation density can be reduced. The introduction of discontinuous changes in composition has been used[88] to obtain abrupt reductions in the inclined dislocation density by forcing much of the mismatch to be taken up by edge dislocations. In Fig. 5.6-7, three distinct networks that consist of a very high concentration of edge dislocations (parallel to the growth plane) can be observed, and there are relatively few dislocations penetrating into the grown regions between them. This layer was grown with composition steps rather than gradual composition grading. Additional work will be required in order to develop techniques that reduce the inclined dislocation densities in graded layers to acceptable levels.

An interesting and potentially useful application of misfit strain during epitaxial growth was demonstrated by Rozgonyi *et al.*[62,65,66] As described in the previous section for $Al_xGa_{1-x}P_yAs_{1-y}$, the room temperature epitaxial layer stress was greatly reduced by the addition of small amounts of P to the solution that was used for the growth of $Al_{0.3}Ga_{0.7}As$ in order to obtain $Al_{0.3}Ga_{0.7}P_yAs_{1-y}$ with $y \approx 0.01$. This addition of small amounts of P permits close control over the lattice mismatch. When the addition of P gives just sufficient mismatch at the growth temperature to initiate dislocation formation at the $GaAs–Al_xGa_{1-x}P_yAs_{1-y}$ interface, a unidirectional array of edge dislocations is observed to form. In many instances, the dislocations of this array originate from threading dislocations in the substrate. When the layer thickness and composition are suitable, the substrate dislocations, which would otherwise simply be grown into the epitaxial layer, appear to be forced by the mismatch strain to bend over and become misfit dislocations. These dislocations then propagate to the edge of the crystal so that the epitaxial layer above the substrate–layer interface is left relatively free of dislocations. If, however, the mismatch at the growth temperature is too large, a crosshatch network of threading dislocations similar to those illustrated in Figs. 5.6-6 and 5.6-7 is observed. In Fig. 5.6-8, an example of the P composition in the liquid at about 800°C and layer thickness for layers with no misfit dislocations, unidirectional arrays, or the crosshatch network are summarized for $Al_{0.34}Ga_{0.66}As_{1-y}P_y$ epitaxial layers. This work with LPE material and the work by Abrahams *et al.*[85,86] with material grown by CVD suggest that techniques for sweeping dislocations out of an epitaxial layer by properly designated growth compositions and grading are possible.

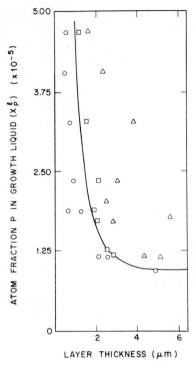

FIG. 5.6-8 Misfit dislocation threshold plot for $Al_{0.34}Ga_{0.66}P_yAs_{1-y}$ grown on GaAs substrates by LPE at $\sim 800°C$. ○—no misfit dislocations, ☐—unidirectional array, and △—crosshatch network (Ref. 62).

Heterostructure Lasers with Compositionally Graded Layers

The motivation for investigating heterostructure lasers with compositionally graded layers has been to utilize ternary or quaternary heterostructure lasers that emit between 1 and 1.4 μm for optical fiber applications or that emit in the visible region of the spectrum. There have been three approaches to compositional grading for heterostructure lasers: (1) step-graded $GaAs_xSb_{1-x}$ layers grown on GaAs substrates so as to make possible a laser with a $GaAs_ySb_{1-y}$ active region; (2) compositionally graded $Ga_xIn_{1-x}As$ layers on GaAs substrates so as to permit lasers with active regions of $Ga_xIn_{1-x}As$; and (3) heterostructures grown on GaP_xAs_{1-x} "substrates" that were grown by compositional grading on GaAs. In the remainder of this section, heterostructure lasers fabricated from several of these heterostructures that have composition or step-grading will be described.

The utilization of the $Al_xGa_{1-x}As_ySb_{1-y}$ quaternary as the wide-energy-gap semiconductor in a DH laser with a $GaAs_ySb_{1-y}$ active region makes possible the achievement of DH lasers with emission in the 1.0–1.1 μm range. The energy gap–lattice constant–composition diagram for the $Al_xGa_{1-x}As_ySb_{1-y}$ system was given in Fig. 5.5-4. The major change in the lattice constant in the quaternary is achieved by varying y. The upper left-hand portion of Fig. 5.5-4 where $E_g \approx 1.2$ eV for $y \approx 0.88$, is the region of interest for the composition of the ternary active region. Compositions with the same y but $x \gtrsim 0.3$ are of interest for the wide-energy-gap part of the heterostructure as indicated in the figure.

Sugiyama and Saito[90] used LPE to grow approximately 20-μm thick layers of $GaAs_xSb_{1-x}$ on GaAs and then grew the DH

$$N–Al_xGa_{1-x}As_ySb_{1-y}|p–GaAs_ySb_{1-y}|P–Al_xGa_{1-x}As_ySb_{1-y},$$

with $x \approx 0.2 - 0.3$ and $y \approx 0.85$. At room temperature, the emission from lasers fabricated from such DH wafers was at 0.980 μm, and the threshold current density $J_{th}(300°K)$ was 8.5×10^3 A/cm^2 for an active layer thickness of 0.8 μm.

Nahory et al[4,91,92] also used LPE to grow step-graded $GaAs_xSb_{1-x}$ layers on GaAs substrates with the successive compositions of $x = 0.975$, 0.942, and 0.907 to provide stress relief. Stripe-geometry devices (Section 7.6) were fabricated by utilizing proton bombardment to provide electrical isolation. For pulsed operation,[92] $J_{th}(300°K)$ was as low as 1.2×10^3 A/cm^2, and for cw operation,[4] $J_{th}(300°K)$ was as low as 2.1×10^3/cm^2. A typical composition for their heterostructure had $x \approx 0.4$ and $y \approx 0.88$, which gave the DH

$$N–Al_{0.4}Ga_{0.6}As_{0.88}Sb_{0.12}|p–GaAs_{0.88}Sb_{0.12}|P–Al_{0.4}Ga_{0.6}As_{0.88}Sb_{0.12}.$$

The emission wavelengths for a number of lasers were in the range of 1.00–1.06 μm, with the best lasers emitting at wavelengths near 1.00 μm. Active layer thicknesses d were as small as 0.3 μm. The highest differential efficiency for pulsed operation was 0.35 (Ref. 92). For the best units, $J_{th}(300°K)/d \approx 4.0 \times 10^3$ A/cm^2-μm.[92]

Although the active-layer thickness of the DH lasers prepared by Nahory et al.[4] was one half that of the lasers prepared by Sugiyama and Saito,[90] the step-graded layers appear to be the major reason for the lower $J_{th}(300°$ K). Presumably the step grading reduced the density of inclined dislocations, so that better crystalline quality was achieved in the lattice-matched DH regions. There was, however, no evidence that inclined dislocations were brought to very low levels by the step-graded layer. These dislocations may cause a serious problem for the reproducible, high yield growth of lasers with long operating life in this system. The initial success suggests that efforts should be made to improve the step-growth process or to grow $GaAs_{0.88}Sb_{0.12}$ bulk crystals for substrates.

Another DH laser with emission in the 1-μm region, which requires a compositionally graded layer, has been investigated by Nuese and Olsen.[93]

TABLE 5.6-1 Heterostructure Lasers on GaP_xAs_{1-x} Substrates

Heterostructure		J_{th}(A/cm^2)	Temperature (°K)	Emission wavelength (μm)	Reference	Comments
$Al_xGa_{1-y}P_yAs_{1-y}$–$Al_xGa_{1-x'}P_yAs_{1-y}$ $x > x'$	DH	1.0×10^4	300	0.845	95	LPE on $GaP_{0.07}As_{0.93}$ substrate
$GaP_{0.4}As_{0.6}{}^a$–$Ga_{0.7}In_{0.3}P_{0.99}As_{0.01}$	SH	1.4×10^4	77	0.636	96	LPE on $GaP_{0.38}As_{0.62}$ substrate
$Ga_{0.63}In_{0.37}P$	homostructure	1×10^5	77	0.590	97	LPE on $GaP_{0.25}As_{0.75}$ substrate
$GaP_{0.32}As_{0.68}{}^a$–$Ga_xIn_{1-x}P_{0.99}As_{0.01}$	SH	—	4.2, 77	—	98	Studied the nitrogen pair lines and nitrogen A-line in GaP_xAs_{1-x}
$Ga_{0.66}In_{0.34}P_{0.99}As_{0.01}$–$Ga_{0.77}In_{0.23}P_{0.79}As_{0.21}{}^a$	DH	2.0×10^4	300	0.647	99	LPE on GaP_xAs_{1-x} substrates
$GaP_{0.3}As_{0.7}{}^a$–$Ga_{0.66}In_{0.34}P$	DH	3.4×10^3	300	0.700	101	CVD on GaP_xAs_{1-x} substrate

^{a} Active layer material.

As discussed in Section 5.4, $Ga_{0.51}In_{0.49}P$ lattice matches to GaAs, and Fig. 5.4-1 shows that $Ga_xIn_{1-x}P$ lattice matches to $Ga_{x'}In_{1-x'}As$ over an extensive range of x and x' with $x < x'$. For the lasers studied by Nuese and Olsen,[93] a $Ga_xIn_{1-x}P$ layer was grown on GaAs by CVD with x varied from 0.51 at the substrate to 0.32. The DH

$$N–Ga_{0.32}In_{0.68}P | p–n \, Ga_{0.84}In_{0.16}As | P–Ga_{0.32}In_{0.68}P$$

was then grown with the $p–n$ junction within the active layer. At room temperature, the emission wavelength for several lasers with nominally the same composition range varied from 1.025 to 1.15 μm, and $J_{th}(300°K)$ was 15×10^3 A/cm^2. The same considerations, as were discussed in Section 5.4 and illustrated in Figs. 5.4-2 and 5.4-3, suggest that high acceptor concentration in the P-layer will improve electron confinement in this DH laser. Subsequent work by Nuese et al.[94] has improved the materials quality and permitted DH lasers with a pulsed $J_{th}(300°K)$ of about 1×10^3 A/cm^2 and an emission wavelength of about 1.0 μm. These lasers have been operated cw at room temperature.

In order to study heterostructure lasers that emit visible radiation, Holonyak and co-workers[95–100] and Kressel et al.[101] have studied a number of ternary and quaternary systems that have been grown on GaP_xAs_{1-x}. The GaP_xAs_{1-x} was grown sufficiently thick by CVD on GaAs to be used as the substrate for subsequent layer growth by LPE or CVD. Emission at wavelengths as short as 0.647 μm has been obtained at room temperature with DH lasers of $Ga_xIn_{1-x}P_yAs_{1-y}$ in which x and y have been varied to change the energy gap while retaining a constant lattice constant.[100] Some of the various heterostructures that have been prepared on CVD grown GaP_xAs_{1-x} substrates are summarized in Table 5.6-1.

5.7 IV–VI BINARY COMPOUNDS AND THEIR SOLUTIONS

Introductory Comments

The initial studies of the IV–VI compounds were based on their applications as infrared detectors of thermal radiation. More recently these materials have been used to prepare injection lasers for applications in ultrahigh-resolution spectroscopy and pollution monitoring.[102] These materials have small energy gaps, typically less than ~ 0.35 eV, and homostructure lasers permit emission from ~ 3 to ~ 30 μm at low temperature. Both SH[103,104] and DH[105–108] lasers have been prepared with $PbTe–Pb_{1-x}Sn_xTe$ heterojunctions. These DH lasers resulted in significantly better performance than was previously obtained with homostructure lasers. A limited amount of work has also been reported with $Pbs–PbS_{1-x}Se_x$ SH and DH lasers.[109,110] The emission wavelength of the IV–VI heterostructure lasers is controlled by both the active-layer composition and the operating temperature. In the work of Walpole *et al.*,[108] temperature tuning of the emission from 15.9 to 8.54 μm was obtained for DH lasers which operated cw up to 114°K.

In contrast to the III–V systems, lattice mismatch with IV–VI heterostructures is not obviously detrimental to either heterostructure preparation or laser operation. It appears that free surfaces or mismatched heterojunction interfaces do not result in readily measurable concentrations of nonradiative recombination centers at the operating temperatures. Also, as described in Chapter 6, the electrical conductivity of the IV–VI compounds is often influenced by lattice vacancies that behave as ionized donors and acceptors. This behavior influences the conditions chosen for epitaxial growth and limits the usefulness of some IV–VI compounds. The epitaxial layers are grown by LPE techniques[104–107] very similar to those described in Chapter 6 for III–V compounds. They are also grown by a modification of the molecular-beam epitaxy (MBE) technique[108,111] that takes into account the different nature of the vapor species from those in III–V systems and the influence of stoichiometry on carrier concentration (Chapter 6). In addition to PbTe–Pb$_{1-x}$Sn$_x$Te lasers with Fabry–Perot cavities,[108] the MBE technique has permitted the preparation of lasers with distributed feedback[111] (Section 7.12). Most of this section will be devoted to summarizing the properties of the IV–VI binary and ternary narrow-gap semiconductors that are relevant to the study of heterostructure lasers. A brief description will also be given of the IV–VI DH lasers that have been prepared and the resulting laser properties.

Binary Properties Relevant to Heterostructure Lasers

The IV–VI compounds of interest for heterostructure lasers are those between Sn and Pb (group IV) and S, Se, and Te (group VI). They crystallize in the rock-salt structure (NaCl). The atoms have six nearest neighbors as shown in Fig. 5.7-1 for PbS. The lattice constant is indicated by a. The lattice constants for the three Pb compounds and SnTe are given in Table 5.7-1.

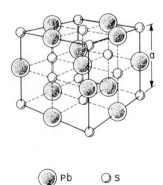

Pb   S

FIG. 5.7-1   The unit cell in PbS for the rock-salt structure. The lattice constant is a.

TABLE 5.7-1   Properties of the IV–VI Binary Compounds

Compound	Lattice constant at 299°K, $a(\text{Å})$	Ref.	Energy gap, $E_g(\text{eV})$ 4°K	Ref.	77°K	Ref.	300°K	Ref.	Density of states effective mass at 4°K, $m_n = m_p$	Ref.	Dielectric constant ε at 77°K	Ref.
PbS	5.9362	a	0.286	c	0.307	c	0.41	d	$0.22m_0$	e	$184\varepsilon_0$	f
PbSe	6.124	a	0.165	c	0.176	c	0.27	d	$0.12m_0$	e	$227\varepsilon_0$	f
PbTe	6.462	b	0.190	c	0.217	c	0.31	d	$0.13m_0$	e	$428\varepsilon_0$	f
SnTe	6.303	a	—		—		—		—		—	

[a] *Powder Diffraction File* (Joint Committee on Powder Diffraction Standards, Swarthmore, Pa., 1975).
[b] R. J. Paff and R. Dalven, unpublished.
[c] D. L. Mitchell, E. D. Palik, and J. N. Zemel, *Phys. Semiconduct.; Proc. Int. Conf., 7th, Paris, 1964* p. 325. Dunod, Paris, 1964.
[d] J. N. Zemel, J. D. Jensen, and R. B. Schoolar, *Phys. Rev.* **140**, A330 (1965).
[e] T. C. Harman and I. Melngailis, "Appl. Solid State Science, Vol. 4," (R. Wolfe, ed.), p. 1. Academic Press, New York, 1974.
[f] R. Dalven, *Infrared Phys.* **9**, 141 (1969).

The band structure of the IV–VI binary compounds[112] can be represented by an energy-versus-momentum wave-vector diagram similar to Fig. 4.2-1 for GaAs. The maximum in the valence band and the minimum in the conduction band occur in the [111] direction at $k = \pi/a$ rather than at $k = 0$ as for the III–V compounds. Therefore, rather than the Γ direct energy gap, these materials have the L direct energy gap. For the Pb binary compounds the conduction band is labeled L_{6^-} and the valence band is labeled L_{6^+}. However, for SnTe, the bands are inverted, and L_{6^+} is the conduction band while L_{6^-} becomes the valence band. Further discussion of the band structure may be found in the reviews by Harman and Melngailis[102] and Dalven.[113] The energy gaps at three temperatures are also given in Table 5.7-1. The temperature dependence of these energy gaps is plotted in Fig. 5.7-2. This figure emphasizes that the temperature dependence of E_g for the IV–VI compounds is opposite to the temperature dependence of E_g for the III–V compounds which was represented by Eq. (5.2-1).

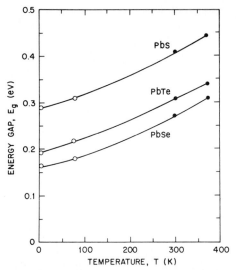

FIG. 5.7-2   Temperature dependence of the direct-energy gap for PbS, PbSe, and PbTe. ○—Ref. 114, ●—Ref. 115.

No data for the electron affinity or for ΔE_c and ΔE_v have been reported. Therefore, it is difficult to consider energy-band diagrams for IV–VI hetero-junctions, although the low injection laser thresholds for DH lasers indicate carrier confinement. The conduction and valence bands are very nearly mirror images. This similarity gives equal electron and hole density of states effective masses as given in Table 5.7-1. The last quantity given in

Table 5.7-1 is the dielectric constant. These values of ε for the IV–VI compounds are an order of magnitude larger than for the III–V compounds. The thermal conductivity for these compounds is about 0.1 W/cm-deg at 77°K.[113] The refractive index at 77°, 300°, and 373°K was measured over an extensive photon energy range by Zemel et al.[114] Results at 77°K are summarized in Fig. 5.7-3. Additional properties are described in Refs. 102, 113–116.

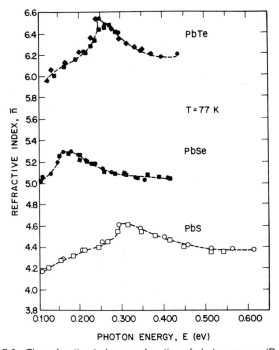

FIG. 5.7-3 The refractive index as a function of photon energy (Ref. 114).

Pb$_{1-x}$Sn$_x$Te

The compositional dependence of the energy gap of Pb$_{1-x}$Sn$_x$Te has been inferred by measurement of the energy of laser emission in homostructure lasers.[117] The results of these measurements are shown in Fig. 5.7-4. From the theoretical band model for Pb$_{1-x}$Sn$_x$Te,[118] the energy gap initially decreases with x as the L_{6-} conduction band and L_{6+} valence band approach each other. At an intermediate composition, E_g goes through zero, the bands invert, and then E_g increases with L_{6+} as the conduction band and L_{6-} as the valence band. By extrapolation of the E_g versus composition data in Fig. 5.7-4, E_g for Pb$_{1-x}$Sn$_x$Te approaches zero for $x \approx 0.35$. At

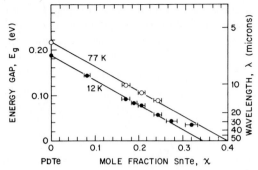

FIG. 5.7-4   Energy gap and laser emission wavelength for $Pb_{1-x}Sn_xTe$ (Ref. 117).

$12°K$, the variation of E_g for $x < 0.35$ may be represented by[102]

$$E_g \text{ (eV)} = 0.19 - 0.543x. \tag{5.7-1}$$

The energy gap is expected to increase linearly again for $x > 0.35$. The refractive indices for $Pb_{1-x}Sn_xTe$ at room temperature for several values of x have been given Jäger and Schubert.[119]

The most successful heterostructure lasers with IV–VI compounds are based on $PbTe–Pb_{1-x}Sn_xTe$ heterojunctions. Groves et al.[106] prepared

$$P–PbTe|n–Pb_{0.88}Sn_{0.12}Te|N–PbTe$$

DH lasers by LPE. The $P–PbTe$ portion of the heterostructure was a $\{100\}$-oriented wafer that was grown by the Bridgman method from a Tl-doped melt. The $n–Pb_{0.88}Sn_{0.12}Te$ layer is the active layer. As given by Eq. (2.2-36), the wavelength in the active layer λ is the free-space wavelength λ_0 divided by the refractive index $\bar{n}$. For a nominal value of $\lambda_0 \approx 10 \, \mu m$ and $\bar{n} \approx 5.0$, the wavelength in the active layer is approximately $2 \, \mu m$. Therefore, active layers in IV–VI DH lasers are generally $\gtrsim 2 \, \mu m$, which is an order of magnitude greater than for typical III–V DH lasers intended for cw operation. With the assumption of a linear compositional dependence of the lattice constant, the lattice mismatch between $PbTe$ and $Pb_{0.88}Sn_{0.12}Te$ at room temperature is only 0.3%. Stripe-geometry devices were prepared by LPE with 50-μm-wide stripes in a MgF_2 coating on the PbTe substrate. These devices operated cw at $77°K$ with $J_{th}(77°K) = 4.2 \times 10^3 \text{ A/cm}^2$. The emission wavelength was $8.35 \, \mu m$, and the power was $\sim 1 \, mW$ at $7.5 \times 10^3 \text{ A/cm}^2$.

Tomasetta and Fonstad also prepared DH lasers by LPE.[105,107] They used both n- and p-type PbTe substrates.[105] The lowest thresholds were obtained for

$$P–PbTe|n–Pb_{0.82}Sn_{0.18}Te|N–PbTe$$

double heterostructures with P–PbTe substrates. The active layer is the n-layer. For an active-layer thickness of 4 μm, the pulsed $J_{th}(77°K)$ was $\sim 1.2 \times 10^3$ A/cm^2. Experimental values of $J_{th}(T)$ were compared with calculated values in Ref. 107.

Walpole et al.[108] prepared asymmetric

$$P–PbTe|n–Pb_{0.78}Sn_{0.22}Te|N–Pb_{0.88}Sn_{0.12}Te$$

DH lasers by MBE on Tl-doped P–PbTe substrates that were grown by the seeded vertical vapor-growth technique. The n–Pb$_{0.78}$Sn$_{0.22}$Te layer is the active layer. The n- and N-layers were doped by adding Bi or TlSe to the vapor sources. The variation with temperature of the emission wavelength and the cw J_{th} are given in Fig. 5.7-5. Walpole et al.[111,120] have also prepared distributed-feedback PbTe-Pb$_{1-x}$SnTe lasers with MBE-grown layers.

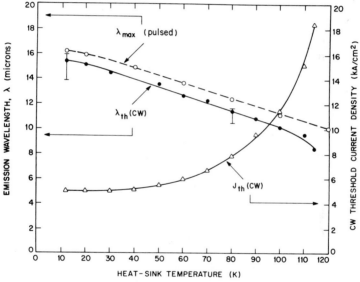

FIG. 5.7-5 Variation of emission wavelength and threshold current density as a function of temperature for PbTe–Pb$_{0.782}$Sn$_{0.218}$Te DH lasers (Ref. 108).

Pb$_{1-x}$Sn$_x$Se

The compositional dependence of the Pb$_{1-x}$Sn$_x$Se energy gap has been assigned from the energy of the laser emission in homojunction lasers.[121] The results at 12°K are shown in Fig. 5.7-6. In this system, E_g goes to zero for $x = 0.15$. In the same manner as for Pb$_{1-x}$Sn$_x$Te, the conduction and valence bands invert as x exceeds 0.15. Also, for $x \leq 0.10$ the temperature coefficient of the energy gap dE_g/dT is positive, but becomes negative for

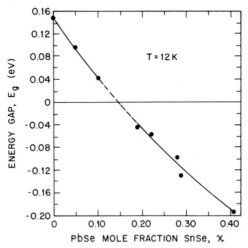

FIG. 5.7-6   Compositional dependence of the direct-energy gap L for $Pb_{1-x}Sn_xSe$ (Ref. 121).

$x \geq 0.19.$[121] Although homostructure lasers have been obtained in the composition range $0 \leq x \leq 0.4$, no heterostructure lasers have been reported for this system. The absence of heterostructure lasers in $Pb_{1-x}Sn_xSe$ is probably due to the similar range in possible emission wavelength as for $Pb_{1-x}Sn_xTe$, where influence of the ionized native defects on the conductivity are not as severe.

$PbS_{1-x}Se_x$

The compositional dependence of the $PbS_{1-x}Se_x$ energy gap has been assigned from the emission energy of electron-beam-pumped Pbs and PbSe lasers at 20°K as[122]

$$E_g(eV) = 0.289 - 0.144x. \qquad (5.7\text{-}2)$$

McLane and Sleger[109] prepared

$$N\text{-}PbS|p\text{-}PbS_{1-x}Se_x|P\text{-}PbS$$

DH lasers by molecular-beam epitaxy. These devices operated cw at 12°K with $J_{th}(12°K) = 60$ A/cm² and had an emission wavelength of 6.1 μm.

Preier et al.[110] prepared PbS–$PbS_{0.6}Se_{0.4}$ DH lasers by MBE on vapor-grown n-type PbS substrates. The n- or p-type active layers were grown by adjusting the compensating Se pressure. Stripe-geometry lasers were fabricated by overgrowth of 100-μm-wide stripes in a MgF_2 coating on the PbS substrate. The best results were obtained for $d \approx 1.0$ μm with cw operation up to 96°K. At 77°K, $J_{th}(77°K) = 400$ A/cm² and the emission wavelength was near 5 μm.

PbS–PbSe

Preier *et al.*[123] prepared PbS–PbSe–PbS DH lasers and obtained cw operation at heat sink temperatures up to 120°K and pulsed operation up to 180°K. The emission wavelength could be temperature tuned from 6.5 to 8.5 μm. Threshold current densities of less than 1×10^3 A/cm^2 were obtained at 77°K with an emission wavelength of $\sim$7.5 μm.

5.8 CONCLUDING COMMENTS

A variety of possible heterostructures for laser emission ranging from about 0.6 to about 15 μm have been described. The attractiveness of each of these heterostructure systems will depend upon the importance of the potential application at a given wavelength and upon how difficult it is to grow a heterostructure wafer of sufficiently high quality. Even for GaAs–Al$_x$Ga$_{1-x}$As heterostructures, there is much to be learned in order to reproducibly prepare lasers with high device yields and long operating life. In the next chapter, a discussion of the phase chemistry that is important to epitaxial growth is presented and is followed by descriptions of several epitaxial growth techniques.

REFERENCES

1. H. Osanai, T. Shioda, T. Moriyama, S. Araki, M. Horiguchi, T. Izawa, and H. Takata, *Electron. Lett.* **12**, 549 (1976).
2. L. G. Cohen and C. Lin, *Appl. Optics* **16**, 3136 (1977).
3. M. Horiguchi, *Electron. Lett.* **12**, 310 (1976).
4. R. E. Nahory, M. A. Pollack, E. D. Beebe, J. C. DeWinter, and R. W. Dixon, *Appl. Phys. Lett.* **28**, 19 (1976).
5. J. J. Hsieh, J. A. Rossi, and J. P. Donnelley, *Appl. Phys. Lett.* **28**, 709 (1976).
6. C. J. Nuese, G. H. Olsen, M. Ettenberg, J. J. Gannon, and T. J. Zamarowski, *Appl. Phys. Lett.* **29**, 807 (1976).
7. A. S. Jordan, A. R. Von Neida, R. Caruso, and C. K. Kim, *J. Electrochem. Soc.* **121**, 153 (1974).
8. H. R. Potts and G. L. Pearson, *J. Appl. Phys.* **37**, 2098 (1966).
9. C. M. H. Driscoll, A. F. W. Willoughby, J. B. Mullin, and B. W. Straughan, "*Gallium Arsenide and Related Compounds, 1974*," p. 275. Inst. of Phys., London, 1975.
10. Y. P. Varshni, *Physica* **34**, 149 (1967).
11. M. Neuberger, "Handbook of Electronic Materials," Vol. 2, III-V Semiconducting Compounds. Plenum Press, New York, 1971.
12. D. D. Sell, H. C. Casey, Jr., and K. W. Wecht, *J. Appl. Phys.* **45**, 2650 (1974).
13. R. E. Fern and A. Onton, *J. Appl. Phys.* **42**, 3499 (1971).
14. D. T. F. Marple, *J. Appl. Phys.* **35**, 1241 (1964).
15. B. O. Seraphin and H. E. Bennett, "Semiconductors and Semimetals" (R. K. Willardson and A. C. Beer, eds.), Vol. 3, p. 499. Academic Press, New York, 1967.
16. P. D. Maycock, *Solid-State Electron.* **10**, 161 (1967).
17. J. A. Van Vechten and T. K. Bergstresser, *Phys. Rev. B.* **1**, 3351 (1970).

18. O. Berolo, J. C. Woolley, and J. A. Van Vechten, *Phys. Rev. B.* **8**, 3794 (1973).
19. H. C. Casey, Jr., D. D. Sell, and M. B. Panish, *Appl. Phys. Lett.* **24**, 63 (1974).
20. G. D. Clark, Jr. and N. Holonyak, Jr., *Phys. Rev.* **156**, 913 (1967).
21. H. C. Casey, Jr., *J. Appl. Phys.* **45**, 2766 (1974).
22. M. A. Afromowitz, *Solid State Commun.* **15**, 59 (1974).
23. S. H. Wemple and M. DiDomenico, Jr., *Phys. Rev. B.* **3**, 1338 (1971).
24. M. A. Afromowitz, *J. Appl. Phys.* **44**, 1292 (1973).
25. M. Neuberger, "Handbook of Electronic Materials," Vol. 7, III-V Ternary Semiconducting Compounds—Data Tables. Plenum Press, New York, 1972.
26. A. Onton, "Festkörperprobleme XIII—Advances in Solid State Physics," p. 59. Pergamon (Vieweg), London and New York, 1973.
27. A. Onton and R. J. Chicotka, *J. Appl. Phys.* **41**, 4205 (1970).
28. M. R. Lorenz and A. Onton, *Proc. Int. Conf. Phys. Semiconduct., 10th, Cambridge, Massachusetts* (S. P. Keller, J. C. Hensel, and F. Stern, eds.), p. 444. U.S. Atomic Energy Comm., Washington, D.C., 1970.
29. F. M. Vorobkalo, K. D. Glinchuk, and V. F. Kovalenko, *Sov. Phys.–Semcond.* **9**, 656 (1975) [Translated from: *Fiz. Tekh. Poluprovodn.* **9**, 998 (1975)].
30. H. Mathieu, D. Auvergne, P. Merle, and K. C. Rustagi, *Phys. Rev. B.* **12**, 5846 (1975).
31. S. M. Bedair, *J. Appl. Phys.* **47**, 4145 (1976).
32. K. Y. Cheng, G. L. Pearson, R. S. Bauer, and D. J. Chadi, *Bull. Am. Phys. Soc.* **21**, 365 (1976).
33. S. Isomura, F. G. D. Prat, and J. C. Woolley, *Phys. Status Solidi (b)* **65**, 213 (1974).
34. M. H. Lee, N. Holonyak, Jr., W. R. Hitchens, and J. C. Campbell, *Solid State Commun.* **15**, 981 (1974).
35. R. J. Nelson and N. Holonyak, Jr., *J. Phys. Chem. Solids* **37**, 629 (1976).
36. A. Onton, M. R. Lorenz, and W. Reuter, *J. Appl. Phys.* **42**, 3420 (1971).
37. B. J. Baliga, R. Bhat, and S. K. Ghandi, *J. Appl. Phys.* **46**, 4608 (1975).
38. R. E. Nahory, M. A. Pollack, and J. C. DeWinter, *J. Appl. Phys.* **46**, 775 (1975).
39. D. Auvergne, J. Camassel, H. Mathieu, and A. Joullie, *J. Phys. Chem. Solids* **35**, 133 (1974).
40. A. G. Thompson, M. Cardona, K. L. Shaklee, and J. C. Woolley, *Phys. Rev.* **146**, 601 (1966).
41. M. G. Craford, G. E. Stillman, J. A. Rossi, and N. Holonyak, Jr., *Phys. Rev.* **168**, 867 (1968).
42. G. A. Antypas and L. W. James, *J. Appl. Phys.* **41**, 2165 (1970).
43. M. B. Thomas, W. M. Coderre, and J. C. Woolley, *Phys. Status Solidi (a)* **2**, K141 (1970).
44. G. A. Antypas and R. L. Moon, *J. Electrochem. Soc.* **121**, 416 (1974).
45. G. A. Antypas and T. O. Yep, *J. Appl. Phys.* **42**, 3201 (1971).
46. J. C. Woolley and J. Warner, *Can. J. Phys.* **42**, 1879 (1964).
47. A. G. Thompson and J. C. Woolley, *Can. J. Phys.* **45**, 255 (1967).
48. W. P. Allred, "Compound Semiconductors". (R. K. Willardson and H. L. Goering, eds.), Vol. 1, Properties of III–V Compounds, p. 187. Reinhold, New York, 1962.
48a. D. V. Lang and R. A. Logan, *Appl. Phys. Lett.* **31**, 683 (1977).
49. B. I. Miller, J. E. Ripper, J. C. Dyment, E. Pinkas, and M. B. Panish, *Appl. Phys. Lett.* **18**, 403 (1971).
50. Zh. I. Alferov, V. M. Andreev, T. Ya. Belousova, V. I. Borodulin, V. A. Gorbylev, G. T. Pak, A. I. Petrov, E. L. Portnoi, N. P. Chernousov, V. I. Shveikin, and I. V. Yashchumov, *Sov. Phys.–Semicond.* **6**, 495 (1972) [*Translated from: Fiz. Tekh. Poluprovodn.* **6**, 568 (1972)].
51. H. Kressel and F. Z. Hawrylo, *Appl. Phys. Lett.* **28**, 598 (1976).
52. D. F. Nelson and E. H. Turner, *J. Appl. Phys.* **39**, 3337 (1968).

53. C. J. Nuese, G. H. Olsen, and M. Ettenberg, *Appl. Phys. Lett.* **29**, 54 (1976).

54. C. J. Nuese, M. Ettenberg, and G. H. Olsen, *Appl. Phys. Lett.* **25**, 612 (1974).

55. C. J. Nuese, A. G. Sigai, J. J. Gannon, and T. Zamerowski, *J. Electron. Mater.* **3**, 51 (1974).

56. B. I. Miller and W. D. Johnston, Jr., *Appl. Phys. Lett.* **25**, 216 (1974).

57. G. Schul and P. Mischel, *Appl. Phys. Lett.* **26**, 394 (1975).

58. C. J. Nuese, R. E. Enstrom, and J. R. Appert, *Device Res. Conf., Ithaca, New York* (June, 1977).

59. T. Yamamoto, K. Saki, S. Akiba, and Y. Suematsu, *IEEE J. Quantum Electron.* **QE-14**, 95 (1978).

60. M. Ettenberg and R. J. Paff, *J. Appl. Phys.* **41**, 3926 (1970).

61. E. D. Pierron, D. L. Parker, and J. B. McNeely, *Acta Crystallogr.* **21**, 290 (1960).

62. G. A. Rozgonyi, P. M. Petroff, and M. B. Panish, *J. Cryst. Growth* **27**, 106 (1974).

63. G. A. Rozgonyi, C. J. Hwang, and T. J. Ciesielka, *J. Electrochem. Soc.* **120**, 333C (1973).

64. R. L. Hartman and A. R. Hartman, *Appl. Phys. Lett.* **23**, 147 (1973).

65. G. A. Rozgonyi and M. B. Panish, *Appl. Phys. Lett.* **23**, 533 (1973).

66. G. A. Rozgonyi, P. M. Petroff, and M. B. Panish, *Appl. Phys. Lett.* **24**, 251 (1974).

67. M. A. Afromowitz and D. L. Rode, *J. Appl. Phys.* **45**, 4738 (1974).

68. R. L. Hartman and R. W. Dixon, *Appl. Phys. Lett.* **26**, 239 (1975).

69. J. C. Dyment, F. R. Nash, C. J. Hwang, G. A. Rozgonyi, R. L. Hartman, H. M. Marcos, and S. E. Haszko, *Appl. Phys. Lett.* **24**, 481 (1974).

69a. R. E. Nahory, M. A. Pollack, E. D. Beebe, J. C. DeWinter, and M. Ilegems, unpublished.

70. M. B. Panish and M. Ilegems, "Progress in Solid State Chemistry, Vol. 7," (H. Reiss and J. O. McCaldin, eds.), p. 39. Pergamon, New York, 1972.

71. M. F. Gratton and J. C. Woolley, *J. Electron. Mater.* **2**, 455 (1973).

72. L. M. Dolginov, L. V. Druzhinina, P. G. Eliseev, M. G. Milvidskii, and B. N. Sverdlov, *Sov. J. Quant Electron.* **6**, 257 (1976) [*Translated from: Kvantovaya Elektron. (Moscow)* **3**, 465 (1976)].

73. A. Onton and R. J. Chicotka, *Int. Conf. Lumininescence, Leningrad* (1972).

74. A. Onton, *J. Lumin.* **7**, 95 (1973).

75. R. L. Moon, G. A. Antypas, and L. W. James, *J. Electron. Mater.* **3**, 635 (1974).

76. A. P. Bogatov, L. M. Dolginov, P. G. Eliseev, M. G. Milvidskii, B. N. Sverdlov, and E. G. Shevchenko, *Sov. Phys.–Semicond.* **9**, 1282 (1976) [*Translated from: Fiz. Tekh. Poluprovodn.* **9**, 1956 (1975)].

77. J. J. Hsieh, *Appl. Phys. Lett.* **28**, 283 (1976).

78. C. C. Shen, Private communication.

79. T. P. Pearsall, B. I. Miller, R. J. Capik, and K. J. Bachmann, *Appl. Phys. Lett.* **28**, 499 (1976).

80. Zh. I. Alferov, I. N. Arcentev, D. Z. Gakbuzov, and V. D. Rumyantsev, *Pis'ma Zh. Tekh. Fiz.* **1**, 406 (1975).

81. W. T. Read, Jr., "Dislocations in Crystals." McGraw-Hill, New York, 1953.

82. J. P. Hirth and J. Lothe, "Theory of Dislocations." McGraw-Hill, New York, 1968.

83. H. Alexander and P. Haasen, "Solid State Physics, Vol. 22," (F. Seitz, D. Turnbull, and H. Ehrenreich, eds.), p. 27. Academic Press, New York, 1968.

84. J. D. Venables and R. M. Broudy, *J. Appl. Phys.* **29**, 1025 (1958).

85. M. S. Abrahams, L. R. Weisberg, C. J. Buiocchi, and J. Blanc, *J. Mater. Sci.* **4**, 223 (1969).

86. M. S. Abrahams and C. J. Buiocchi, *J, Appl. Phys.* **45**, 3315 (1974).

87. J. W. Matthews, S. Mader, and T. B. Light, *J. Appl. Phys.* **41**, 3800 (1970).

88. J. W. Matthews and A. E. Blakeslee, *J, Cryst. Growth* **27**, 118 (1974).

89. J. F. Black, C. J. Summers, and B. Sherman, *Appl. Phys. Lett.* **19**, 28 (1971).

90. K. Sugiyama and H. Saito, *Jpn. J. Appl. Phys.* **11**, 1057 (1972).
91. R. E. Nahory and M. A. Pollack, *Appl. Phys. Lett.* **27**, 562 (1975).
92. R. E. Nahory, M. A. Pollack, and J. K. Abrokwah, *J. Appl. Phys.* **48**, 3988 (1977).
93. C. J. Nuese and G. H. Olsen, *Appl. Phys. Lett.* **26**, 528 (1975).
94. C. J. Nuese, G. H. Olsen, M. Ettenberg, J. J. Gannon, and T. J. Zamerowski, *Appl. Phys. Lett.* **29**, 807 (1976).
95. R. D. Burnham, N. Holonyak, Jr., H. W. Korb, H. M. Macksey, D. R. Scifres, J. B. Woodhouse, and Zh. I. Alferov, *Appl. Phys. Lett.* **19**, 25 (1971).
96. J. J. Coleman, W. R. Hitchens, N. Holonyak, Jr., M. J. Ludowise, W. O. Groves, and D. L. Keune, *Appl. Phys. Lett.* **25**, 725 (1974).
97. W. R. Hitchens, N. Holonyak, Jr., M. H. Lee, J. C. Campbell, J. J. Coleman, W. O. Groves, and D. L. Keune, *Appl. Phys. Lett.* **25**, 352 (1974).
98. J. J. Coleman, N. Holonyak, Jr., M. J. Ludowise, R. J. Nelson, P. D. Wright, W. O. Groves, D. L. Keune, and M. G. Craford, *J. Appl. Phys.* **46**, 4835 (1975).
99. J. J. Coleman, N. Holonyak, Jr., M. J. Ludowise, P. D. Wright, R. Chin, W. O. Groves, and D. L. Keune, *Appl. Phys. Lett.* **29**, 167 (1976).
100. J. J. Coleman, N. Holonyak, Jr., M. J. Ludowise, and P. D. Wright, *J. Appl. Phys.* **47**, 2015 (1976).
101. H. Kressel, G. H. Olsen, and C. J. Nuese, *Appl. Phys. Lett.* **30**, 249 (1977).
102. T. C. Harman and I. Melngailis, "Applied Solid State Science, Vol. 4" (R. Wolfe, ed.), p. 1 Academic Press, New York, 1974.
103. J. N. Walpole, A. R. Calawa, R. W. Ralston, T. C. Harman, and J. P. McVittie, *Appl. Phys. Lett.* **23**, 620 (1973).
104. L. R. Tomasetta and C. G. Fonstad, *Appl. Phys. Lett.* **24**, 567 (1974).
105. L. R. Tomasetta and C. G. Fonstad, *Appl. Phys. Lett.* **25**, 440 (1974).
106. S. H. Groves, K. W. Nill, and A. J. Strauss, *Appl. Phys. Lett.* **25**, 331 (1974).
107. L. R. Tomasetta and C. G. Fonstad, *IEEE J. Quant.* Electron. **QE-11**, 384 (1975).
108. J. N. Walpole, A. R. Calawa, T. C. Harman, and S. H. Groves, *Appl. Phys. Lett.* **28**, 552 (1976).
109. G. F. McLane and K. J. Sleger, *J. Electron. Mater.* **4**, 465 (1975).
110. H. Preier, M. Bleicher, W. Riedel, and H. Maier, *Appl. Phys. Lett.* **28**, 669 (1976).
111. J. N. Walpole, A. R. Calawa, S. R. Chinn, S. H. Groves, and T. C. Harman, *Appl. Phys. Lett.* **29**, 307 (1976).
112. P. J. Lin and L. Kleinman, *Phys. Rev.* **142**, 478 (1966).
113. R. Dalven, *Infrared Phys.* **9**, 141 (1969).
114. J. N. Zemel, J. D. Jensen, and R. B. Schoolar, *Phys. Rev.* **140**, A330 (1965).
115. D. L. Mitchell, E. D. Palik, and J. N. Zemel, *Phys. Semicond.*; *Proc. Int. Conf., 7th, Paris, 1964* p. 325.
116. D. L. Carter and R. T. Bate, eds. "The Physics of Semimetals and Narrow-Gap Semiconductors." Pergamon, Oxford, 1971.
117. J. F. Butler and T. C. Harman, *IEEE J. Quant. Electron.* **5**, 50 (1969).
118. J. O. Dimmock, I. Melngailis, and A. J. Strauss, *Phys. Rev. Lett.* **16**, 1193 (1966).
119. H. Jäger and G. Schubert, *Infrared Phys.* **13**, 29 (1973).
120. J. N. Walpole, A. R. Calawa, S. R. Chinn, S. H. Groves, and T. C. Harman, *Appl. Phys. Lett.* **30**, 524 (1977).
121. T. C. Harman, A. R. Calawa, I. Melngailis, and J. O. Dimmock, *Appl. Phys. Lett.* **14**, 333 (1969).
122. C. E. Hurwitz, A. R. Calawa, and R. H. Rediker, *IEEE J. Quant. Electron.* **1**, 102 (1965).
123. H. Preier, M. Bleicher, W. Riedel, and H. Maier, *J. Appl. Phys.* **47**, 5476 (1976).

6.1 INTRODUCTION

Preparation of the various heterostructure lasers requires the development of heteroepitaxial growth processes for the growth of very thin multilayers of the solid solutions that were discussed in the preceeding chapter. The various procedures that are used for epitaxial growth of the semiconductor layers in heterostructures are based upon an understanding of the chemistry of the growth process. The controlled incorporation of impurities to obtain desired conductivities requires consideration of the chemical equilibria between the vapor or liquid and the solid. There are three epitaxial growth techniques that are of interest. Growth on single-crystal substrates from metallic solutions in a graphite boat, which is called liquid-phase epitaxy (LPE), is the most commonly used process for heterostructure lasers. A new technique in which beams of atoms and molecules from effusion ovens in an ultrahigh-vacuum system impinge on a heated substrate has been developed. This technique is called molecular-beam epitaxy (MBE). Chemical-vapor deposition (CVD) is epitaxy by the transport of reactant species in a flowing gas stream to the substrate where the deposition reaction occurs. In this chapter, discussions of the phase equilibria, impurity incorporation, and the LPE, MBE, and CVD growth techniques for heterostructure lasers are presented.

Section 6.2 gives a moderately detailed chemical–thermodynamic treatment of the phase equilibria of binary and ternary III–V systems. For the ternary, the emphasis is on the Al–Ga–As system. A more limited discussion of quaternary III–V systems is also presented. As given in Table 4.3-1, there are a number of different impurity elements that may be used to obtain the desired conductivity type and carrier concentration in GaAs. Some of the chemical constraints involved in their incorporation are described in Section 6.3. In Section 6.4, the phase equilibria in IV–VI systems are discussed briefly.

These discussions of phase equilibria and dopant incorporation are particularly important for an understanding of the advantages and limitations of LPE. This technique has evolved from the GaAs LPE described by Nelson,[1] and the demonstration by Woodall[2,3] that high-quality LPE $Al_xGa_{1-x}As$ could be grown on GaAs. A major portion of this chapter (Section 6.5) is devoted to GaAs–$Al_xGa_{1-x}As$ LPE and the horizontal-slider technique that is frequently used for the growth of heteroepitaxial wafers. Growth is usually from a stagnant solution with the rate-limiting step being diffusion of the components in the liquid. The morphology of the resulting epitaxy is strongly dependent upon the kinetic mechanism of attachment of atoms at the growing surface, the details of which are poorly understood. The LPE layers are characterized by a variety of morphological detail pertinent to laser studies. Several of these details are described and discussed in Section 6.5.

The search for a growth technique suitable for the preparation of both DH lasers and more complex opto-electronic structures resulted in the development of MBE.[4,5] This thin-film growth technique was demonstrated by Arthur,[4] and Cho and Casey[6] developed device-quality layers. Molecular-beam epitaxy is described in Section 6.6. With MBE, GaAs–Al$_x$Ga$_{1-x}$As DH lasers with threshold current densities that approach the values of comparable geometry LPE DH lasers have been obtained.[7] A molecular-beam deposition technique has significant advantages over LPE in dimensional control and versatility. Furthermore, it is far more amenable to the preparation of optical integrated circuits, and structures with uniform dimensions over large areas. As a highly nonequilibrium technique, the phase-equilibria constraints are somewhat relaxed, and the growth of lattice-matched heterostructures of crystalline solid solutions other than Al$_x$Ga$_{1-x}$As becomes feasible. However, growth of these other solid solutions will require better control over atomic and molecular beam intensities than has yet been achieved.

In the most commonly used CVD techniques, the halide[8] and hydride[9] processes, the group V element in the vapor reacts with a group III halide to yield the III–V compound. The discussion of CVD layer deposition for heterostructure lasers is presented in Section 6.7. Chemical-vapor deposition with halide and hydride processes is extensively used for the growth of GaP$_x$As$_{1-x}$ for light-emitting diodes, but only limited use has been made for heterostructure lasers. For layers containing Al, there are several difficulties that result from the high reactivity of Al. It is difficult to grow well-controlled alloy compositions, and unwanted impurities such as oxygen are readily incorporated. If these are the only limitations, then the use of CVD for the preparation of other solid solutions can be expected to be extensively investigated. Low threshold heterostructure lasers have already been reported for wafers grown by the hydride CVD process. Nuese et al. have obtained cw room-temperature operation with GaAs–Ga$_{0.51}$In$_{0.49}$P (Ref. 10) and Ga$_x$In$_{1-x}$As–Ga$_y$In$_{1-y}$P (Ref. 11) DH lasers. The most recent new technique by which low threshold lasers have been grown is by the organometallic decomposition (OMD–CVD) technique used by Dupuis and Dapkus[11a] to prepare GaAs–Al$_x$Ga$_{1-x}$As DH lasers. Chemical-vapor deposition, although less restricted by compositional limitations imposed by liquidus–solidus phase boundaries, will require precision in compositional control beyond what is usually achieved if lattice–matching structures such as those described in Chapter 5 are to be reproducibly grown.

6.2 PHASE EQUILIBRIA IN III–V SYSTEMS

Introductory Comments

In general, the liquidus compositions that are in equilibrium with the 1:1 III–V compounds constitute the major part of the III–V phase diagram. Thus, a large degree of compositional variation is possible in the components of the liquid or vapor from which a crystal is grown, while still maintaining equilibrium with the desired compound. This predominance of the III–V solid phase and the close stoichiometry of these compounds are important factors that help to make III–V compounds potentially so useful. There are a large range of conditions for the binary compounds or solid solutions where the solid phase is stable and where the crystal properties essential to application in electronic and optoelectronic devices can be varied. It should be recalled that there is a tendency for chemical compounds to form with small whole number ratios of the constituent elements. These ratios are the stoichiometric compositions. The small deviations from stoichiometry that always occur are referred to as nonstoichiometry.

In this part of Chapter 6, a discussion of the phase equilibria between the solid and liquid phases in III–V systems is presented. This discussion is primarily important for crystal growth by LPE. However, the calculated chemical activities of the solid solution components are needed also for equilibrium calculations used for CVD, which is discussed in Section 6.7. The thermodynamic model most frequently used for III–V systems is presented in moderate detail for binary systems. This model is also applied to Al–Ga–As as an example for a ternary system, and its application to quaternary solid solutions is introduced briefly. The application of these thermodynamic considerations to the Al–Ga–As system is particularly useful because of the present technological importance of LPE $Al_xGa_{1-x}As$. For other III–V solid solution systems, LPE may or may not be the most desirable growth technique.

Binary III–V Systems

The liquidus–solidus phase diagram of most binary III–V compounds can be represented by the very simple case shown in Fig. 6.2-1. In this figure, most of the diagram for two phase equilibria represents the equilibrium between the liquidus and the congruently melting solid AC. Congruent melting is the melting of a compound at a fixed temperature at which the solid and liquid have the same composition. The melting temperature of the compound AC is T_F. The temperatures T_1 and T_2 are the temperature for

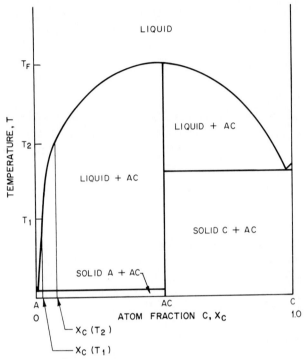

FIG. 6.2-1 Schematic representation of the liquidus–solidus equilibrium in a system with a large AC primary phase field.

the equilibrium between the solid phase and the compositions $X_C(T_1)$ and $X_C(T_2)$ on the liquidus curve. At a given temperature, $X_A + X_C = 1$. The group III element is A, and the III–V compound AC can be in equilibrium with liquid solutions that are extremely dilute in C. As will be described in Section 6.5, this feature of III–V phase diagrams is the basis for liquid-phase epitaxy of III–V compounds from a liquid that consists primarily of the group III element. A derivation of the thermodynamic relationships that describe the binary phase equilibria follows.[12]

At temperature T, the general equilibrium for solid AC in equilibrium with a liquid solution of A and C is

$$A(\ell) + B(\ell) \rightleftarrows AC(s). \tag{6.2-1}$$

At equilibrium, the Gibbs free energy change for a reaction is zero. Since the Gibbs free energy is the chemical potential μ, the equilibrium for this reaction may be expressed as

$$\mu_A(T) + \mu_C(T) - \mu_{AC}(T) = 0. \tag{6.2-2}$$

In Eq. (6.2-2), the subscripts A and C denote the liquid, the subscript AC the solid, and the T in parentheses the temperature. The chemical potential is the partial-molal free energy at constant temperature and pressure. More detailed treatments of the relationships among the thermodynamic quantities used in this discussion can be found in representative textbooks.[13,14]

At a given temperature the chemical potential of constituent i may be written as

$$\mu_i = \mu_i{}^0 + RT \ln a_i = \mu_i{}^0 + RT \ln \gamma_i X_i, \qquad (6.2\text{-}3)$$

where a_i, X_i, and γ_i are, respectively, the chemical activity, mole fraction, and activity coefficient of component i. The superscript ^{0} is used to designate the thermodynamic quantity for a pure component (not in solution). For the pure solid AC, the activity a_{AC} is unity, and

$$\mu_{AC} = \mu_{AC}^0. \qquad (6.2\text{-}4)$$

Equation (6.2-2) may now be written as

$$\mu_A{}^0(T) + RT \ln[\gamma_A(T)X_A(T)] + \mu_C{}^0(T) + RT \ln[\gamma_C(T)X_C(T)] - \mu_{AC}^0(T) = 0. \qquad (6.2\text{-}5)$$

For the arbitrary temperatures T_1 and T_2 and with $T_2 > T_1$, the chemical potential change between T_2 and T_1 may be obtained by evaluating Eq. (6.2-5) at T_2 and T_1. The difference between these expressions at T_2 and T_1 is

$$\mu_A{}^0(T_2) - \mu_A{}^0(T_1) + \mu_C{}^0(T_2) - \mu_C{}^0(T_1) - \mu_{AC}^0(T_2) + \mu_{AC}^0(T_1) \equiv \Delta\mu^0$$
$$= -RT_2 \ln[\gamma_A(T_2)\gamma_C(T_2)X_A(T_2)X_C(T_2)]$$
$$+ RT_1 \ln[\gamma_A(T_1)\gamma_C(T_1)X_A(T_1)X_C(T_1)]. \qquad (6.2\text{-}6)$$

It is more convenient to express the left-hand side of Eq. (6.2-6), which deals with pure components only, by thermodynamic quantities that may be numerically evaluated. The chemical potential of component i is by definition the partial-molal free energy of that component. Then at constant pressure and composition, the partial molal entropy of component i, $\bar{S}_i$, is[15]

$$\left(\frac{\partial \mu_i}{\partial T}\right) = -\bar{S}_i, \qquad (6.2\text{-}7)$$

where $\bar{S}_i$ is the partial molar entropy of component i. For a pure component, μ_i is a function of temperature only, and Eq. (6.2-7) may be written between T_2 and T_1 to give

$$\mu_i{}^0(T_2) - \mu_i{}^0(T_1) = -\int_{T_1}^{T_2} S_i{}^0(T)\,dT, \qquad (6.2\text{-}8)$$

where S_i^0 is the entropy of pure component i. For a reversible process,[16]

$$dS = (C_P/T)\,dT, \tag{6.2-9}$$

so that for a pure component in which there is no phase change in i between T_2 and T

$$S_i^0(T) = S_i^0(T_2) + \int_{T_2}^{T} \frac{C_{P,i}^0}{T}\,dT. \tag{6.2-10}$$

In Eq. (6.2-10), $C_{P,i}^0$ is the heat capacity at constant pressure for pure component i. Combining Eqs. (6.2-8) and (6.2-10) gives

$$\mu_i^0(T_2) - \mu_i^0(T_1) = S_i^0(T_2)(T_1 - T_2) - \int_{T_1}^{T_2}\int_{T_2}^{T} \frac{C_{P,i}^0}{T'}\,dT'\,dT, \tag{6.2-11}$$

where $(T_1 - T_2)$ is a multiplicative term times S_i^0 at T_2. When Eq. (6.2-11) is evaluated for $i =$ A, C, and AC, the left side of Eq. (6.2-6) becomes

$$\Delta\mu^0 = \Delta S^0(T_2)(T_1 - T_2) - \int_{T_1}^{T_2}\int_{T_2}^{T} \frac{\Delta C_P^0}{T'}\,dT'\,dT, \tag{6.2-12}$$

where $\Delta S^0(T_2) = S_A^0(T_2) + S_C^0(T_2) - S_{AC}^0(T_2)$ and $\Delta C_P^0 = C_{P,A}^0 + C_{P,C}^0 - C_{P,AC}^0$. By setting T_2 equal to T_F and noting that $X_A = X_C = 0.5$ at T_F, the right side of Eq. (6.2-6) may be equated to the right side of Eq. (6.2-12) to give

$$RT_1 \ln[\gamma_A(T_1)\gamma_C(T_1)X_A(T_1)X_C(T_1)] - RT_F \ln[\gamma_A(T_F)\gamma_C(T_F)/4]$$

$$= -\Delta S^0(T_F)(T_F - T_1) - \int_{T_1}^{T_F}\int_{T_F}^{T} \frac{\Delta C_P^0}{T'}\,dT'\,dT. \tag{6.2-13}$$

Except for the specification of no phase transformations in A, C, or AC in the temperature range of T_F to T_1, no simplifying assumptions have been made in the derivation of this liquidus equation.

The liquidus equation in the form given in Eq. (6.2-13) cannot be used to obtain the liquidus, $X_C(T)$, without an evaluation of the activity coefficients, the heat capacities, and $\Delta S^0(T_F)$. Since ΔC_P^0 may be shown to be small[17] compared to the other terms, the integral term may be neglected. Although activity coefficients are frequently obtained from vapor pressure or electrical measurements, such methods have not been feasible for III–V systems. The next step in this derivation is to consider the representation of the activity coefficients by a quantity called the interaction parameter $\alpha(T)$. The III–V liquid is considered to be an unassociated solution belonging to the class of binary mixtures called *simple* by Guggenheim.[14] He defined *simple* solutions as solutions with their excess Gibbs free energy of mixing

G^E given by[18]

$$G^E = \alpha(T)X_i(1 - X_i). \qquad (6.2\text{-}14)$$

For a two component system, the excess chemical potential of component A, $\mu_A{}^E$, is simply the nonideal part of μ_A given in Eq. (6.2-3):

$$\mu_A{}^E = RT \ln \gamma_A. \qquad (6.2\text{-}15)$$

Also, it has been shown[19] that

$$\mu_A{}^E = G^E - X_C(\partial G^E/\partial X_C). \qquad (6.2\text{-}16)$$

Evaluation of Eq. (6.2-16) with Eq. (6.2-14) with $X_i = X_C$ gives

$$\mu_A{}^E = \alpha(T)X_C{}^2. \qquad (6.2\text{-}17)$$

Equating Eqs. (6.2-15) and (6.2-17) then gives

$$RT \ln \gamma_A = \alpha(T)X_C{}^2 = \alpha(T)(1 - X_A)^2 \qquad (6.2\text{-}18)$$

for $X_A + X_C = 1$. In a similar manner,

$$RT \ln \gamma_C = \alpha(T)X_A{}^2 = \alpha(T)(1 - X_C)^2. \qquad (6.2\text{-}19)$$

Introduction of Eqs. (6.2-18) and (6.2-19) into Eq. (6.2-13) gives the liquidus equation of a simple liquid solution with a binary compound as

$$RT \ln[X_C(1 - X_C)] + \Delta S^0(T_F)(T_F - T) + RT_F \ln 4$$
$$+ \alpha(T)[2X_C{}^2 - 2X_C + 1] - \alpha(T_F)/2 = 0 \qquad (6.2\text{-}20)$$

for the arbitrary temperature $T = T_1$. As previously described, the integral term in Eq. (6.2-13) has been neglected because $\Delta C_P{}^0$ is small.

The liquidus equation represented by Eq. (6.2-20) may be reduced further by adding and subtracting $RT \ln 4$ to give

$$RT \ln[4X_C(1 - X_C)] + [\Delta S^0(T_F) + R \ln 4](T_F - T)$$
$$+ \alpha(T)[2X_C{}^2 - 2X_C + 1] - \alpha(T_F)/2 = 0. \qquad (6.2\text{-}21)$$

In this equation, $\Delta S^0(T_F)$ is the difference in entropy between the solid AC and its components in their pure liquid state. An ideal entropy of fusion ΔS_F^{ID} is defined as the entropy difference between the solid AC and its components A and C forming a hypothetical ideal equimolal solution A–C. Ideal random mixing of the components A and C contributes[20] an entropy term of $-R[0.5 \ln 0.5 + 0.5 \ln 0.5] = (R/2) \ln 4$ per gram atom AC or $R \ln 4$ per mole AC. Thus,

$$\Delta S^0(T_F) + R \ln 4 = \Delta S_F^{ID}, \qquad (6.2\text{-}22)$$

where ΔS_F^{ID} is the ideal entropy of fusion.

Experimentally it has been found that for many III–V binary systems $\alpha(T)$ has a linear temperature dependence[21] which may be expressed as

$$\alpha(T) = a + bT, \qquad (6.2\text{-}23)$$

where a and b are constants. Substitution of Eqs. (6.2-22) and (6.2-23) into Eq. (6.2-21) gives

$$0.5\{RT\ln[4X_C(1 - X_C)] + (\Delta S_F^{ID} - b/2)(T_F - T)\}$$
$$= -(a + bT)(0.5 - X_C)^2. \qquad (6.2\text{-}24)$$

The excess entropy of mixing at constant pressure and composition is given by

$$S^E = -\partial G^E/\partial T. \qquad (6.2\text{-}25)$$

With Eq. (6.2-23) in Eq. (6.2-14), Eq. (6.2-25) gives S^E as $-b/4$ per gram atom AC or $-b/2$ per mole AC at T_F. Since the entropy of fusion is the sum of the ideal and excess entropy, the entropy of fusion ΔS_F may be written as

$$\Delta S_F = \Delta S_F^{ID} - b/2. \qquad (6.2\text{-}26)$$

In Eq. (6.2-24), replacement of $(a + bT)$ by $\alpha(T)$ and substitution of Eq. (6.2-26) gives

$$\alpha(T) = -0.5\{RT\ln[4X_C(1 - X_C)] + \Delta S_F(T_F - T)\}/(0.5 - X_C)^2. \qquad (6.2\text{-}27)$$

An equation similar to Eq. (6.2-27) was derived by Vieland[22] for regular solutions with a different procedure. With regular solutions the interaction parameter is a constant. The analysis given above is most applicable to the higher-melting-temperature III–V systems and may be inappropriate at low temperatures because of association in the liquid.

The experimental liquidus data for GaAs, GaP, and InP are given in Fig. 6.2-2 for these three systems of particular interest. A semilogarithmic plot of the liquidus curve is used here to permit representation of the very dilute solutions of the group V elements. The experimental data used in these plots were considered[23] to be the most reliable in the available literature. Each experimental point was used to determine a value of $\alpha(T)$ at each X and T by Eq. (6.2-27) and the resulting $\alpha(T)$ has been plotted in Fig. 6.2-3. The values of of ΔS_F are given in Table 6.2-1. The best linear curve through the points in Fig. 6.2-3 has been used with Eq. (6.2-27) to calculate the solid line through the data of Fig. 6.2-2. The use of Eq. (6.2-27) for the liquidus frequently introduces some degree of uncertainty into the calculations because frequently the entropy of fusion is not well known. The effect of uncertainty in ΔS_F is to introduce some arbitrariness into the values of a and b in Eq. (6.2-23) while maintaining the same functional relationship for $\alpha(T)$. As a result of this uncertainty when ΔS_F is not well known, ΔS_F and

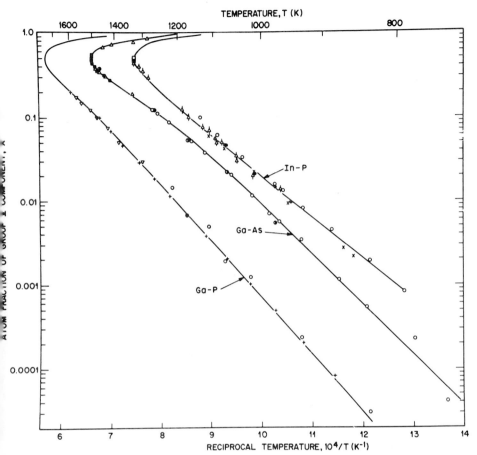

FIG. 6.2-2   Liquidus composition versus reciprocal temperature for Ga–As, Ga–P, and In–P. Experimental data were used for the determination of the individual points, and each point represents a set of experimental data (Ref. 23). The original references are given in Ref. 23. As described in the text, the solid line drawn through the data was obtained with Eq. (6.2-27) with the $\alpha(T)$ determined in Fig. 6.2-3.

$\alpha(T)$ should be tabulated together with the understanding that a modification of one implies a modification of the other. Sets of values of T_F, ΔS_F, and $\alpha(T)$ are given in Table 6.2-1. A more detailed discussion of the reported experimental data for several III–V systems is given in Ref. 21. The binary phase diagrams[21] of the lower temperature III–V systems are given in Fig. 6.2-4.

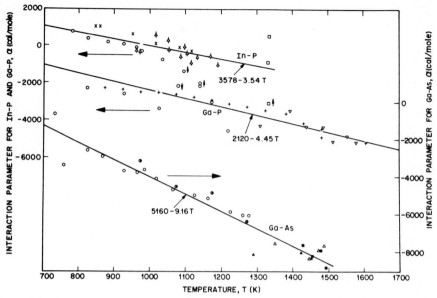

FIG. 6.2-3 The interaction parameter $\alpha(T)$ for the Ga–P, In–P, and Ga–As experimental liquidus data of Fig. 6.2-2 by Eq. (6.2-27) (Ref. 23).

Ternary III–V Systems

It is clear that the chemical thermodynamics and phase equilibria of ternary III–V crystalline solid solutions are a particular concern because of the importance of $Al_xGa_{1-x}As$ to heterostructure laser studies. For this reason, the Al–Ga–As system is considered as a representative example. The 900°C liquidus isotherm for the Al–Ga–As system is given in Fig. 6.2-5 with the triangular coordinates generally used for ternaries. This figure serves as a typical example of the shape of a liquidus isotherm in the group-III-rich region of an A^{III}–B^{III}–C^V system. The designation of composition is illustrated in Fig. 6.2-6. The relative distance of the point D from each corner represents the composition in terms of A, B, and C. With an appropriately drawn grid, the composition can be read directly from the sides of the triangle as illustrated. Thus it can be seen that the composition at point D is 60 % A, 10% B, and 30% C. When a liquidus isotherm such as that of Fig. 6.2-5 is given, each point on the curve represents a composition in equilibrium with some solid phase at some isothermal temperature. In this case, the solid is $Al_xGa_{1-x}As$, and the composition of the solid in equilibrium

TABLE 6.2-1 Temperature of Fusion, Entropy of Fusion,
and Interaction Parameter for Binary III–V Systems

Compound	Temperature of fusion, $T_F(°K)$	Ref.	Entropy of fusion, ΔS_F(cal/mole-°K)	Ref.	Interaction parameter, $\alpha(T)$(cal/mole)	Ref.
AlP	2803	a	15.0	g	$1,750 - 2.0T$	o
AlAs	2043	b	15.6	g	$-6,390 - 5.5T$	p
AlSb	1333	c	14.74	k	$12,300 - 10T$	g
GaP	1740	d, e	17.3	l	$2,120 - 4.45T$	q
GaAs	1511	d, f	16.64	m	$5,160 - 9.16T$	q, p
GaSb	983	g	15.80	k	$4,700 - 6.0T$	g
InP	1335	h	15.2	n	$3,578 - 3.54T$	q
InAs	1215	i	14.52	m	$3,860 - 10.0T$	g
InSb	798	j	14.32	k	$3,400 - 12T$	g

[a] W. Kischio, *J. Inog. Nucl. Chem.* **27**, 750 (1965).

[b] L. M. Foster and J. E. Scardefield, *J. Electrochem. Soc.* **118**, 495 (1971).

[c] H. Welker, *Z. Naturforsch.* **8a**, 248 (1953).

[d] D. Richman, *J. Phys. Chem. Solids* **24**, 1131 (1963).

[e] A slightly higher value (1743°K) was used in the calculations of Ilegems and Panish[o] and Panish.[q]

[f] W. Koster and B. Thoma, *Z. Metalk.* **46**, 291 (1955).

[g] M. B. Panish and M. Ilegems, "Progress in Solid State Chemistry," (H. Reiss and J. O. McCaldin, eds.), Vol. 7, p. 39. Pergamon, New York, 1972.

[h] K. J. Bachman and E. Buehler, *J. Electrochem. Soc.* **121**, 835 (1974).

[i] T. S. Liu and C. A. Peretti, *Trans. Am. Soc. Metals* **45**, 677 (1953).

[j] T. S. Liu and C. A. Peretti, *Trans. Am. Soc. Metals* **44**, 539 (1952).

[k] B. D. Lichter and P. Sommelet, *Trans. AIME* **245**, 99 (1969).

[l] No entropy of fusion data. Estimated from $\Delta S_F^{GaP} = \Delta S_F^{Si} + \Delta S_F^{Ge} + R \ln 4$. See Panish and Ilegems[g] and Panish.[q]

[m] B. D. Lichter and P. Sommelet, *Trans. AIME* **245**, 1021 (1969).

[n] No entropy data. Estimated from $\Delta S_F^{InP} = \Delta S_F^{Si} + \Delta S_F^{Grey Sn} + R \ln 4$. See Panish and Ilegems[g] and Ilegems and Panish.[o]

[o] M. Ilegems and M. B. Panish, *J. Crystal Growth* **20**, 77 (1973). No binary Al–P phase data other than T_F. $\alpha(T)$ curve fit to Al–Ga–P ternary.

[p] M. B. Panish and M. Ilegems, unpublished. No binary Al–As phase data other than T_F. $\alpha(T)$ curve fit to ternary Al–Ga–As phase data as described in the part of Section 6.2 on ternary III–V systems.

[q] M. B. Panish, *J. Crystal Growth* **27**, 6 (1974).

with a composition of the liquid is represented by a "tie line" as illustrated by the dashed line. The tie line connects the corresponding liquid and solid compositions at a given temperature. Frequently, a three-dimensional plot of the type given in Fig. 6.2-7 is used to represent the generalized liquidus surface compositions as a function of temperature.

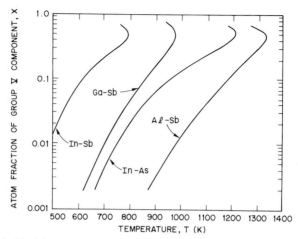

FIG. 6.2-4 Liquidus composition versus temperature for In–Sb, Ga–Sb, In–As, and Al–Sb (Ref. 21).

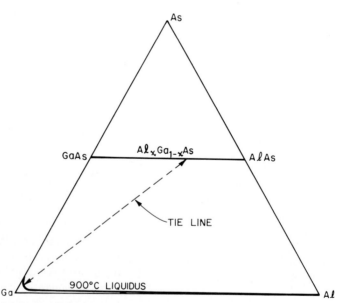

FIG. 6.2-5 The 900°C Al–Ga–As liquidus isotherm. The tie line is drawn from $X = 0.01$ to the equilibrium solid $Al_{0.63}Ga_{0.37}As$.

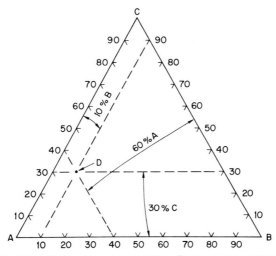

FIG. 6.2-6 Triangular representation of ternary compositions.

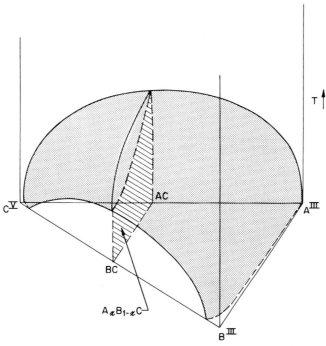

FIG. 6.2-7 Schematic representation of the liquidus and solidus surfaces in the phase diagram of an A^{III}–B^{III}–C^V system at temperatures greater than any eutectic temperatures in the system. The shaded area shows the ternary liquidus compositions that may be in equilibrium with a solid composition. The cross hatch shows all solidus compositions. As with Fig. 6.2-5, tie lines can be drawn that show the solid composition in equilibrium with any given liquid composition.

As with the binary systems, the general equilibrium is expressed in terms of chemical potentials:

$$\mu_{Al}(T) + \mu_{As}(T) - \mu_{AlAs}(T) = 0, \qquad (6.2\text{-}28a)$$

and

$$\mu_{Ga}(T) + \mu_{As}(T) - \mu_{GaAs}(T) = 0, \qquad (6.2\text{-}28b)$$

where the subscripts Al, Ga, and As denote the liquid and the subscripts AlAs and GaAs the solid. Now, however, there are two such equations and the chemical potential of the ternary solid is not that of a pure binary compound. The ternary crystalline solid solution $Al_xGa_{1-x}As$ is considered to be a binary mixture of $(1 - x)$ moles of GaAs and x moles of AlAs so that $\mu_{GaAs}(T)$ and $\mu_{AlAs}(T)$ are the chemical potentials of the components of that solid solution. This assignment can be made even though molecules of GaAs and AlAs are not the actual entities. In this case, the mixing of Ga and Al atoms on the group III sublattice in the presence of only As atoms in the As sublattice is mathematically equivalent to considering the solid solution as a mixture of GaAs and AlAs molecules.

As shown by Ilegems and Pearson,[24] an extension of the derivation for the liquidus in binary systems can be made for the ternary systems. By Eq. (6.2-3), the chemical potential of each binary component of the solid is

$$\mu_{AlAs} = \mu^0_{AlAs} + RT \ln[\gamma_{AlAs}(T)x(T)], \qquad (6.2\text{-}29a)$$

and

$$\mu_{GaAs} = \mu^0_{GaAs} + RT \ln\{\gamma_{GaAs}(T)[1 - x(T)]\}, \qquad (6.2\text{-}29b)$$

where x is the AlAs mole fraction. Equations (6.2-2) and (6.2-3) with A replaced by Al and then Ga and C replaced with As become

$$\mu^0_{Al}(T) + RT \ln[\gamma_{Al}(T)X_{Al}(T)] + \mu^0_{As}(T) + RT \ln[\gamma_{As}(T)X_{As}(T)]$$
$$- \mu^0_{AlAs}(T) - RT \ln[\gamma_{AlAs}(T)x(T)] = 0, \qquad (6.2\text{-}30a)$$

and

$$\mu^0_{Ga}(T) + RT \ln[\gamma_{Ga}(T)X_{Ga}(T)] + \mu^0_{As}(T) + RT \ln[\gamma_{As}(T)X_{As}(T)]$$
$$- \mu^0_{GaAs}(T) - RT \ln\{\gamma_{GaAs}(T)[1 - x(T)]\} = 0, \qquad (6.2\text{-}30b)$$

where X represents liquid composition and x solid composition. As for the binary case with Eq. (6.2-5), Eq. (6.2-30a) is evaluated at T_1 and T_2, and the difference between the resulting expressions gives an equation equivalent to Eq. (6.2-6) except for the additional terms for the solid solution. A similar procedure is followed with Eq. (6.2-30b). Then, following the procedure used for treating the entropy in the binary case with Eqs. (6.2-7)–(6.2-13) and with the $\Delta C_p{}^0$ terms neglected, the liquidus equation at the arbitrary temperature T may be written as

$$RT \ln\left(\frac{\gamma_{Al}(T)\gamma_{As}(T)X_{Al}(T)X_{As}(T)}{\gamma_{AlAs}(T)x(T)}\right) - RT_F^{AlAs} \ln\left(\frac{\gamma_{Al}(T_F^{AlAs})\gamma_{As}(T_F^{AlAs})}{4\gamma_{AlAs}(T_F^{AlAs})x(T_F^{AlAs})}\right)$$
$$+ \Delta S_{AlAs}^0(T_F^{AlAs})(T_F^{AlAs} - T) = 0 \qquad (6.2\text{-}31a)$$

plus an identical equation with Al replaced by Ga to give Eq. (6.2-31b). Note that in Eq. (6.2-31a) for $T = T_F^{AlAs}$, $\gamma_{AlAs}x = 1$. By the addition and subtraction of $RT \ln 4$ as was done for the binary case to obtain Eq. (6.2-21), and with Eq. (6.2-22) for the ideal entropy of fusion, Eq. (6.2-31a) becomes

$$RT \ln\left(\frac{4\gamma_{Al}(T)\gamma_{As}(T)X_{Al}(T)X_{As}(T)}{\gamma_{AlAs}(T)x(T)}\right) - RT_F^{AlAs} \ln[\gamma_{Al}(T_F^{AlAs})\gamma_{As}(T_F^{AlAs})]$$
$$+ \Delta S_F^{ID,AlAs}(T_F^{AlAs} - T) = 0, \qquad (6.2\text{-}32a)$$

and a similar equation with Al replaced by Ga gives Eq. (6.2-32b).

For simple solutions with a linear temperature–dependent $\alpha(T)$, as given in Eq. (6.2-23), Eqs. (6.2-18) and (6.2-19) give

$$RT \ln[\gamma_{Al}^{s\ell}(T)\gamma_{As}^{s\ell}(T)] = \tfrac{1}{2}\alpha_{Al-As}(T) = \tfrac{1}{2}(a_{Al-As} + b_{Al-As}T), \qquad (6.2\text{-}33a)$$

where α_{Al-As}, a_{Al-As}, and b_{Al-As} are the interaction constants for the component pair Al–As. The superscript $s\ell$ indicates that the liquid is stoichiometric Al–As so that $X_{As}^{s\ell} = X_{Al}^{s\ell} = 0.5$. The difference between Eq. (6.2-33a) evaluated at the melting point T_F^{AlAs} of AlAs and the arbitrary temperature T gives

$$RT_F^{AlAs} \ln[\gamma_{Al}^{s\ell}(T_F^{AlAs})\gamma_{As}^{s\ell}(T_F^{AlAs})] - RT \ln[\gamma_{Al}^{s\ell}(T)\gamma_{As}^{s\ell}(T)]$$
$$= \tfrac{1}{2}b_{Al-As}(T_F^{AlAs} - T). \qquad (6.2\text{-}34a)$$

As shown by Eq. (6.2-26), the term $\tfrac{1}{2}b_{Al-As}$ represents the difference between the real and ideal AlAs entropy of fusion for the simple solution model. By substituting Eq. (6.2-26) into Eq. (6.2-32a) and by using Eq. (6.2-34a) for $\tfrac{1}{2}b_{Al-As}$, Eq. (6.2-32a) becomes

$$RT \ln\left(\frac{4\gamma_{Al}(T)\gamma_{As}(T)X_{Al}(T)X_{As}(T)}{\gamma_{AlAs}(T)x(T)}\right) - RT \ln[\gamma_A^{s\ell}(T)\gamma_{As}^{s\ell}(T)]$$
$$+ \Delta S_F^{AlAs}(T_F^{AlAs} - T) = 0. \qquad (6.2\text{-}35a)$$

By rearranging terms,

$$\left(\frac{4\gamma_{Al}(T)\gamma_{As}(T)X_{Al}(T)X_{As}(T)}{\gamma_{Al}^{s\ell}(T)\gamma_{As}^{s\ell}(T)}\right)\exp\left(\frac{\Delta S_F^{AlAs}}{RT}(T_F^{AlAs} - T)\right)$$
$$= \gamma_{AlAs}(T)x(T). \qquad (6.2\text{-}36a)$$

There is a corresponding derivation that begins with Eq. (6.2-32b) and gives

$$\left(\frac{4\gamma_{Ga}(T)\gamma_{As}(T)X_{Ga}(T)X_{As}(T)}{\gamma_{Ga}^{ol}(T)\gamma_{As}^{ol}(T)}\right)\exp\left(\frac{\Delta S_F^{GaAs}}{RT}(T_F^{GaAs} - T)\right)$$

$$= \gamma_{GaAs}(T)[1 - x(T)]. \tag{6.2-36b}$$

These equations represent the relationship between the ternary liquidus and solid composition at a given temperature T. The assumptions that have been made are that the term in $\Delta C_p{}^0$ can be neglected and that the binary liquid solutions Al–As and Ga–As can be represented as simple liquids with linear temperature-dependent α's.

To evaluate the liquid and solid compositions with Eqs. (6.2-36a and b), expressions in terms of simple-solution interaction parameters and composition must be obtained for the liquid activity coefficients. The general relation between the activity coefficients γ_i, the compositions X_i, and binary interaction parameters α_{ij} for multicomponent simple solutions at temperature T has been given by Jordan as[25]

$$RT\ln\gamma_i = \sum_{\substack{j=1 \\ i\neq j}}^{m} \alpha_{ij}X_j^2 + \sum_{\substack{k=1 \\ k<j,j\neq i,i\neq k}}^{m} \sum_{j=1}^{m} X_k X_j(\alpha_{ij} + \alpha_{ik} - \alpha_{kj}). \tag{6.2-37}$$

For the ternary liquid Al–Ga–As,

$$RT\ln\gamma_{As} = \alpha_{Al-As}X_{Al}^2 + \alpha_{Ga-As}X_{Ga}^2 + (\alpha_{Al-As} + \alpha_{Ga-As} - \alpha_{Al-Ga})X_{Al}X_{Ga}, \tag{6.2-38a}$$

$$RT\ln\gamma_{Ga} = \alpha_{Ga-As}X_{As}^2 + \alpha_{Al-Ga}X_{Al}^2 + (\alpha_{Ga-As} + \alpha_{Al-Ga} - \alpha_{Al-As})X_{Al}X_{As}, \tag{6.2-38b}$$

$$RT\ln\gamma_{Al} = \alpha_{Al-As}X_{As}^2 + \alpha_{Al-Ga}X_{Ga}^2 + (\alpha_{Al-As} + \alpha_{Al-Ga} - \alpha_{Ga-As})X_{Ga}X_{As}. \tag{6.2-38c}$$

The interaction parameters α_{Al-As}, α_{Ga-As}, and α_{Al-Ga} are for the subscripted component binary pairs. Equations (6.2-38a–c) are used to eliminate the activity coefficients from Eqs. (6.2-36a, b). The liquidus compositions are related through mass conservation as expressed by

$$X_{Al} + X_{Ga} + X_{As} = 1. \tag{6.2-39}$$

The right sides of Eqs. (6.2-36a, b) contain the composition and activity coefficients of the binary components (AlAs and GaAs) of the solid solution. For a number of III–V systems, it has been found that a regular or simple solution treatment may be used to adequately represent the solid solution.[21] Then for $Al_x Ga_{1-x}As$, Eq. (6.2-18) gives

$$RT\ln\gamma_{AlAs} = \alpha_{AlAs-GaAs}x^2, \tag{6.2-40a}$$

and

$$RT \ln \gamma_{\text{GaAs}} = \alpha_{\text{AlAs–GaAs}}(1 - x)^2. \qquad (6.2\text{-}40b)$$

These two equations permit elimination of activity coefficients γ_{AlAs} and γ_{GaAs} in Eqs. (6.2-36a, b).

There are three interaction parameters, two independent liquid compositions, two temperatures of fusion, two entropies of fusion, and one solid composition involved in the evaluation of the ternary phase diagram with Eqs. (6.2-36a, b), (6.2-38a–c), (6.2-39), and (6.2-40a, b). The temperatures of fusion, $T_{\text{F}}^{\text{GaAs}}$ and $T_{\text{F}}^{\text{AlAs}}$, are taken from the literature and are given in Table 6.2-1. The assignment of the entropy of fusion for GaAs, $\Delta S_{\text{F}}^{\text{GaAs}}$, was given in the preceding part of this section, while the entropy of fusion for AlAs, $\Delta S_{\text{F}}^{\text{AlAs}}$, was estimated as described in Ref. 21. These ΔS_{F} values are also given in Table 6.2-1. The $\alpha_{\text{Ga–As}}$ interaction parameter was obtained from the Ga–As liquidus as described in the preceding part of this section. For Al–Ga, a value of 104 cal/mole for $\alpha_{\text{Al–Ga}}$ has been used. This value was obtained[24] from the Al–Ga liquidus. It may be somewhat low in view of direct calorimetric measurements.[26] For the initial evaluation, $\alpha_{\text{AlAs–GaAs}}$ is taken as zero so that $\gamma_{\text{GaAs}} = \gamma_{\text{AlAs}} = 1$ in Eqs. (6.2-36a, b). With these values, a reasonably good fit is obtained to the available experimental liquidus and solidus compositions to give the remaining interaction parameter, $\alpha_{\text{Al–As}}$. The good fit with $\alpha_{\text{AlAs–GaAs}} = 0$ suggests the near ideality of the Al–Ga–As solid solution. This near ideality apparently results from the nearly equal Al and Ga covalent radii. With this nominal value of $\alpha_{\text{Al–As}}$, a two parameter fit to the experimental liquidus and solidus at each temperature is obtained by varying $\alpha_{\text{Al–As}}$ and $\alpha_{\text{AlAs–GaAs}}$. The resulting interaction parameters together with the quantities necessary for calculation of the Al–Ga–As phase diagram are summarized in Table 6.2-2.

TABLE 6.2-2 Parameters for Calculation of the
Al–Ga–As Phase Diagram[a]

$T_{\text{F}}^{\text{GaAs}} = 1511°\text{K}$
$T_{\text{F}}^{\text{AlAs}} = 2043°\text{K}$
$\Delta S_{\text{F}}^{\text{GaAs}} = 16.64 \text{ cal/mole-}°\text{K}$
$\Delta S_{\text{F}}^{\text{AlAs}} = 15.6 \text{ cal/mole-}°\text{K}$
$\alpha_{\text{Ga–As}} = 5160 - 9.16T \text{ cal/mole}$
$\alpha_{\text{Al–As}} = -6390 - 5.5T \text{ cal/mole}$
$\alpha_{\text{Al–Ga}} = 104 \text{ cal/mole}$
$\alpha_{\text{GaAs–AlAs}} = 400 \text{ cal/mole at } 973°\text{K}$
$\alpha_{\text{GaAs–AlAs}} = -3892 + 4T \text{ cal/mole from } 1073° \text{ to } 1273°\text{K}$

[a] For references, see Table 6.2-1 and the text.

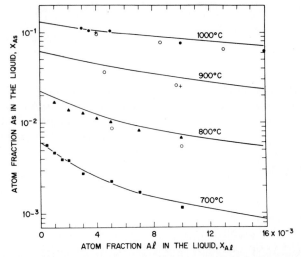

FIG. 6.2-8   Liquidus isotherms in the Al–Ga–As system (Ref. 27). The original references for the experimental data are given in Ref. 27. The solid lines drawn through the data
were obtained by the equations and parameters described in the text.

With these parameters, the liquidus curves of Fig. 6.2-8 and the solidus
compositions as a function of the liquidus in Fig. 6.2-9 are obtained.[27] It is
necessary to plot these figures semilogarithmically in order to permit representation of the very small Al and As concentrations in the liquid over the useful solid composition range. When these plots are used, it is understood that
Eq. (6.2-39) holds, and for the liquid, the specification of X_{Al} and temperature completely specifies the liquid composition. With the parameters in
Table 6.2-2, a good fit to the solidus data is obtained, but a slightly poorer
fit to the liquidus data results than for the assumption of an ideal solid
$(\gamma_{AlAs} = \gamma_{GaAs} = 1)$. Since the most common way to prepare solutions for
liquid-phase epitaxy in the Al–Ga–As system is to saturate a Ga–Al solution
with As by the addition of GaAs, it is more important to be able to predict
the solidus than the liquidus curves. A summary of the calculated composition data are given in Table 6.2-3. The calculated and experimental phase
diagrams for a large number of III–V ternary systems are given in Ref. 21.

Although the phase equilibrium considerations discussed above are most
readily applicable to the Al–Ga–As system for liquid-phase epitaxy, it is
illustrative to consider briefly several of the other III–V systems that show
potential for laser heterostructures. In Section 5.5 the heterostructure

$$N-(Al_{x'}Ga_{1-x'})_{0.51} In_{0.49}P|n- \text{ or } p-(Al_xGa_{1-x})_{0.51} In_{0.49}P|$$
$$P-(Al_{x'}Ga_{1-x'})_{0.51} In_{0.49}P$$

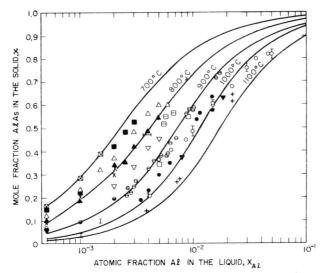

FIG. 6.2-9 Solidus compositions in $Al_xGa_{1-x}As$ as a function of liquidus composition (Ref. 27). The original references for the experimental data are given in Ref. 27. The solid lines drawn through the data were obtained by the equations and parameters described in the text.

with $x' > x$ and $x \lesssim 0.4$ was described. This DH lattice matches to a GaAs substrate and would be expected to yield low-threshold-injection lasers that emit well into the visible region of the spectrum.

Figure 6.2-10 shows estimated[21] liquidus–solidus curves for Al–In–P. This figure is analogous to Fig. 6.2-9 for Al–Ga–As except that complete curves cannot be drawn entirely in the group-III-rich region of the phase diagram. The "pseudobinary liquidus–solidus" shown in Fig. 6.2-10 consists of all liquidus compositions containing 50 atomic percent P. For reasonable temperatures ($<1000°C$) and $Al_xIn_{1-x}P$ compositions ($x \approx 0.5$) for LPE of lattice matched structures to GaAs, this plot in the Al-In-P system shows that x/X_{Al} is more than 100 times greater than in the Al-Ga-As system. This large x/X_{Al} ratio will be a source of extensive difficulty for the growth of epitaxial layers containing Al, In, and P by any near-equilibrium technique, and particularly by LPE. Compositional control and thus lattice parameter control will be very difficult because of extreme sensitivity of the system to the presence of Al. In LPE the large x/X_{Al} ratio also means that the growing solid in LPE will rapidly deplete Al from the liquid, and epitaxial layers without extensive composition grading will be very difficult to achieve. In addition, the very small amounts of Al that transfer from one LPE solution to another will drastically perturb the growth. This behavior of the Al–In–P

TABLE 6.2-3 Liquidus and Solidus
Compositions for Al–Ga–As and
$Al_xGa_{1-x}As^a$

Temperature, $T(^\circ C)$	Liquidus		Solidus
	$X_{Al}(\%)$	$X_{As}(\%)$	x
700	0.0	0.63	0.0
700	0.05	0.54	0.16
700	0.10	0.46	0.29
700	0.20	0.36	0.47
700	0.30	0.29	0.59
700	0.40	0.24	0.66
700	0.60	0.16	0.75
800	0.0	2.27	0.0
800	0.05	2.09	0.09
800	0.10	1.92	0.17
800	0.20	1.65	0.31
800	0.30	1.44	0.41
800	0.40	1.28	0.49
800	0.60	1.04	0.60
800	1.00	0.75	0.73
900	0.0	6.02	0.0
900	0.05	5.79	0.05
900	0.10	5.57	0.09
900	0.20	5.17	0.18
900	0.30	4.81	0.26
900	0.40	4.47	0.33
900	0.60	3.90	0.45
900	1.00	3.09	0.60
1000	0.00	12.35	0.0
1000	0.05	12.14	0.03
1000	0.10	11.93	0.05
1000	0.20	11.51	0.10
1000	0.30	11.11	0.15
1000	0.40	10.71	0.20
1000	0.60	9.97	0.29
1000	1.00	8.65	0.45

^{a} Calculated with the parameters of Table
6.2-2.

ternary implies similar difficulties for the Al–Ga–In–P quaternary and has, in fact, been confirmed by quaternary phase calculations[28] such as those briefly introduced below. Similar difficulties, although not quite so severe, are expected for LPE growth of the $InP|(Al_xGa_{1-x})_{0.47}In_{0.53}As|InP$ DH described in Section 5.5. Quaternary phase calculations[28] show that the ratio x/X_{Al} at useful compositions is a factor of ten or more greater than for Al–Ga–As.

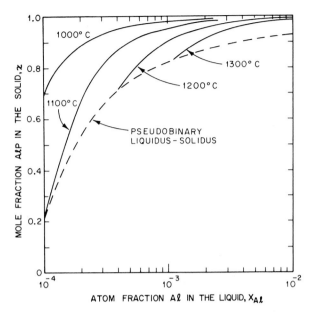

FIG. 6.2-10 Solidus composition in $Al_xIn_{1-x}P$ as a function of the liquidus composition (Ref. 21).

Quaternary III–V Systems

The thermodynamic treatment that has already been presented for binary and ternary III–V systems has been extended to quaternary solid solutions.[29,30] Again, the liquid may be treated as a "simple" solution with linear temperature-dependent interaction coefficients between the different binary pairs of elements. These interaction coefficients have been determined independently in studies of binary systems. There are, however, two types of quaternary solid solutions that must be carefully distinguished.

In the simplest case, the mixing of different constituents is restricted to only one of the sublattices, as in $(A_x^{III}B_{1-x}^{III})_yC_{1-y}^{III}D^V$, and the mixture may be described thermodynamically as a ternary mixture of AD, BD, and CD. The treatment is entirely analogous to the simpler systems described above. If the mixing occurs on both sublattices, as with $A_x^{III}B_{1-x}^{III}C_y^VD_{1-y}^V$, the situation is much more complex because treatment of the solution as a mixture of four binary compounds AD, BD, AC, and BC is not straightforward. This latter case is most simply treated by taking the quaternary solid to be a binary mixture of ternary compounds.[29] These calculations have been used to obtain initial estimates of the P concentration in the liquid necessary to give lattice-matching values of in stress compensated $GaAs–Al_xGa_{1-x}P_yAs_{1-y}$

heterostructures. Jordan and Ilegems[30] have shown that this latter approach is thermodynamically consistent and have given a detailed thermodynamic analysis of the treatment of the $A_x^{III}B_{1-x}^{III}C_y^V D_{1-y}^V$ solid as a regular mixture of binary components. Only a limited amount of experimental quaternary III–V phase data are available for comparison to the simple solution model. Sankaran *et al.*[31] give some liquidus–solidus compositions of $Ga_x In_{1-x} P_y As_{1-y}$ for the lattice-matching solid to InP. However, their thermodynamic calculations, which apparently do not take into account the additional complexities of $A_x^{III}B_{1-x}C_y^V D_{1-y}^V$ systems, do not predict the experimental data well.

6.3 IMPURITY INCORPORATION IN III–V COMPOUNDS

Introductory Comments

In this section, a brief description of the solution of impurities in III–V compounds is presented. For GaAs with the commonly used impurity elements, many of the more complicated interactions occur at impurity concentrations in excess of $\sim 1 \times 10^{18}$ cm^{-3} which is higher than generally required for heterostructure lasers. Therefore, these high-concentration interactions, such as complex formation, are only briefly mentioned. The most useful elements for controling conductivity type and concentration of shallow donors and acceptors in III–V compounds are from column IIB (Zn, Cd), IVA (Si, Ge, Sn), and VIA (S, Se, Te) of the periodic table. The group IIB elements are believed to incorporate into the III–V lattice primarily by substituting for the group III element on its lattice site. Group IIB elements are deficient in valence electrons needed to form the covalent bonds and are therefore acceptors. Conversely, the group VIA elements incorporate primarily on group V lattice sites. They have one more valence electron than is necessary to form the covalent bonds and (except for oxygen) are shallow donors. The group IVA elements are amphoteric. That is, they may be incorporated on either lattice site, becoming donors when on the group III lattice site and acceptors when on the group V lattice site. The solubility on a particular lattice site is highly variable and depends upon the host compound and its stoichiometry. Therefore, solubility at equilibrium depends upon the growth temperature and partial pressures (or liquidus compositions) of the various components during growth. For heterostructures grown by molecular-beam epitaxy, Be, Mn, and Mg, are the useful acceptors. In the discussion that follows, impurity incorporation by diffusion will not be considered because impurities are usually incorporated into heterostructures during growth of the layers. A detailed summary of diffusion in the III-V compounds has been given by Casey and Pearson.[32]

Perhaps the most direct approach to the study of impurity incorporation is the measurement of the solubility parameters resulting from incorporation at or near equilibrium. An attempt is then made to infer the equilibrium incorporation mechanism at the growth temperature. A complete description is always impossible because electrical and optical properties are usually obtained only near or below room temperature while incorporation occurs at the growth temperature. Thus annealing effects such as reactions among the various defect entities and precipitation during growth and cooling must be inferred. Also, if the growth technique results in incorporation under conditions far from equilibrium, the equilibrium behavior may only be useful as a guideline to the actual behavior. The effect of impurities on the electrical and optical properties was introduced in Sections 2.3, 2.5, 3.5, 3.7, and 4.3.

The basic terminology for impurity incorporation can be established by consideration of the equilibrium constant for chemical equilibria. For the generalized equilibrium reaction

$$lL + mM + \cdots \rightleftarrows qQ + rR + \cdots, \tag{6.3-1}$$

where $L, M, \ldots, Q, R, \ldots$ may be components in the gaseous, liquid, or solid state, and $l, m, \ldots, q, r, \ldots$ are the number of moles of each component required for the balanced chemical reaction. The change in the Gibbs free energy ΔG^0 when each component is in its standard state is given by[33]

$$\Delta G^0 = -RT \ln(a_Q{}^q a_R{}^r \cdots / a_L{}^l a_M{}^m \cdots). \tag{6.3-2}$$

At constant temperature ΔG^0 is a constant, so that there is an equilibrium constant K for the reaction defined as

$$K_{eq} = a_Q{}^q a_R{}^r \cdots / a_L{}^l a_M{}^m \cdots, \tag{6.3-3}$$

where $a_i = \gamma_i X_i$ as defined in Eq. (6.2-3) for liquid and solid solutions.

Although each impurity and each host compound present different problems, a reasonable approach is to describe the behavior of several commonly used impurities in GaAs and $Al_x Ga_{1-x} As$. Very little information is available for impurity incorporation in most III–V solid solutions, but the properties may, to some extent, be inferred from the properties of the binary end components. The experimental and thermodynamic treatment of the equilibrium incorporation of impurities in semiconductors considers incorporation during slow growth of the solid from the liquid. The properties of both the liquid and solid must be included in the analysis. Thurmond and Kowalchik[34] showed that the binary liquid phase of Ge or Si with many other elements may be described as simple solutions with linear temperature dependent interaction parameters, although they used somewhat different terminology. That treatment has been extended to III–V binary systems plus an impurity,[35–39] ternary III–V systems plus one impurity,[40] and a binary III–V system plus two impurities.[41] In all of these analyses, the activity coefficients of the components of the liquid are obtained from binary interaction parameters expressed by Eq. (6.2-23).

Reiss and Fuller[42] showed that the ionization of impurities in semiconductors led to departures from the solid solubility expected on the basis of the simple thermodynamic concepts. They demonstrated that the solubility of Li in Si was also dependent on the position of the Fermi level in the semiconductor bulk, where the Fermi level is the electron (or hole) chemical potential.[43] This result suggests that the thermodynamic treatments usually applied to Eq. (6.3-1), with the components $L, M, \ldots, Q, R \ldots$ being only atoms or chemical components, may now include all impurities and lattice defects as well as holes and electrons. Detailed analysis of chemical reactions with impurities, lattice vacancies, and electrons and holes has been given by Kröger[44] and Van Gool.[45]

Extension of the Reiss and Fuller[42] concepts to the incorporation of singly ionized substitutional impurities in extrinsic GaAs leads to a prediction of a square-root dependence of the amount of impurity in the solid on the amount in the liquid. The square-root dependence is observed for Zn in GaAs (Ref. 46) and GaP (Ref. 47), but a linear dependence is observed for Te (Ref. 48), Sn (Ref. 49), and Ge (Ref. 50) in GaAs. Whether there is a concentration range where there is a linear or a square-root dependence between the amount of impurity in the liquid and in the solid is determined by whether the Fermi level at the surface or in the semiconductor bulk enters the solubility equilibrium relationships. The results of Zschauer and Vogel[51] show that the impurity diffusivity in the solid divided by the width of the surface space-charge region must exceed the growth rate in order for the liquid phase to be in equilibrium with the semiconductor bulk. This criterion is apparently met for the rapidly diffusing Zn in GaAs or GaP but not for the slowly diffusing Te, Sn, or Ge in GaAs and InP. Therefore, it is necessary to consider the conditions established by Zschauer and Vogel[51] for the influence of the surface or bulk Fermi level on the impurity incorporation.

The Surface Space-Charge Layer

The analysis by Zschauer and Vogel[51] suggests that D/L_s (diffusivity D and intrinsic Debye length L_s) must exceed the growth rate v by about a factor of ten for the semiconductor bulk to be in equilibrium with the liquid phase. Furthermore, when D/L_s is less than v by about a factor of ten, the liquid is in equilibrium with the surface of the solid. For growth rates between these limits, the impurity incorporation is growth rate dependent.

The Debye length was given in Eq. (3.5-14) as

$$L_s = (kT\varepsilon/q^2 n)^{1/2}. \tag{3.5-14}$$

With $n_i = 5 \times 10^{17}$ (Ref. 52), $\varepsilon = 1.1 \times 10^{-12}$ F/cm, L_s at 1000°C is $\sim 10^{-6}$ cm. The actual width of the space-charge layer depends on both temperature and impurity density in the solid. Therefore, it is not entirely clear that the intrinsic Debye length (L_s for $n = n_i$) is the correct quantity to use for the space-charge layer width when the concentration in the solid is varied under extrinsic conditions.

The surface space-charge layer at the solid–liquid interface for an n-type semiconductor is shown in Fig. 6.3-1. This space-charge layer at the surface of the solid is due to surface states that result from disruption of the lattice periodicity by the surface and the unsaturated or dangling bonds of the surface atoms.[54] The surface states result in levels within the energy gap which are characteristic of the surface, and they tend to compensate the donors (or acceptors) and control the position of the Fermi level at the surface. The significant quantities are the barrier height ϕ_{Bn}, which is the separation in energy of the Fermi level and the conduction-band edge at the surface, and the width w of the space-charge layer. Because of the high density of conduction electrons in the liquid, this interface is considered to behave as a metal-semiconductor Schottky barrier. It has been observed[55,56] that the position of the Fermi level at the surface remains at a fixed energy

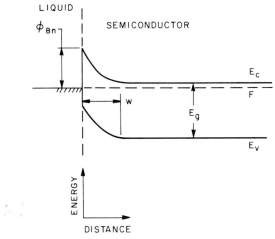

FIG. 6.3-1 Energy-band diagram for a liquid n-type semiconductor interface with a surface space-charge layer width w. The separation between the valence band E_v and the conduction band E_c is the energy gap E_g. The Fermi level is F and the barrier height ϕ_{Bn} is the position of F at the liquid–semiconductor interface (Refs. 48 and 53).

above the valence band as the temperature varies:

$$E_g(T) - \phi_{Bn}(T) = \text{constant}, \qquad (6.3\text{-}4)$$

where $E_g(T)$ is the temperature-dependent energy gap and was given in Table 5.2-2 for the III–V compounds. At room temperature, $\phi_{Bn} \approx 0.90$ eV (Ref. 55) for GaAs.

Tellurium in GaAs

For the incorporation of Te in GaAs at 1000°C by LPE, $D \approx 10^{-13}$ cm^2/ sec (Ref. 32), $L_s \approx 10^{-6}$ cm, and $v \approx 10^{-6}$ cm/sec. Therefore, $D/L_s v$ is approximately 0.1, and the liquid should be in equilibrium with the surface rather than the semiconductor bulk. The diffusivity will be much smaller at lower temperature where LPE layers are generally grown. The reaction for Te incorporation during LPE growth may then be described by[48,53]

$$\text{Te}(\ell) + V_{As} \rightleftarrows \text{Te}(s)^+ + e^-. \qquad (6.3\text{-}5)$$

In this reaction, Te in the liquid $\text{Te}(\ell)$ is taken to react with an As vacancy V_{As} to give an ionized-substitutional donor on an As site $\text{Te}(s)^+$ and a free carrier electron e^-. The equilibrium relationship [see Eq. (6.3-3)] may be written as

$$K_1(T) = \gamma_{Te}^s C_{Te} \gamma_n n / \gamma_{Te} X_{Te} X_{V_{As}}, \qquad (6.3\text{-}6)$$

where γ_n is the activity coefficient of electrons in the solid, n the electron concentration, and γ_{Te}^s and C_{Te} the activity coefficient and concentration of $\text{Te}(s)^+$ on As sites. The quantities γ_{Te} and X_{Te} are the activity coefficient and atom fraction for Te in the liquid. It is convenient to express C_{Te} in units of atoms/cm^3 and the concentrations of the composition in the liquid, X_{Te} and X_{Ga}, as atom fractions. Because the vacancy concentrations are believed to be very small, the As vacancy activity coefficient has been taken as unity, and the arsenic vacancy atom fraction is $X_{V_{As}}$.

In Eq. (6.3-6) it is more convenient to write the As vacancy concentration in terms of the Ga activity. The GaAs decomposition reaction is given by

$$\text{GaAs}(s) \rightleftarrows \text{Ga}(\ell) + \text{As}(\ell), \qquad (6.3\text{-}7)$$

and the equilibrium constant is

$$K_2(T) = a_{Ga} a_{As}. \qquad (6.3\text{-}8)$$

The reaction for the formation of As vacancies is

$$\text{As}_{As} \rightleftarrows \text{As}(\ell) + V_{As}, \qquad (6.3\text{-}9)$$

and the equilibrium constant is

$$K_3(T) = a_{As} X_{V_{As}}. \qquad (6.3\text{-}10)$$

In the reaction of Eq. (6.3-9), As_{As} represents As on As sites in the solid, and its concentration remains constant. Combining Eqs. (6.3-8) and (6.3-10) gives

$$X_{V_{As}} = K_3(T)a_{Ga}/K_2(T). \tag{6.3-11}$$

Therefore, $X_{V_{As}}$ in Eq. (6.3-6) may be represented by Eq. (6.3-11) and Eq. (6.3-6) becomes

$$K_4(T) = \gamma_{Te}^a C_{Te}\gamma_n n/\gamma_{Te}X_{Te}\gamma_{Ga}X_{Ga}, \tag{6.3-12}$$

where γ_{Ga} and X_{Ga} are the activity coefficient and atom fraction of Ga in the liquid.

For a discussion of the incorporation reaction, it is useful to simplify Eq. (6.3-12). For the experimental data to be considered here, the solid solutions of Te in GaAs are dilute with maximum concentrations of about 5×10^{19} cm^{-3} (0.1 atomic %). Therefore, Henry's law (see Ref. 57 for an introduction to Henry's law) should be obeyed, and γ_{Te}^a is taken as constant. Since the Te concentrations in the liquid are quite low, and X_{Ga} is essentially constant at 0.88 atom fraction, γ_{Te} and $\gamma_{Ga}X_{Ga}$ may also be taken as constant. Treatment of the electron activity coefficient by Hwang and Brews[58] shows that γ_n is relatively constant at a value of approximately 0.4 at 1000°C in the concentration range considered here. Equation (6.3-12) reduces to the simple expression

$$K_5(T) = C_{Te}n/X_{Te} \tag{6.3-13}$$

for no complex formation occurring in the solid at the growth temperature, and with the Te concentration in excess of the intrinsic-carrier concentration n_i.

The electron concentration was given by Eq. (4.3-25) with the exponential approximation for the Fermi–Dirac function, and the electron concentration at the surface $n(0)$ will be given by

$$n(0) = N_c\exp(-\phi_{Bn}/kT). \tag{6.3-14}$$

At high temperature, it is necessary to consider the electron distribution between the direct and indirect conduction-band minima as represented in Section 4.3 by Eq. (4.3-24) in order to evaluate the conduction band effective density of states N_c. Equation (6.3-13) may now be written as

$$C_{Te} = K_5(T)X_{Te}/N_c\exp(-\phi_{Bn}/kT), \tag{6.3-15}$$

and hence C_{Te} varies linearly with X_{Te} at a given temperature. This predicted linear dependence is demonstrated by a portion of the 1000°C solid solubility isotherm shown in Fig. 6.3-2. The data shown in this figure were obtained from LPE layers grown in a closed system and were doped with radioactive Te^{129m}. The agreement between Eq. (6.3-15) and the experimental data verify

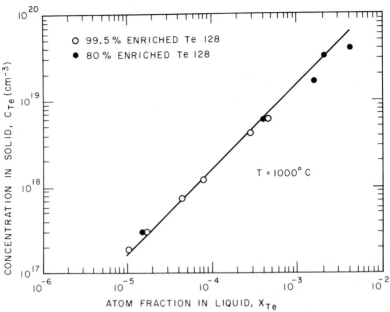

FIG. 6.3-2   A portion of the 1000°C solid–solubility isotherm for Te in GaAs (Refs. 48 and 53).

that when $D/L_s \ll v$, it is the position of the Fermi level at the surface rather than in the semiconductor bulk that dominates the impurity incorporation.

Because of the linear dependence of C_{Te} upon X_{Te}, a distribution coefficient, which is defined as the atomic fraction in the solid to that in the liquid, may be assigned at each temperature. Kang and Greene[59] determined the distribution coefficient in an open system between 700° and 850°C by measuring the electron concentration and assuming that $C_{Te} = n$. Milvidskii and Pelevin[60] determined the distribution coefficient at the GaAs melting point by chemical analysis. Figure 6.3-3 is a plot of data from Refs. 48, 59, and 60, and illustrates the interesting result that the distribution coefficient increases as the temperature is decreased. Note that the distribution coefficient goes from greater than unity at low temperature to less than unity at high temperature. Similar behavior has been observed for Se in GaAs.[61]

It should be pointed out that for group VIA elements as impurities in GaAs, the amount of impurity in the solid begins to exceed the electrically active donor concentration for impurity concentrations above approximately 1×10^{18} cm^{-3}.[48,60,62] Equation (6.3-15) suggests that the impurity concentration incorporated at the surface is greater than the impurity equilibrium in the crystal interior because $n(0)$ at the surface is less than n within the

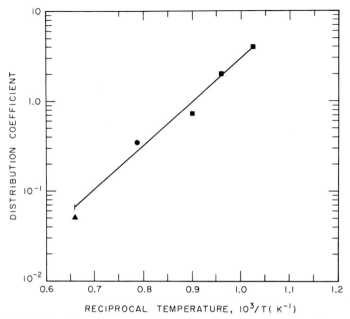

FIG. 6.3-3   The distribution coefficient of Te in GaAs as a function of temperature.
● Ref. 48; ■ Ref. 59; ▲ Ref. 60.

crystal. Therefore, once the impurity is grown into the bulk material away from the surface space-charge region, there is a thermodynamic driving force to reduce the impurity concentration by the formation of complexes or precipitates, even at the growth temperature. Vieland and Kudman[62] obtained an approximately cube-root relationship between the Se in the solid and the free electron concentration above $\sim 5 \times 10^{18}$ Se atoms/cm^3. A theoretical model for the formation of electrically inactive complexes has been given by Schottky.[63] Transmission-electron micrographs have been used to study these electrically active complexes.[64,65] Fortunately, heterostructure lasers require $n \lesssim 1 \times 10^{18}$ cm^{-3}, and these problems that occur at high impurity concentrations can be avoided. It is important, however, to be aware that they exist.

There are many more publications on the group VIA impurities in GaAs and other III–V compounds than have been discussed here. A particularly interesting study was Te in InP.[66] Here Rosztoczy et al.[66] have shown that C_{Te} in the extrinsic range varies linearly with X_{Te} for InP grown from solution. Therefore, Te incorporation in InP can also be considered to be controlled by the equilibrium between the liquid and the solid surface.

Zinc in GaAs

Zinc in GaAs is an example of the incorporation of a rapidly diffusing impurity. At Zn concentrations in excess of 10^{18} cm^{-3} at 1000°C, $D > 10^{-11}$ cm^2/sec (Ref. 32). Therefore, with $L_s \approx 10^{-6}$ cm^{-1} and $v \approx 10^{-6}$ cm/sec, $D/L_s v > 10$, and the liquid phase should be in equilibrium with the semi-conductor bulk. The incorporation of Zn in the liquid Zn(ℓ) into a Ga vacancy V_{Ga} as a singly-ionized substitutional acceptor Zn(s)$^-$ on a Ga site plus a hole e$^+$ is represented by[46]

$$Zn(\ell) + V_{Ga} \rightleftarrows Zn(s)^- + e^+. \tag{6.3-16}$$

The equilibrium relation for Eq. (6.3-16) may be written as

$$K_6(T) = \gamma_{Zn}^s C_{Zn} \gamma_p p / \gamma_{Zn} X_{Zn} X_{V_{Ga}}, \tag{6.3-17}$$

where γ_p is the activity coefficient of holes in the solid, p is the hole concentration, and γ_{Zn}^s and C_{Zn} are the activity coefficient and concentration of Zn(s)$^-$ on Ga sites. The quantities γ_{Zn} and X_{Zn} are the activity coefficient and atom fraction for Zn in the liquid. Again the vacancy activity coefficient has been taken as unity, and the Ga vacancy atom fraction is $X_{V_{Ga}}$.

The reaction for the formation of Ga vacancies is

$$Ga_{Ga} \rightleftarrows Ga(\ell) + V_{Ga}, \tag{6.3-18}$$

where Ga_{Ga} represents Ga on Ga sites in the solid. The equilibrium constant for the reaction is

$$K_7(T) = X_{V_{Ga}} a_{Ga}. \tag{6.3-19}$$

Combining Eqs. (6.3-8) and (6.3-19) gives

$$X_{V_{Ga}} = K_7(T) a_{As} / K_2(T). \tag{6.3-20}$$

With Eq. (6.3-20), Eq. (6.3-17) becomes

$$K_8(T) = \gamma_{Zn}^s C_{Zn} \gamma_p p / \gamma_{Zn} X_{Zn} \gamma_{As} X_{As}, \tag{6.3-21}$$

where γ_{As} and X_{As} are the activity coefficient and atom fraction of As in the liquid.

Equation (6.3-21) may be simplified by assuming Henry's law applies for Zn in the solid so that γ_{Zn}^s may be taken as constant and included in $K_8(T)$ as $K_8'(T)$. For extrinsic conditions ($p > n_i$) and fully ionized Zn in the solid, the condition of electrical neutrality may be expressed by $C_{Zn} = p$. The solid solubility of Zn is then given by

$$C_{Zn} = [K_8'(T) \gamma_{Zn} X_{Zn} \gamma_{As} X_{As} / \gamma_p]^{1/2}. \tag{6.3-22}$$

At a given temperature, the variation of X_{As} with X_{Zn} may be obtained from the liquidus isotherm of the Ga–As–Zn ternary phase diagram[67] which is shown for 1000°C by the insert in Fig. 6.3-4. Jordan's[39] analysis of the Zn and arsenic pressure measurements by Shih *et al.*[68] permits evaluation of γ_{Zn} and γ_{As}. The complete solid solubility along the 1000°C liquidus isotherm, as calculated by Eq. (6.3-22) with $\gamma_p = 1$, is given by the dashed line in Fig. 6.3-4. The double-valued solid solubility curve results from the fact that the liquidus isotherm is also double valued in Zn composition (see the insert of Fig. 6.3-4). At high concentrations, the experimental solid solubility exceeds C_{Zn} obtained from Eq. (6.3-22) and indicates that γ_p is less than unity in this region. When the values of γ_p from Ref. 69 are used in Eq. (6.3-22), the solid line shown in Fig. 6.3-4 is obtained and is in agreement with the experimental data. It should also be noted that $\gamma_{Zn}\gamma_{As}X_{As}/\gamma_p$ is constant for $X_{Zn} < 0.1$ atom fraction and the concentration dependence of the amount of Zn in the solid on the amount in the liquid is given by

$$C_{Zn} = [K_8''(T)X_{Zn}]^{1/2}, \tag{6.3-23}$$

which is the square-root dependence of the Zn concentration for equilibrium between the liquid and semiconductor bulk. The Zn solubility for Ga-rich isotherms at temperatures between 600° and 1000°C is summarized in Fig. 6.3-5.[47]

A discussion of the concentration dependence of the ionization energy for impurities was given in Section 3.5, and no neutral Zn is expected at high concentrations. As opposed to Te in GaAs, it appears that most of the Zn in GaAs is electrically active, even at high concentrations.[70]

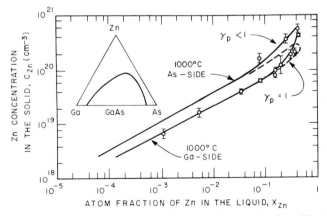

FIG. 6.3-4   The Zn concentration in the solid versus the atom fraction of Zn in the liquid along the Ga–As–Zn 1000°C liquidus isotherm. The 1000°C liquidus isotherm is shown by the inset (Ref. 53).

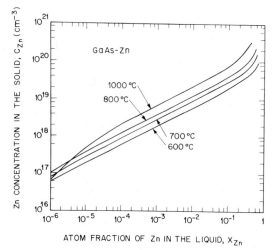

FIG. 6.3-5 The Zn concentration in GaAs versus the atom fraction of Zn in the liquid along the 600°, 700°, 800°, and 1000°C Ga-rich liquidus isotherms in the Ga–As–Zn system. These isotherms were calculated by Jordan (Ref. 47).

Group IVA Impurities in GaAs

The group IVA elements Si, Ge, and Sn are all useful impurities in GaAs for preparation of heterostructure lasers. Carbon is only found as a residual, undesired impurity in epitaxial layers.[71] The other group IV elements are important impurities in liquid-phase epitaxy (LPE) and molecular-beam epitaxy (MBE) because they have low vapor pressures, low diffusivities, and small impurity ionization energies (see Table 4.3-1). As compared to Te or Zn, relatively high Ge and Sn concentrations in the liquid are required in order to obtain useful impurity concentrations in the solid. These properties permit the use of liquid solutions for LPE that contain easily weighable quantities of Ge and Sn, and they do not, as do Zn and Te, cross contaminate the other solutions by vapor transport. Because the group IVA impurities can be donors when substitutional on Ga sites and acceptors when substitutional on As sites, they are amphoteric dopants. As described below, Si can give heavily-doped, closely compensated n- or p-type LPE GaAs layers. Germanium gives relatively uncompensated p-type LPE layers, while Sn gives relatively uncompensated n-type LPE layers. Further discussion of dopants for MBE layers will be given in Section 6.6.

The variation of the hole concentration in GaAs at room temperature with the amount of Ge in the liquid used to grow the GaAs at 800° (Ref. 72) and 900°C (Ref. 50) is shown in Fig. 6.3-6. The total Ge in the solid was also determined by Rosztoczy and Wolfstirn.[50] Except at $p > 2 \times 10^{18}$ cm^{-3} at

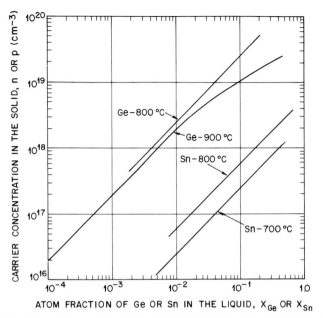

FIG. 6.3-6 The upper curves are the room-temperature hole concentration in GaAs versus the atom fraction of Ge in the liquid along the 800° (Ref. 72) and 900°C (Ref. 50) Ga-rich liquidus isotherms. The lower curves are the room temperature electron concentration in GaAs versus the atom fraction of Sn in the liquid along the 700° and 900°C Ga-rich liquidus isotherms (Ref. 49).

900°C, there is a linear dependence between the amount of Ge in the liquid and solid. The diffusivity of Ge in GaAs is believed to be small. Therefore, the liquid should be in equilibrium with the surface and give the linear dependence as observed. Germanium is extensively used as an acceptor for both the active layer and the p-type $Al_xGa_{1-x}As$ confining layer in GaAs–$Al_xGa_{1-x}As$ DH lasers. Rosztoczy et al.[66] obtained data for Ge in InP where it incorporates primarily as a shallow donor. A linear dependence between the amount in the liquid and the solid was also observed. The variation of the electron concentration in GaAs at room temperature with the amount of Sn in the liquid at growth temperatures of 700° and 800°C is shown along with the data for Ge in Fig. 6.3-6 (Ref. 49). The distribution coefficient for Sn can be seen to be a factor of 50 less than for Ge. References to other results for Sn in GaAs may be found in Ref. 49. The linear dependence of n on X_{Sn} for GaAs (Fig. 6.3-6) and InP (Ref. 66) indicates that in both of these cases equilibrium between the liquid and surface dominates at the growth rates used.

Silicon-doped GaAs grown by LPE can give LED's with external electroluminescent efficiencies in excess of 20%.[73] Similar results have been obtained for Si-doped $Al_xGa_{1-x}As$ with $x < 0.1$.[74] This high external efficiency is related to the reduced self-absorption that results from close compensation at high Si concentrations. The incorporation of Si in GaAs as a donor, acceptor, or both has been found to depend on both the amount of Si in the melt and the growth temperature.[75,76] Figure 6.3-7 shows that the conductivity type varies with the growth temperature and Si concentration in the liquid.[77] The carrier concentration can vary from $\sim 10^{16}$ cm^{-3} to $\sim 5 \times 10^{18}$ cm^{-3} while the total Si concentration is $\sim 3 \times 10^{19}$ cm^{-3} (Ref. 78). There is evidence that both Si_{Ga} (donors) and Si_{As} (acceptors) are present in Si-doped GaAs.[75,79] These Si species, however, do not account for all of the Si present in the crystal. It may be inferred from photoluminescence studies and Hall measurements for as-grown and annealed samples that there are several other unidentified Si-containing species in the solid.[75,79,80] Since Si-doped laser-active layers have high Si concentrations, these layers contain many Si species that are not well understood. Nevertheless, $GaAs–Al_xGa_{1-x}As$ DH

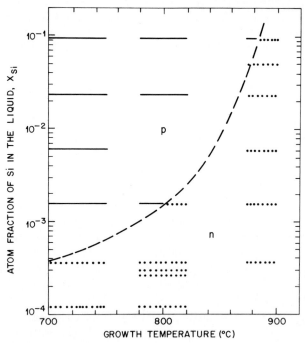

FIG. 6.3-7 Effect of growth temperature and Si concentration in the liquid on the behavior of Si in GaAs.———p-type; · · · n-type (Ref. 77).

heterostructure lasers with Si-doped active layers have low threshold current densities unless the heteroepitaxial wafer is subjected to annealing at temperatures in excess of $\sim 700°$C.

Impurities in Al$_x$Ga$_{1-x}$As

Studies of the incorporation of impurities in Al$_x$Ga$_{1-x}$As have been made for Te and Ge (Ref. 81) and Sn (Ref. 40). As shown in Fig. 4.3-3, the acceptor ionization energy was found to increase for $x > 0$, and for Te the donor ionization energy increased abruptly for $x \gtrsim 0.25$.[81] The donor ionization energy for Sn in Al$_x$Ga$_{1-x}$As (Ref. 40) behaved similarly to Te. The larger impurity ionization energies mean that the impurity is only partially ionized at room temperature and larger impurity concentrations are necessary in order to obtain the same resistivities as for GaAs. For Sn in Al$_x$Ga$_{1-x}$As at the usual values of $x > 0.25$ in heterostructure lasers, values of electron concentrations only up to $\sim 5 \times 10^{17}$ cm^{-3} may be achieved.[40] To obtain larger free carrier concentrations, the required Sn levels in the liquid become so large that the Sn becomes the major component of the Al–Ga–As–Sn quaternary liquid from which the Sn-doped Al$_x$Ga$_{1-x}$As layers are grown. This large Sn composition has deleterious effects on the LPE growth and results in a practical limitation on the layer resistivity. The liquidus isotherms for the Al–Ga–As–Sn system may be found in Ref. 40.

6.4 PHASE EQUILIBRIA IN IV–VI SYSTEMS

General Discussion

Temperature–composition projections of Pb–Te, Sn–Te, Pb–S, and Pb–Se liquidi show that, as with the III–V systems, the largest part of the phase diagram consists of the liquidus in equilibrium with the binary IV–VI compound. The departures from stoichiometry are relatively small. However, unlike the III–V compounds, the lattice vacancies behave as donors and acceptors and are present in sufficient concentrations to influence the crystal conductivity. Another striking difference between the phase chemistry of these compounds and that of the III–V compounds is the nature of the vapor in equilibrium with the binary solid. In all cases the metal-rich liquid is in equilibrium with a vapor that consists primarily of binary IV–VI molecules.

The phase equilibria have been reviewed by Novoselova.[82] A set of temperature–composition–stoichiometry–partial pressure diagrams for Pb–Te that is typical of these systems is given in Fig. 6.4-1. The Pb–Te liquidus is given in the $T–X$ diagram of Fig. 6.4-1a. The solid curve of Fig. 6.4-1a was calculated by Ilegems and Pearson[83] to fit the experimental data

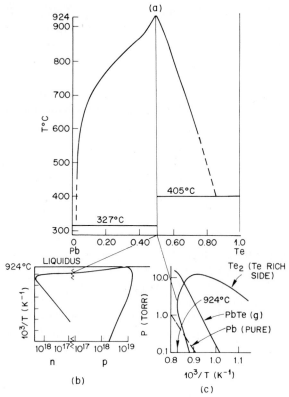

FIG. 6.4-1   (a) The liquidus of the Pb–Te primary phase field (Ref. 83). (b) The solid existence region of PbTe as represented by the electron concentration n and hole concentration p (Ref. 87). (c) Partial pressures of Te_2 and PbTe in equilibrium with the Pb- and Te-rich Pb–Te liquidus (Ref. 89). The vapor pressure of pure Pb is included for comparison.

of Miller and Komarek[84] and Lugscheider *et al.*[85] In this calculation, Ilegems and Pearson[83] assumed an almost completely associated liquid. Jordan's[86] associated regular solution model was used. The peaking at 50 atomic percent Te is characteristic of an associated liquid. The existence region of the solid is sufficiently narrow that it cannot be represented in part (a), and therefore this region around the 50 atomic percent Te composition has been expanded[87] and is shown in Fig. 6.4-1b. These data are the carrier concentrations calculated from Hall coefficient measurements at 77°K for various isothermal annealing temperatures. It is believed that the Pb vacancies are shallow donors and the Te vacancies are shallow acceptors and represent the solidus region.[87,88] The solidus nonstoichiometry boundary is based on the carrier concentration because the departure from stoichiometry is too small to permit its determination by chemical analysis.

The equilibrium vapor pressures of the various species that correspond to the liquidus and solidus of Fig. 6.4-1a, b are shown in Fig. 6.4-1c.[89] A wide range of pressures can be in equilibrium with the PbTe solid phase. These curves show the Te_2 partial pressure in equilibrium with the liquid and solid from the Pb-rich region, through the melting point, and up into the Te-rich region. There should be a curve for the Pb pressure that corresponds to this curve, but it has not been determined. The maximum Pb pressure in the Pb-rich region will be near the vapor pressure of pure Pb and will be much less than the pressure over pure Pb as the concentration of Te in the equilibrium liquid increases. Note that the pressure of PbTe(g) is greater than the pressure of Pb over the entire composition range and greater than the pressure of Te_2 in the Pb-rich region. These pressure relationships have important implications for chemical-vapor transport and molecular-beam epitaxy growth. In these cases, PbTe(g) will usually be the major mass transporting species even though the crystal stoichiometry (and thus the carrier concentration) are determined by the partial pressures of Pb and Te_2.

The phase diagrams of the IV–VI ternary systems have not been studied in detail. They are somewhat similar to the III–V phase diagrams and exhibit a very large composition region in which the $A_x^{IV}B_{1-x}^{IV}C^{VI}$ compound is in equilibrium with the liquid. Stoichiometry, and thus both conductivity type and carrier concentration may be adjusted by annealing under appropriate partial pressures of the component elements. For the binary compounds, these annealing procedures yield, as the limit, the existence range of the compound. For the ternaries, the annealing has usually been done either in the presence of a mixture metal at the same ratio as the compound, or in the presence of excess group VI element. In either case, the stoichiometry and thus the carrier concentration that are obtained are not representative of the liquidus–solidus existence field limits of the solid. Curves that are obtained in this manner are referred to here as *meta-solidus curves* in order to distinguish them from data that represent the actual liquidus–solidus equilibrium.

$Pb_{1-x}Sn_xTe$

Since both the lead and tin tellurides crystallize with NaCl (rock salt) lattice structure, and their lattice parameters differ by only about 2%, it is not surprising that they form a complete series of solid solutions. Phase diagrams[90] and phase calculations[83] have been reported. Meta-solidus curves in Fig. 6.4-2 with the stoichiometry reported as carrier concentrations have been constructed by Harman[87,91] with his own annealing data and also with the data of Brebrick and Gubner for PbTe[88] and Calawa et al.[92]

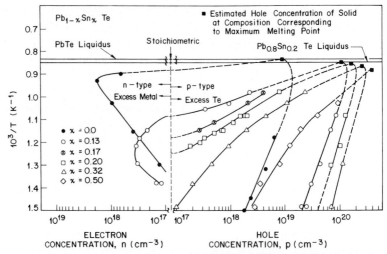

FIG. 6.4-2 Carrier concentration from Hall measurements at 77°K as a function of isothermal annealing temperature for PbTe and $Pb_{1-x}Sn_xTe$ at several values of x. The latter are the meta-solidus curves discussed in the text (Refs. 87 and 91).

These curves illustrate how carrier concentration can be adjusted in the bulk material. The equilibrium curves, if available, would be expected to show the same general features although differing somewhat in shape and position.

The effects of impurities as dopants in $Pb_{1-x}Sn_xTe$ are strongly masked by the ionized native defects. In general, group 1A and 1B impurities are acceptors when substitutional and donors when interstitial. Group IIIB elements are donors, except for Tl which is an acceptor. Frequently, the $PbTe–Pb_xSn_{1-x}Te$ heterostructure lasers are not doped, and the native defects are utilized to give the proper conductivity type.

$Pb_{1-x}Sn_xSe$

Since SnSe does not have the rock-salt structure, a complete series of solid solutions does not exist over the entire composition range, and, depending upon the temperature, the maximum attainable value of x is between 0.4 and 0.5. The only condensed phase data available are the binary-phase diagrams,[93] the pseudobinary liquidus-solidus equilibria, and meta-solidus curves.[87,91]

Doping studies for this system have not been reported, presumably because of the very high native defect concentration of $10^{18}–10^{19}$ cm^{-3}. Control of carrier concentration with impurities can be achieved only with material grown or annealed at low temperatures ($\lesssim 650°C$) if there is a highly soluble impurity available.

PbS$_{1-x}$Se$_x$

Both of the end components of this system have the rock-salt structure, and there is a complete series of solid solutions. Liquidus–solidus equilibria have been studied only along the PbS–PbSe pseudobinary.[94] There is only a small amount of information about the existence field of the solid, which consists primarily of the existence fields of the end components and metastability curves for a few ternary compositions.[87,91]

6.5 LIQUID-PHASE EPITAXY

General Discussion

In the most general terms, liquid-phase epitaxy (LPE) is the growth of an oriented crystalline layer of material from a saturated or supersaturated liquid solution onto a crystalline substrate. For the epitaxy described here, the growth occurs on a single-crystal substrate that has similar enough crystal structure and lattice dimensions to the growing layer to permit the continuation of the coherent crystal structure. Most frequently, and in all cases described here, the major constituent of the liquid solution is one of the major components of the solid, and the phase equilibria are such that the liquid solution from which growth occurs is relatively dilute in all components but one.

It is useful to use the binary system A–C of Fig. 6.2-1 and the hypothetical ternary system A–B–C of Fig. 6.2-7 in order to illustrate the thermodynamic basis of LPE. Consider the case where the epitaxial growth of the binary compound AC is a near equilibrium situation. It is simply the growth onto a substrate of an amount of solid AC equivalent to the loss of $X_C(T_2) - X_C(T_1)$ atom fraction of C (and the same amount of A) from the liquid solution (see Fig. 6.2-1) as the result of cooling from T_2 to T_1. The situation is somewhat more complex for the equilibrium ternary. The ternary illustrated in Fig. 6.2-7 is representative of the class of ternaries in which A and B are group III elements and C is a group V element. This figure is expanded in Fig. 6.5-1 to show only the group III rich region between two close isotherms. Each isothermal phase diagram (see Fig. 6.2-5) represents a cut through the liquidus and solidus surfaces. The compositions of liquid A–B–C that can be in existence at a given temperature with the solid A$_x$B$_{1-x}$C are completely represented by the liquidus curve and the corresponding tie lines. When growing the ternary, the liquid solution at (2) in Fig. 6.5-1 is cooled to (1) and a solid richer in A than the liquid will precipitate as the epitaxial solid. As the epitaxial layer grows during cooling from T_2 to T_1, its composition will follow curve b as the composition of the liquid follows curve a.

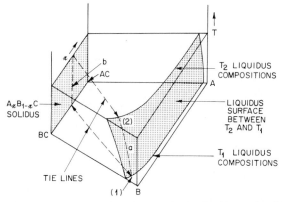

FIG. 6.5-1 Three-dimensional phase diagram for the liquidus and solidus of a ternary A^{III}–B^{III}–C^V in equilibrium with the solid solution $A_x B_{1-x} C$ where $0 \leq x \leq 1$. Only the portion of the system in which $X_A + X_B > X_C$ between two closely lying temperatures T_2 and T_1 is shown. The triangular composition diagram for ternary systems was described in Fig. 6.2-6.

Since useful phase diagrams can be obtained from interpretation of a limited amount of experimental data as previously described in Section 6.2, the discussion of LPE would be complete if that were the only consideration. Although determined ultimately by equilibrium considerations, LPE growth is also greatly influenced by other factors. These are limitations to the arrival of constituents at the growing interface (usually in stagnant and isothermal solutions), supersaturation of the solution during growth, nucleation and the mechanism of growth at the surface, and convection as the result of compositional and temperature gradients. In addition, when heterostructures are grown, there is always thermodynamic instability between the solution and the crystal surface when a new layer is started, i.e., at the heterojunction.

Thermodynamic instability between the crystal surface and the liquid solution must always exist if the only solid phase that can be in equilibrium with the liquid is different in composition from the composition of the crystal in contact with the solution. This situation is well illustrated by the Al–Ga–As system. In Fig. 6.2-5, the 900°C liquidus isotherm is shown by the usual triangular composition diagram. Also shown is one tie line connecting the composition of the solid in equilibrium with the 900°C liquidus composition containing 1.0 atomic percent Al. Clearly the only solid that can be in equilibrium with the liquid containing 1.0 atomic percent Al at 900°C is $Al_{0.63}Ga_{0.37}As$ which is very different in composition from the GaAs substrate usually used. In a system initially composed of such a solution in contact with GaAs at 900°C, the solution and solid will eventually react to completely dissolve the GaAs. Then the system will consist of a liquid at a composition on the isotherm but with less Al than the starting solution. It will be in equilibrium with $Al_xGa_{1-x}As$ and no GaAs will be present. Panish *et al.*[95] suggested that a very thin surface layer of $Al_xGa_{1-x}As$ rapidly forms on the GaAs when it is in contact with the Al–Ga–As liquid at the liquidus temperature. This layer protects the substrate and layer growth may continue if the system is cooled. Unfortunately, this rapid protection of the substrate seems to occur in only one other III–V system, the all indirect energy gap $Al_xGa_{1-x}P$ on GaP.[96,97] Substrate instability has been observed with several other III–V systems:[28] Ga–In–P and Ga–In–As solutions in contact with GaAs, In–Ga–As–P solutions in contact with InP, and Ga–As–P solutions in contact with GaAs and GaP. Therefore, seed instability with slow cooling at near equilibrium growth conditions is the rule for III–V systems and not the exception. This result does not mean that LPE cannot be done with combinations of liquid and solid where such thermodynamic instability is important. It means that special precautions, usually requiring growth from supersaturated solutions are necessary. The step-cooling procedures described in the following part of this section are particularly applicable.

Throughout the discussions of Chapter 5 where many III–V heterostructures were considered for lasers, the importance of a sufficiently good lattice match to prevent extensive inclined dislocation formation was emphasized. With $Al_xGa_{1-x}As$, a good lattice match occurs for all x and small variations of x cause no mismatch problem. However, consider the growth of $Ga_xIn_{1-x}P$ on GaAs. This ternary is well represented by the hypothetical diagram of Fig. 6.5-1 with A as Ga, and B as In. At equilibrium the solid surface will change composition (curve b) as the solution is cooled. This situation is further aggravated because diffusion in the liquid limits the arrival of Ga from the bulk of the liquid so that curve b drifts even further toward BC. It is not unreasonable to expect that in this situation x will vary by as much as 1% in a thin multilayer structure. Stringfellow[98] has pointed out that for $Ga_xIn_{1-x}P$, which is intended to lattice match GaAs, a lattice mismatch shift of $x = \pm 0.01$ is sufficient to prevent epitaxial-crystal growth. However, for $Ga_xIn_{1-x}P$ on GaAs (Ref. 98) and $GaAs_ySb_{1-y}$ on GaAs (Ref. 99), there is a tendency for lattice-match growth to occur, even from solutions expected to yield a slightly unmatched crystal within this range of x of about $\pm 1\%$. This effect, which has been called "pulling," is not well understood and is not observed for $In_xGa_{1-x}P_yAs_{1-y}$ on InP (Ref. 100).

Virtually all the discussion presented in this section deals with LPE of III-VI compounds. When considering the growth of IV–VI heterostructures by LPE, some of the problems described above for III–V systems may not be significant. The much longer laser emission wavelengths permit optical confinement with much thicker active regions. Also, growth conditions much further from equilibrium, such as step cooling described below, may be used to overcome substrate dissolution. Furthermore, a lattice match, although presumably desirable, is less essential. If epitaxy can be achieved, small variations in composition as the result of high distribution coefficients should not be detrimental to laser operation of IV–VI lasers as would be expected for III–V lasers. A more serious problem is the high concentration of vacancies that behave as donors and acceptors and influence the crystal conductivity as described in Section 6.4. These defects make conductivity control difficult with IV–VI compounds and restrict the range of conditions under which laser structures can be grown.

Uniform Cooling and Step Cooling

There are several ways that phase equilibria can be employed as the starting point for liquid-phase epitaxy. In the most commonly used technique for the growth of GaAs–$Al_xGa_{1-x}As$ heterostructures, the GaAs substrate crystal is brought into contact with the equilibrated solution at T_2 and then slowly cooled, together with the solution, to T_1. It is convenient to designate this procedure as a "uniform cooling" (UC) technique. The equilibrium situation has already been described for the hypothetical binary and ternary of Figs. 6.2-1 and 6.5-1, but that situation actually never occurs. In epitaxial growth of both the binary and ternary III–V compounds, diffusion in the liquid is not rapid enough for the components at any distance from the growing surface to reach equilibrium with it. In addition to compositional variations already described, diffusion limitations result in slower growth than expected at equilibrium.

There are several descriptions of diffusion limited epitaxial growth for the binary III–V compounds.[101–105] One of the simplest was given by Hsieh.[101] He assumed that the binary solution A–C is deep, stagnant, isothermal, and precipitates AC only on the AC substrate which provides all necessary nucleation sites. Growth is assumed to be limited by the diffusion of component C to the growing surface and the change in solubility with temperature. The example considered by Hsieh[101] was GaAs, so that component C would be As as represented in Fig. 6.2-1. In the layer growth model, the variation of the As concentration is of interest because As is the more dilute component and is considered to be the solute.

The amount of solute per unit area M_t that leaves the solution in time t during growth on the substrate is

$$M_t = \int_0^t D \left[\frac{\partial C_{As}^\ell(z, t)}{\partial z} \right]_{z=0} dt, \qquad (6.5-1)$$

where D is the diffusivity. Rather than atom fraction, the usual convention in the solution of the diffusion equation is to use the concentration C_{As}^ℓ

which is the number of As atoms per unit volume in the liquid. The spatial coordinate is z, and $z = 0$ is taken as the substrate surface because the layer thickness is so small compared to the solution that the growing layer thickness may be neglected. The resulting epitaxial layer thickness is

$$d = M_t/C_{As}^a, \tag{6.5-2}$$

where C_{As}^a is the concentration of component C in the solid. To evaluate M_t, Hsieh obtained $C_{As}^\ell(z, t)$ by solving the one-dimensional diffusion equation[106]

$$D[\partial^2 C_{As}^\ell(z, t)/\partial z^2] = \partial C_{As}^\ell(z, t)/\partial t. \tag{6.5-3}$$

The initial concentration of $C_{As}^\ell(z, 0)$ in the liquid at T_2 is given by the liquidus of Fig. 6.2-2 for GaAs. Hsieh assumed that the slope of the liquidus curve at T_2 is given by

$$dT/dC_{As}^\ell = (T_2 - T_1)/[C_{As}^\ell(T_2) - C_{As}^\ell(T_1)] \equiv \text{constant} = m. \tag{6.5-4}$$

For uniform cooling, the boundary conditions are $C_{As}^\ell(z, 0) = C_{As}^\ell(T_2)$ and $C_{As}^\ell(0, t) = C_{As}^\ell(T_2) - (R/m)t$, where R is the cooling rate. The solution of these equations for d is

$$d = (4/3)(R/C_{As}^a m)(D/\pi)^{1/2} t^{3/2}. \tag{6.5-5}$$

In Fig. 5.2-2, it may be seen that there are four Ga and four As atoms per unit cell so that $C_{As}^a = 4/a_0^3$. The lattice constant for GaAs as a function of T was given in Fig. 5.5-1.

Although uniform cooling is the most commonly used technique at present for growth of $Al_x Ga_{1-x}As$ heterostructures, a more recent approach that shows promise of providing improved interfaces is the step-cooling technique. The solution is saturated at some temperature T_2, separated from the saturating source, cooled to T_1, and brought into contact with the substrate at T_1. The temperature difference $T_2 - T_1 = \Delta T$ must be small enough that nucleation of crystallites in the solution does not occur. Two simple variations of this technique are: (1) to hold the solution and substrate at T_1 (SC1), or (2) to maintain the same cooling rate after growth starts, as was used in the supersaturation step (SC2). Hsieh[101] has compared the growth rate for UC, SC1, and SC2. His solutions of the diffusion equations with the same assumptions as for UC, but with the boundary conditions $C_{As}^\ell(z, 0) = C_{As}^\ell(T_2)$ and $C_{As}^\ell(0, t) = C_{As}^\ell(T_1)$ gives the thickness of the layer grown by SC1 as

$$d = (2\Delta T/C_{As}^a m)(D/\pi)^{1/2} t^{1/2}. \tag{6.5-6}$$

The sum of Eqs. (6.5-5) and (6.5-6) gives d for SC2 as

$$d = (1/C_{As}^a m)(D/\pi)^{1/2} [2\Delta T t^{1/2} + (4/3)R t^{3/2}]. \tag{6.5-7}$$

Hsieh[101] compared the thickness of LPE layers of GaAs grown on GaAs substrates from GaAs solutions at 800°C with the predicted d from Eqs. (6.5-5)–(6.5-7). The calculated curves and experimental data of Hsieh[101] are shown in Fig. 6.5-2. In all cases, D for As in the liquid was found to be in the range $4–5.2 \times 10^{-5}$ cm²/sec. These values of D were determined by Hsieh with Eqs. (6.5-5)–(6.5-7) and a measured d. Dawson[107] obtained $D \approx 8 \times 10^{-5}$ cm²/sec in a similar manner. Except at long growth times, where the finite thickness of the solution perturbs the experiments, the data and calculated curves agree very well. Hsieh has also shown that identical considerations describe the LPE growth of InP from In–P solutions.[100] Similar treatments have not been reported for ternary systems such as Al–Ga–As. In addition, for the SC1 process Zschauer has shown that the effective distribution coefficient for an impurity,[107a] or even for a major component such as Al in $Al_xGa_{1-x}As$,[107b] is invariant with time for an infinitely deep solution.

Examination of Fig. 6.5-2 reveals that with step cooling it may be more difficult to grow the very thin (0.1 μm) layers necessary for some heterostructure lasers than with uniform cooling. Probably the primary advantage of

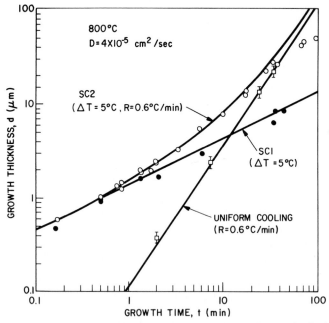

FIG. 6.5-2 Epitaxial layer thickness d as a function of growth time t for GaAs epitaxial layers grown by the uniform cooling, step-cooling 1, and step-cooling 2 techniques. The curves are calculated from Eqs. (6.6-5)–(6.6-7) (Ref. 101).

step cooling over uniform cooling is the possibility of rapid initial growth, presumably from many nucleation sites, which results from the greater driving force for crystal growth from the supersaturated solution. Smoother layers may be expected if this assumption is true. Hsieh[101] compared layers of GaAs grown on GaAs substrates by UC, SC1, and SC2 and found that the SC layers are indeed smoother. Rode and Sobers[108] have used a modified SC1 technique for the growth of GaAs–$Al_xGa_{1-x}As$ heterostructures and found that an improvement in the uniformity of layer thickness is also achieved. They attributed the improvement to a decrease in cooling-induced convection. Another potential advantage of the SC technique is the possibility of suppressing the interaction of the growth solution with an unstable substrate. A similar technique has, in fact, been used for the LPE of $Ga_{0.51}In_{0.49}P$ on GaAs (Ref. 98), and Hsieh et al.[109] have used SC2 for the growth of the InP–$In_xGa_{1-x}P_yAs_{1-y}$–InP DH laser which was described in Section 5.5. The results of studies of the interface smoothness for GaAs–$Al_xGa_{1-x}As$ show that there is sufficient roughness in most uniformly cooled DH lasers to cause losses due to scattering.[110] This roughness may result from instability of the GaAs to the Al–Ga–As solution and SC growth procedures may reduce such scattering losses.

Constitutional Supercooling

Rode[102] used a model for LPE growth of GaAs that is essentially identical to that of Hsieh, except that m was not taken to be constant, and a finite liquid solution depth was considered. Numerical computer simulation was used for the LPE growth. Those simulations gave further insight into the growth dynamics. For these calculations, Rode[102] used $D = 4.1 \times 10^{-5}$ cm^2/sec. Similar calculations were made by Dawson[107] with $D = 8 \times 10^{-5}$ cm^2/sec. Figure 6.5-3 shows the development of supersaturation normal to the growing surface for typical growth conditions used for heteroepitaxy by the UC method. Frequently growth of the first layer of a heterostructure is initiated from a slightly undersaturated solution. In a stagnant solution, the prevailing dynamic situation for a slightly undersaturated solution for growth by UC method is represented by Fig. 6.5-4. A solution step cooled from 800° to 790°C for the growth of a layer by the SC1 method is represented by Fig. 6.5-5.

The development of supersaturation gradients such as those shown in Figs. 6.5-3–6.5-5 has important implications in addition to those already discussed. In metal systems, such "constitutional supercooling" leads to growth instability at the liquid–solid interface.[103] These growth instabilities are the result of nucleation of crystallites or dendrites near or at the growing surface, from lateral composition or thermal gradients, or nonsmoothness of

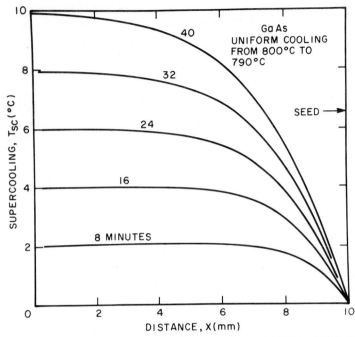

FIG. 6.5-3 Development of supersaturation in a stagnant solution during growth of GaAs on a GaAs substrate for typical heterostructure laser growth conditions. At the start of the growth, the solution is taken to be in equilibrium with the solid. Solution depth is 10 mm, $D = 4.1 \times 10^{-5}$ cm^2/sec, and $R = 0.25$°C/min (Ref. 102).

the starting surface. Such instability in all-metal systems leads to characteristic nonsmooth growth patterns. Minden[111] did a detailed analysis to predict the required temperature gradient in the liquid that is necessary to prevent supersaturation from occurring during LPE. The resulting requirement was a gradient of some tens of degrees per centimeter with the substrate at the lower temperature. Such a gradient is difficult to achieve in a liquid metal solution for the usual conditions for multiple LPE of heterostructure lasers.

Because of these effects of constitutional supercooling, it is useful to consider briefly some observations of Crossley and Small.[112] These observations permit the qualitative evaluation of the importance of growth instability, due to constitutional supercooling, on the growth of III–V heterostructures. Crossley and Small[112] described the morphology of single GaAs LPE layers and suggest that it developed in three stages. A first stage occurs where surface morphology depends upon the condition of solution

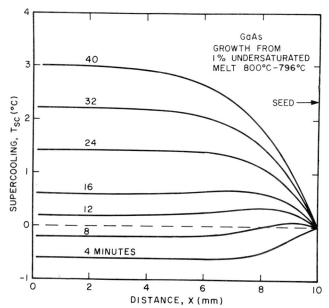

FIG. 6.5-4 Same as Fig. 6.5-3 but with solution initially undersaturated by 1% of the liquidus As concentration. In this figure $R = 0.10°C/min$ and initial temperature is 800°C. The positive slope of the As profile indicates dissolution of the seed located at $x = 10$ mm for the first 5 min of the run (Ref. 102).

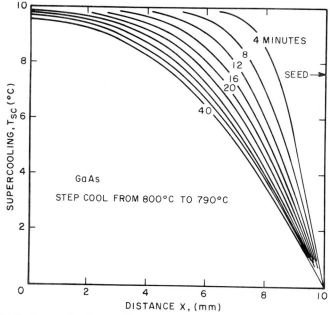

FIG. 6.5-5 Supersaturation profile in a stagnant solution during growth by the SCI method (Ref. 102).

saturation as it contacts the seed. The second stage results in smoothing from the initial nucleation sites. In the third stage, roughening that may result from constitutional supercooling instability occurs. For LPE of GaAs on GaAs from Ga solutions under conditions similar to those used for multiple layer LPE, they showed that the third stage does not occur until after 15–25 μm of growth.

Crossley and Small's qualitative observations of the initial development of single layers of GaAs when grown from solutions that are undersaturated, at or very near saturation, or supersaturated are given in Table 6.5-1. These observations suggest the following behavior. At the high supersaturation characteristic of SC, nucleation occurs readily over the entire crystal surface giving relatively smooth growth. In situations where the growth occurs from a solution at or very near saturation, there is very little initial driving force for growth. In this case, nucleation may occur only at a few scattered sites, and seed preparation and pretreatment may be critical. A substrate surface that has been subjected to a small amount of dissolution apparently has a high concentration of nucleation sites so that smooth growth is possible as the solution near the surface changes from under saturated to supersaturated during cooling.

The solutions usually used for LPE of III–V compounds will in fact withstand supercooling much greater than those usually encountered during LPE of thin structures without growth of dendrites or spurious nucleation.[113] Constitutional supercooling instability is probably not an important cause of surface roughness in those cases. Crossley and Small's[112] observation that stage three requires extensive growth is consistent with our own observations that cellular growth characteristics of constitutional supercooling instability is never observed in the growth of heterostructure lasers.

The other class of undesirable effects that result from the supersaturation gradients is caused by the requirements of multiple LPE where each layer

TABLE 6.5-1 Development of GaAs LPE Layers at 800°C from Undersaturated, Saturated, and Supersaturated Solutions (Ref. 112)

Growth condition	Appearance
Inserted seed into 4°C undersaturated solution—no cooling.	Rough (etched).
Inserted seed into 4°C undersaturated solution—cooling sufficient to grow $\lesssim 1$ μm.	Smooth layers "sweeping" across surface.
Inserted seed with solution at saturation. Cooling at 0.5°C/min.	Island growth: Very prominent 2 min (1.5 μm). Smoothing but still observable at 6 min ($\sim$5 μm).
Inserted seed into 5°C supersaturated solution.	Smooth, terraced growth.

must be grown from a separate solution. In an isothermal or near isothermal furnace, each solution is subjected to the same temperature changes during a run whether or not it is being used at a particular time. With the UC method, a solution starts at saturation at the beginning of a run, but is intended to grow some layer beyond the first and will become supersaturated while earlier layers are grown. Unless care is taken to relieve this supersaturation, each layer past the first will start its growth from a supersaturated solution.

This supersaturation of the multiple LPE solutions results in an unpredictable rapid growth rate. Dawson[107] also observed a tendency toward poor surface nucleation, leading to a rough surface. For the UC technique, Dawson suggested that a precursor seed be used ahead of the growth seed. Then, while one layer is being grown, the supersaturation of the following solutions in the immediate vicinity of the bottom of the solution is being relieved. Although the use of the precursor seed improves the situation, this technique does not eliminate the supersaturation profile in the bulk of the solution. The supersaturation profile will influence the growth of subsequent layers. The active layer in GaAs–Al$_x$Ga$_{1-x}$As heterostructures is frequently the second or third layer to be grown and is always the thinnest layer. Therefore, the previous cooling history of that solution will certainly affect the reproducibility in thickness of that layer even with the precursor seed. Presumably beyond some critical supersaturation, nucleation improves and smooth growth again results. Then, the previous cooling history during growth will be expected to be less important because the previous cooling will have caused a relatively small part of the total supersaturation. There is very little work reported for SC multiple-layer LPE.

Apparatus and Procedures for Multiple-Layer LPE

All LPE procedures depend upon utilization of the fixed relationship between temperature and solubility as predicted by the phase diagram and upon the dynamic processes of diffusion, convection, and nucleation that are system and procedure dependent. The details of the apparatus and procedures used by different workers vary considerably. In general, these growth techniques have evolved in a semi-empirical way, each with a particular combination of furnace geometry, boat geometry, and gross time–temperature parameters. In this part of Section 6.5, the apparatus and procedures used by several workers for multiple-layer LPE are described. The selection of examples is intended to cover a range of experimental studies, but not to be all-inclusive.

The use of LPE for III–V compounds is generally acknowledged to have started with Nelson's[1] studies of the homoepitaxy of GaAs and also Ge. His apparatus is shown in Fig. 6.5-6. A saturated Ga–As solution was brought into contact with a GaAs seed by tipping the solution. The apparatus was

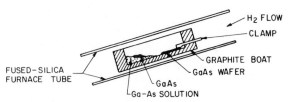

FIG. 6.5-6   The tipping apparatus used by Nelson for the epitaxial growth of GaAs on GaAs from Ga-rich solutions (Ref. 1).

slowly cooled, and an epitaxial layer was grown on the seed during cooling. In the evolution of this single-layer technique to multilayered crystal growth applications, the tipping was replaced by alternate means of translation of one solution onto the seed after another in order to sequentially grow a number of layers.

A recent version[114] of a multiple LPE apparatus for the growth of GaAs–Al$_x$Ga$_{1-x}$As heterostructures by the uniform cooling technique is shown in Fig. 6.5-7. The solution and seed holder is a massive split graphite barrel with a graphite slider. A photograph of an actual graphite boat is

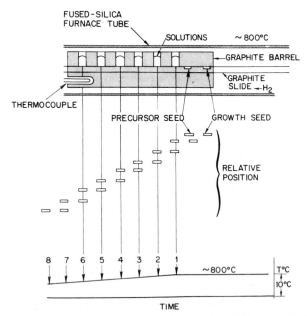

FIG. 6.5-7   Schematic representation of a multiple-layer LPE apparatus (top) with the relative positions for the precursor and growth seeds and solutions during layer growth. The temperature profile is shown at the bottom (Ref. 114).

shown in Fig. 6.5-8. The barrel has six (or more if desired) solution chambers, and the slider has two slots for the precursor seed and the substrate growth seed. These seeds are brought into contact with the solutions by motion of the barrel over the slider. The graphite boat is inside a fused-silica tube in an atmosphere of H_2. The fused-silica tube is within a heat-pipe thermal liner[115] in the furnace. A well-controlled furnace without a heat-pipe is also quite satisfactory. An approximate temperature–time profile and the relative seed solution positions are also shown in Fig. 6.5-7. The heat-pipe is oversized, and the graphite boat is placed near one end so that the vertical gradient in the system is very small (but not measured), while a small horizontal gradient ($\sim 0.1°C/cm$) remains outside the graphite boat. This gradient is somewhat reduced by the thermal conductivity of the graphite and the growth solutions.

The starting point for deciding upon the solution compositions necessary to yield the desired solid composition of a given layer is usually the phase diagram. For example, the first solution may be intended for growth at 800°C of the N–$Al_{0.3}Ga_{0.7}As$ layer of a DH laser. The Al–Ga–As phase data of Figs. 6.2-8 and 6.2-9 serve as a first approximation to determine the solution composition and show that the solution should contain $X_{Al} = 2 \times 10^{-3}$, $X_{As} = 1.7 \times 10^{-2}$, and $X_{Ga} = 1 - X_{Al} - X_{As}$. If the donor impurity is to be Te, small amounts are added to the liquid to obtain the desired carrier concentration, but no adjustment of the Al concentration of the liquid is necessary. If the donor impurity is to be Sn, which has a very low distribution coefficient, then the Al concentration in the liquid must be modified from that of the Al–Ga–As ternary to that for the Al–Ga–As–Sn quaternary.[41] In this case, for $x = 0.3$ and $N = 1 \times 10^{17}$ cm^{-3}, the solution will contain

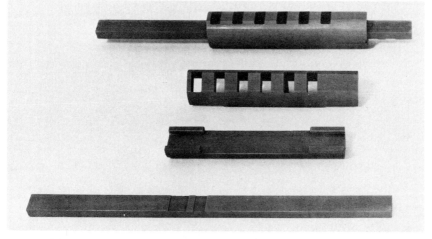

FIG. 6.5-8   Assembled graphite boat (top) and disassembled boat (lower).

$X_{Sn} \approx 0.1$, $X_{Al} \approx 1.6 \times 10^{-3}$, $X_{As} \approx 1.7 \times 10^{-2}$, and $X_{Ga} = 1 - 0.1 - 1.6 \times 10^{-3} - 1.7 \times 10^{-2}$. If the laser active layer is to be Ge-doped GaAs with $p = 5 \times 10^{17}$ cm^{-3}, then the second solution will contain $X_{As} = 2 \times 10^{-2}$ from Fig. 6.2-2, $X_{Ge} = 2 \times 10^{-3}$ from Fig. 6.3-6, and the balance will be Ga. For the Ge-doped $Al_{0.3}Ga_{0.7}As$ third layer with $P = 3 \times 10^{17}$ cm^{-3}, the third solution will contain $X_{Al} = 2 \times 10^{-3}$, $X_{As} = 1.7 \times 10^{-2}$, $X_{Ge} \approx 1.2 \times 10^{-2}$, and the balance will be Ga. Because the amount of Ge added to the second and third solutions is small, the binary data for Ga–As or the ternary data for Al–Ga–As may be used. The liquidus–solidus (hole concentration) data for Ge in $Al_xGa_{1-x}As$ have not been published. It is expected, however, that somewhat more Ge will be needed in the liquid for the third solution than would have been needed to achieve the same hole concentration in GaAs, since the Ge acceptor level in $Al_{0.3}Ga_{0.7}As$ is several times larger than in GaAs (see Fig. 4.3-3a). The amount of Ge given in this example for the P-layer was determined experimentally.

The weight of each element i needed in each solution is readily detemined from the definition

$$X_i = N_i/(N_1 + N_2 + \cdots + N_n), \tag{6.5-8}$$

where N_i, the number of moles of each of the n components in the solution, is the weight of the element divided by its molecular weight. For the apparatus of Fig. 6.5-7, each solution contains 3 gm (4.3×10^{-2} moles) of Ga. Using the first solution as an illustrative example with the compositions specified above as $X_{Sn} = 0.1$, $X_{Al} = 1.6 \times 10^{-3}$, $X_{As} = 1.7 \times 10^{-2}$, and $X_{Ga} = 0.881$, it is readily seen that $N_{Sn} + N_{Ga} + N_{Al} + N_{As} \approx N_{Ga} + N_{Sn}$. Therefore, by Eq. (6.5-8),

$$X_{Ga} = N_{Ga}/(N_{Ga} + N_{Sn}), \tag{6.5-9}$$

and

$$X_{Sn} = N_{Sn}/(N_{Ga} + N_{Sn}). \tag{6.5-10}$$

These equations give

$$N_{Ga} + N_{Sn} = N_{Ga}/X_{Ga} = N_{Sn}/X_{Sn}, \tag{6.5-11}$$

or

$$N_{Sn} = (N_{Ga}/X_{Ga})X_{Sn}. \tag{6.5-12}$$

Thus, for the solution described, $N_{Sn} = 4.9 \times 10^{-3}$ moles, and $N_{Ga} + N_{Sn} = 4.8 \times 10^{-2}$ moles. The weight of Sn, w_{Sn}, to be added to the 3 gm of Ga is then $N_{Sn}M_{Sn} = 0.58$ gm, where M_{Sn} is the molecular weight of Sn which is 118.7 gm/mole. Similarly,

$$w_{Al} = N_{Al}M_{Al} = X_{Al}(N_{Ga} + N_{Sn})M_{Al}$$
$$= 1.6 \times 10^{-3} \times 4.8 \times 10^{-2} \times 27.0 = 2.0 \times 10^{-3} \text{ gm,}$$

and

$$w_{As} = X_{As}(N_{Ga} + N_{Sn})M_{As} = 1.7 \times 10^{-2} \times 4.8 \times 10^{-2} \times 74.9$$
$$= 6.1 \times 10^{-2} \text{ gm.}$$

At the start of a run, two GaAs wafers are placed into the slider immediately after having been polished in a Br_2–methanol solution. The growth face is $\{100\}$. To achieve the solution compositions described above, the weighed quantities of Ga plus dopants are placed in the solution chambers and the system is flushed with H_2 and heated at 800°C for about 15 hr. The apparatus is then rapidly cooled and the necessary amount of Al is added to each solution through a gas lock to prevent contamination by air. The boat is briefly heated to dissolve the Al and is cooled again. The As concentration in each solution is automatically brought to the proper value by adding chunks of GaAs to each cold solution through the gas lock. Then, when heated to the starting temperature, each solution dissolves only as much GaAs as is needed to give the equilibrium liquidus composition. For a typical run, the starting temperature is 800°C. To initiate the run, the apparatus is brought to 800°C and held there for about 2 hr to permit the solutions to equilibrate.

The growth procedure consists of a series of steps in which a solution composition very close to saturation, but apparently not quite saturated, is achieved in each solution when the growth seed is brought into contact with it. The growth procedure is begun by bringing the first GaAs seed, the precursor seed, into contact with the first solution by holding the seeds fixed and moving the barrel up the temperature gradient. Then, a time–temperature program as illustrated in Fig. 6.5-7 is initiated. For a cooling rate of ~ 0.05°C/min, the p-type active layer of ~ 0.15-μm thickness is grown in 10 sec, while the next P–$Al_{0.3}Ga_{0.7}As$ layer of ~ 1.5-μm thickness is grown in 10 min. If difficulty is experienced in obtaining a continuous active layer, an increase in growth rate may be necessary.

In addition to reducing the supersaturation of each solution in the vicinity of the seed, this procedure is intended to provide for a small undersaturation as a result of the small temperature gradient. In effect, each solution encounters a seed that is slightly above the solution temperature. Unfortunately, as with most of these growth techniques, the precise details of the environment of each solution cannot be specified. Even with this

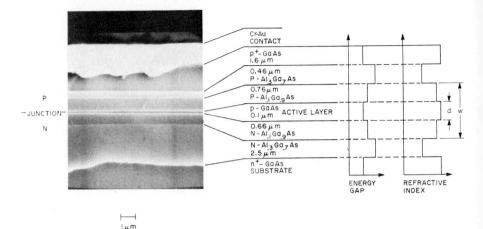

FIG. 6.5-9 Scanning-electron photomicrograph of the selectively etched surface of the SCH laser. The layer thickness, Al composition, and conductivity type are indicated for each layer. A representative variation in the energy gap and refractive index is also shown. The active-layer thickness is *d* and the optical-waveguide thickness is *w* (Ref. 114).

procedure, the degree of under or supersaturation that is present at the crystal surface when the seed and solution come together is not known.

The apparatus of Fig. 6.5-7 has been used for the growth of GaAs–$Al_xGa_{1-x}As$ DH and separate-confinement heterostructure (SCH) lasers. A cross section of an SCH laser grown in this manner is illustrated in Fig. 6.5-9. An interesting feature is the first rough interface that is then followed by smooth growth. The rough interface is due to a deliberately induced undersaturation of the first solution in contact with the substrate as a result of a small temperature increase just before the seed was placed under that solution. This behavior is consistent with the observations of Crossley and Small.[112]

The boat with thin-walled solution wells used by Dawson[107] for the growth of the single layers for the As diffusivity studies with Rode,[102] and for the growth of GaAs–$Al_xGa_{1-x}As$ DH wafers is shown in Fig. 6.5-10. Dawson used a nominally isothermal furnace with horizontal temperature

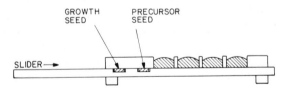

FIG. 6.5-10 Multiple-layer LPE graphite boat used by Dawson (Ref. 107).

gradients of $\leq 0.5°C$ along the length of the boat. The loading and growth procedures are similar to those described above. The seed is kept in contact with the solution for 10 min before cooling. This procedure yields acceptably smooth grown layers and laser quality heterostructures.

Rode and Sobers[108] suggested that the excess edge growth frequently observed in LPE layers during solution epitaxy results from the high radiant heat loss of the graphite compared to the liquid surface during cooling. The resulting cool walls presumably cause convective cells to be formed. The convective cells result in transport of As from the "excess" GaAs at the top of the solution to the edges of the growth region more rapidly than diffusive transport to the rest of the crystal surface. Based upon this idea, a modification of the step-cooling growth procedure was introduced. The solutions are rapidly cooled to 5°C of supersaturation (starting at 778°C) out of contact with the precursor or growth seed. The smallest cooling rate available with their equipment, 0.03°C/min, was established to offset variation in furnace temperature, and the solutions are held 10 min in this condition to allow convection to damp out. Then the two seeds were sequentially placed under each solution in the usual manner. Because their constant temperature control allowed variation of ± 0.02–$0.03°C/min$, the very small cooling rate in effect produced a "constant" temperature. The dominant driving force for growth was the solute stored by supersaturation in the bulk of the solution by the original 5°C of supercooling, and not the 0.03°C/min cooling rate to any significant extent. Appreciable reduction in edge growth was obtained.

Another variation of the horizontal boat technique that has been used by several workers (see, for example, Ref. 116) is to drastically reduce the depth of the solution by wedging it between the seed and a graphite slider. Apparently this procedure was intended as an aid to thin layer growth by reducing the solution volume from which solute could originate. Such an approach may also be useful for suppression of convection and edge growth.

Thompson and Kirkby[117] have used a graphite boat in which rotary motion is used to transport seeds from solution to solution for the growth of GaAs–$Al_x Ga_{1-x} As$ heterostructures. The rotary boat is placed into a three-zone vertical furnace as illustrated in Fig. 6.5-11. With the seed at the hottest region, vertical temperature gradients are obtained by regulation of the three zones while maintaining radial temperature uniformity. The objective is apparently to reduce the gradient of supersaturation throughout the solution in order to improve layer thickness control. With this approach, they have been able to prepare SCH laser structures with active regions as thin as 400 Å.

The growth procedure Thompson and Kirby[117] used with the vertical-rotary apparatus is quite different from the procedures that are commonly

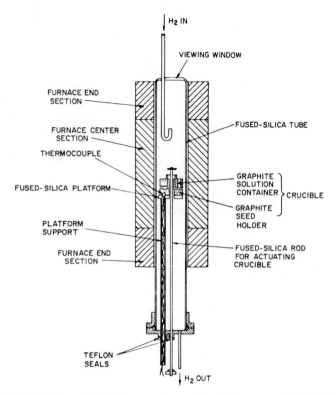

FIG. 6.5-11 Vertical multiple LPE apparatus used by Thompson and Kirkby (Ref. 117).

used with horizontal-slider arrangements. No precursor seed is used and an unsaturated Ga–As solution is employed immediately before growth to slightly etch the surface of the substrate. The vertical gradient when measured in the H_2 is 2.5°C/cm. Growth starts at about 850°C with a cooling rate of 0.2°C/min. Before growth, the solutions which contain excess GaAs are brought to 20°C above the growth temperature and cooled rapidly by 10°C. The temperature is decreased by an additional 10°C at 0.2°C/min and growth is initiated by rotary motion of the seed to a position under each solution for the desired period of growth. The solutions are reused.

The growth of $Al_xGa_{1-x}As$ by this technique appears to be diffusion limited. However, the GaAs grows more rapidly than expected and some convection may occur. The first use of the solutions gives greater growth thickness and Al composition in the solid than subsequent runs because the saturating solid floating on the solutions becomes covered with $Al_xGa_{1-x}As$. Although the temperature gradient was empirically adjusted to give a near linear growth rate, the precise growth rate is somewhat dependent upon the previous cooling history of the solution. This behavior means that the negative temperature gradient has not completely relieved the constitutional supercooling throughout the solution. Nevertheless, the use of vertical gradients provides another parameter that may, with careful control, provide added reproducibility for the growth of LPE heterostructures.

Liquid-phase epitaxial techniques in which the solution used for the growth of a layer is pushed out by the solution for the subsequent layer have also been described.[118,119] The advantages of this procedure over the more usual techniques described above are the prevention of the exposure of the layer surface between growth solutions and easier multilayer growth at temperatures lower than the usual 750–825°C growth temperatures. A disadvantage is the formation of graded composition regions between the layers. Alferov et al.[119] have used this technique with a complex LPE apparatus and have described the formation and control of the graded layers.

Reinhart and Logan[120,121] have introduced modifications to the horizontal-slider LPE technique in order to grow heterostructure lasers coupled to waveguides. These modifications permitted the growth of wafers for the composition-coupled laser[120] (CCL) and the taper-coupled laser[121] (TCL). The CCL is a DH laser contiguous to a passive waveguide with an energy gap larger than the laser active region. The TCL is a DH laser in which the active layer tapers to zero thickness so that the radiation is coupled into an adjacent passive waveguide. The TCL as a distributed Bragg reflector laser is illustrated in Fig. 7.12-7. For the growth of the CCL, a thin graphite spacer that does not quite reach the seed separates a solution well into two halfs. The graphite boat is similar to the one represented in Fig. 6.5-7, and a solution well with a graphite spacer is illustrated in Fig. 6.5-12a. Solutions

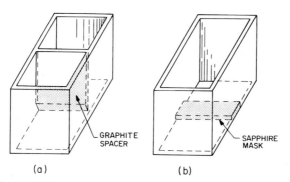

(a)   (b)

FIG. 6.5-12 (a) Solution well with graphite spacer for the growth of composition-coupled lasers. (Ref. 120). (b) Solution well with sapphire spacer used for the growth of taper-coupled lasers (Ref. 121). These solution wells are used with multiple-layer LPE apparatus that is similar to the apparatus shown in Fig. 6.5-7.

that differ in Al composition are on each side of the spacer. They join at the seed under the spacer so that there is an Al composition gradient at the spacer location in any layer grown from the divided solution wells. The growth procedure is similar to that illustrated in Fig. 6.5-7. An interesting feature of layers grown from the wells with the spacer is an increased layer thickness at the spacer that is apparently due to cooling of the solution by the spacer and the resultant convection. For structures with a taper in the layer thickness, as in the TCL, one of the solution wells contains a thin sapphire mask as shown in Fig. 6.5-12b. This mask is separated from the seed by about 70 μm. When a layer is grown from that solution well, the layer edges in the region that are masked by the sapphire are tapered smoothly to zero thickness over a distance of 100 to 150 μm. A variation of the LPE technique is Peltier-induced LPE. In this process, the interface region of the seed and solution is cooled by the Peltier effect obtained when current is passed through the seed–solution interface. The furnace temperature is not changed. Daniele et al.[121a] have used this process to grow GaAs–Al$_x$Ga$_{1-x}$As laser structures that compare in quality to those prepared by normal LPE.

Surface Morphology of LPE III–V Layers

Difficulty in achieving control over smoothness of the epitaxial layer is one of the most vexing problems associated with liquid-phase epitaxy. There are several distinct types of surface features. Inadequate nucleation results in surface features designated as island growth. Surface terracing is related to the substrate misorientation from some (usually {100}) low index crystal faces. It is the most frequently observed surface feature. The so-called meniscus lines are related to the mechanical solution removal.

As summarized previously in Table 6.5-1, insertion of the seed with the growth solution at saturation can result in island growth. A typical surface with this feature is shown in Fig. 6.5-13. It probably results from the presence of an insufficient number of nucleation sites. The islands appear to grow at the expense of newer sites because they presumably locally deplete the solution of solute. They are faceted, and the orientation of the facets depends upon the orientation of the growth surface. Qualitatively, it appears that smoother layers grow on solution-etched surfaces,[112,114,117] although the surface features described below also occur. Apparently, the solution-etched surfaces have sufficient nucleation sites. Some workers have also noted that island formation may occur when the crystal surface is oxidized, either accidentally[122] or deliberately.[123] It may be taken as a general rule that improved morphology results from increased precautions against contamination by air or water vapor.

The surface features that are most frequently observed on III–V LPE layers are terraces such as those illustrated for a DH wafer in Fig. 6.5-14a,b.[124]

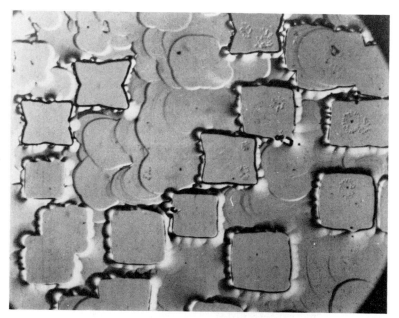

FIG. 6.5-13   Island growth during LPE (Ref. 107).

Part (a) is a Nomarski photomicrograph of the as-grown surface of a GaAs–Al$_x$Ga$_{1-x}$As DH laser wafer. Part (b) shows the photoluminescence emission from the 0.15 μm thick GaAs active layer. These terraces consist of steps with long treads and relatively small risers. Typically, the treads are 100 μm long, while the risers are approximately 200 Å high. The nature of these terraces on layers that are grown on nominally {111} or {100} oriented substrates has a sensitive dependence upon slight ($\sim 0.5°$) mis-orientation.[124–126] The angle between the risers and the tread surface is usually quite small ($\sim 1°$).[126] This small angle, combined with the several hundred angstroms riser height, suggests that the riser consists of a group of atomic steps.

Rode[126] and Dawson[127] observed that the nominal {111}A, {111}B, and {100} surfaces exhibit terrace formation and are the surfaces that are known to form two-dimensional surface structures under ultrahigh vacuum conditions.[128,129] The formation of these surface structures in which the periodicity of the surface layer of atoms differs from that of the crystal bulk is usually referred to as surface reconstruction. Surface reconstruction is associated with a singularity in surface energy as a function of orientation at the low-index orientation. For convenience such surfaces can be referred to as singular. Terrace formation is not observed for GaAs LPE at about

NOMINALLY ORIENTED (100)

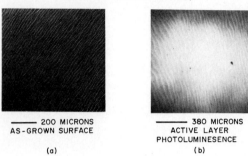

——— 200 MICRONS	——— 380 MICRONS
AS-GROWN SURFACE	ACTIVE LAYER
	PHOTOLUMINESENCE
(a)	(b)

CRITICALLY ORIENTED (100)

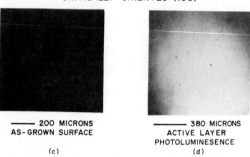

——— 200 MICRONS	——— 380 MICRONS
AS-GROWN SURFACE	ACTIVE LAYER
	PHOTOLUMINESENCE
(c)	(d)

FIG. 6.5-14 Liquid-phase epitaxial GaAs–Al$_x$Ga$_{1-x}$As DH laser wafers grown at 775°C. Parts (a) and (b) are nominal {100} ± 0.1° oriented substrates. Parts (c) and (d) are critically oriented {100} + 0.8 ± 0.1° substrates. The as-grown surfaces in parts (a) and (c) were photographed with Nomarski phase-contrast microscopy and are the GaAs surface of a N-p-P-p$^+$ structure. In parts (b) and (c), the top surface is Al$_x$Ga$_{1-x}$As of a N-p-P-P$^+$ structure (Ref. 124).

780°C on substrates with nominally {110}, {211}A, {211}B, and {511} orientation. None of these surfaces reconstruct in high vacuum.[128–130] The latter orientations are not usually used for multiple-layer LPE of heterostructure lasers because they do not have suitable etching and cleaving properties for mirror formation. Also, it has been experimentally observed that it is difficult to achieve planar layers with these orientations.

Rode [131] has considered a model for epitaxial growth on a surface slightly misoriented from the singular orientation to explain the origin of the growth terraces and to suggest a method for their elimination. In his analysis, an attractive interaction between monatomic steps is found that is due to elastic energy stored in the substrate as a result of lattice mismatch between

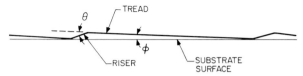

FIG. 6.5-15   Schematic representation of surface terrace on low index substrate.

the reconstructed crystal surface and the bulk crystal. From that analysis, a surface misorientation that can be used to obtain planar growth can be inferred. For the surface terrace illustrated in Fig. 6.5-15, the tread is the singular surface when ϕ is zero, so that the substrate misorientation is ϕ. The riser is misoriented from the tread, and thus the singular plane by the angle θ. Rode's analysis[131] of terrace formation suggests that for a given nominal low index surface, θ is approximately constant for given growth conditions independent of misorientation from that nominal surface. It can be seen in Fig. 6.5-15 that the surface may be expected to become all tread when ϕ goes to zero or, as Rode claims, when the misorientation angle ϕ is made to be the angle θ.

Rode's model[131] is supported by the experimental observation[124] illustrated in Fig. 6.5-14c, d. These pictures illustrate the suppression of terrace formation on GaAs–$Al_xGa_{1-x}As$ DH wafers by critical misorientation from the {100} surface by 0.8°. The experimental observations for wafers grown at 775°C show that the critical value for misorientation decreases with x for the growth of $Al_xGa_{1-x}As$. The critical angle also decreases with increasing temperature so that at about 850°C for {100} surfaces of GaAs the critical angle is $\pm 0.1°$. For near {111}A surfaces, the critical angle is much greater than for {100} surfaces at all temperatures. The formation of growth terraces can cause layer thickness variations in DH wafers that seriously degrade laser yield and reproducibility. Also, the nonplanar interfaces cause optical scattering and increase the laser threshold current.[110]

The last feature to be discussed is the meniscus line, so-called because it appears to represent the contour of the trailing edge of the liquid as it moved across the crystal during the sliding procedure. Although this feature is not observable by the unaided eye, it may readily be observed on smooth, relatively unterraced LPE GaAs or $Al_xGa_{1-x}As$ surfaces by phase-constant microscopy.[132–134a] A number of such lines are usually seen, and as illustrated in Fig. 6.5-16, they are roughly parallel and spaced about $100 \pm 50 \mu m$ apart. The meniscus lines occur at each interface in a multilayered structure. Logan and Rode[133] and Small et al.[134] report that the meniscus line profile is S-shaped and has a width of about 1 μm. The meniscus line consists of a peak that rises above the plane of the crystal surface by several hundred angstroms and then a valley that falls below the surface. Apparently, each

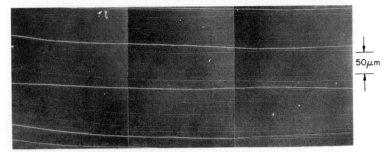

FIG. 6.5-16 Nomarski phase-contrast photomicrograph of meniscus lines on the surface of a GaAs LPE layer (Ref. 132).

line forms when the trailing edge of the liquid stops momentarily as the solution is being removed from the seed. The mechanism by which the meniscus line forms is not understood. However, it can be a significant enough feature to seriously perturb the behavior of injection lasers when it traverses the active region. Multiple-layer wafers that are lapped at a shallow angle to magnify the layer thickness show that the active layer can be excessively thin or nonexistent adjacent to a meniscus line. Small et al.[134a] account for this by suggesting that the nucleation can be dominated by the meniscus line during the growth of very thin layers. Then, islandlike growth occurs along one side of the meniscus line. A common procedure to obtain lasers from wafers with meniscus lines is to fabricate the stripe-geometry lasers parallel to the meniscus lines. Since the usual stripe is approximately 10 μm wide and the meniscus line spacing is about 100 μm, a significant fraction of the fabricated lasers will not have perturbed active regions if a large fraction of the space between the meniscus lines has filled in.

6.6 MOLECULAR-BEAM EPITAXY

General Discussion

Molecular-beam epitaxy (MBE) is a growth technique in which epitaxial layers are grown by impinging thermal beams of molecules or atoms upon a heated substrate under ultrahigh vacuum conditions. For III–V compounds, MBE differs from those procedures usually called "evaporation" techniques because for MBE the beam intensities of the constituents are separately controlled so that sticking coefficient differences may be taken into consideration. It differs from conventional chemical-vapor deposition (CVD) since it is an ultrahigh vacuum rather than a near atmospheric pressure technique. As a result, kinetic processes characteristic of the components on a freely evaporating surface are important rather than boundary layer transport properties characteristic of flowing gas systems used for CVD. One unique feature of MBE is the slow growth rate of $<0.1–2$ μm/hr that permits very precise layer thickness control over a large area. Because the solid–solution composition is controlled by the evaporation oven temperature, the composition can be continuously varied.

The successful use of MBE to produce heterostructures in the GaAs–$Al_xGa_{1-x}As$ system is a direct consequence of the studies by Arthur[4,135,136] of the reaction kinetics of Ga and As_2 on heated GaAs surfaces. He observed that the sticking coefficient of arsenic from As_2 beams projected onto the heated GaAs substrate is negligible unless Ga had previously been deposited on the GaAs substrate. In that case, the sticking coefficient of arsenic was proportional to the Ga coverage of the surface. This result suggested that the As_2 molecules could only be absorbed if they reacted with Ga atoms to form GaAs on the surface. Then the simultaneous deposition of Ga and As_2 is expected to yield stoichiometric GaAs. If the arsenic deposition rate is greater than the Ga rate, the excess arsenic is not expected to stick, and the rate of GaAs layer growth will be proportional to the Ga arrival rate.

In a series of studies that started in 1969 and are still underway, Cho and co-workers further elaborated the fundamentals of III–V MBE and its use for growth of layers useful for semiconductor devices. They studied the surface morphology,[5,137–140] doping,[141–144] photoluminescence[139,141,142] and electrical properties[6,141] of MBE layers, primarily GaAs and $Al_xGa_{1-x}As$. These studies led to MBE growth of layers for microwave devices,[145,146] passive waveguides,[147–149] and heterostructure lasers[7,150,151] by Cho and co-workers, and to distributed-feedback lasers.[152,153] Studies of the growth of MBE GaAs–$Al_xGa_{1-x}As$ heteroepitaxy also led to the study of the quantum states of confined carriers in very thin layered (50–200 Å) multiple-layer heterostructures by Dingle et al.[154–156] and to the preparation of superlattices by Ludeke et al.[157] for the study of resonant tunneling.[158] Monolayer GaAs–AlAs structures were prepared and studied by Gossard et al.[159] Molecular-beam epitaxy was used by Walpole et al.[160–162] for the growth of PbTe–$Pb_xSn_{1-x}Te$ heterostructure lasers and by McLane and Sleger[163] and by Preier et al.[164] for the growth of PbS–PbS_xSe_{1-x} heterostructure lasers. A detailed description of MBE is given in the review article by Cho and Arthur.[165]

Growth of III–V Compound Layers and Heterostructures

The molecular and atomic beams that impinge upon the heated substrate are usually generated by heating the source material in a container that has an orifice. This container is called an effusion oven and is represented schematically in Fig. 6.6-1.[166] In the simplest case, only a single effusion oven is used as the source of Ga and As_2. The oven contains Ga and GaAs,

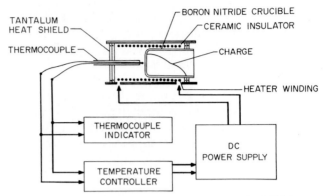

FIG. 6.6-1   Schematic representation of an effusion oven for MBE layer growth (Ref. 166).

and the partial pressures of the various species within the oven are near their equilibrium partial pressures[167] shown in Fig. 6.6-2. The beam source arrangements may increase in complexity depending upon whether separate Ga or As source ovens are used. When crystalline solid solutions and doped crystals are being grown, there is often an effusion oven for each dopant and for each group III and group V element.

The beam flux F of a given species at the orifice of an ideal effusion oven is related to the pressure P within the oven. The number of atoms striking a unit area per second within the oven can be taken as F and is[168]

$$F = (1/4)n\bar{v}, \tag{6.6-1}$$

where n is the number of atoms or molecules per unit volume and $\bar{v}$ is the average velocity. For a Maxwellian distribution,[168]

$$\bar{v} = (8kT/\pi m)^{1/2}, \tag{6.6-2}$$

where m is the atom or molecule mass and is given by the molecular weight divided by Avogadro's number (6.0×10^{23}). Since the pressure is related to n by[168]

$$P = nkT, \tag{6.6-3}$$

the flux may be written as

$$F(\text{atoms/cm}^2\text{-sec}) = 1.01 \times 10^6 \, P(\text{atm})/(2\pi mkT)^{1/2}, \tag{6.6-4}$$

with $k = 1.38 \times 10^{-16}$ erg-K^{-1}. The factor 1.01×10^6 converts dynes/cm^2 to atmospheres. The flux outside the orifice spreads with a cosine distribution. Ideal effusion ovens have an orifice whose area is small compared to the area of the vaporizing source, and whose diameter is small compared to the mean free path within the oven. The ovens usually used for MBE

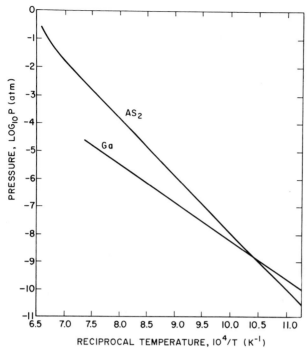

FIG. 6.6-2   The equilibrium vapor pressures of Ga and As_2 along the Ga-rich liquidus of the GaAs system. The As_4 pressure is negligible by comparison to the As_2 pressure (Ref. 167).

are not ideal because the orifice is too large. Equation (6.6-4) is, however, representative of the flux achieved at the orifice.

For growth of GaAs–$Al_xGa_{1-x}As$ heterostructures, the Ga beam flux at the substrate surface is 10^{12}–10^{14} atoms/cm²-sec. The arrival rate of arsenic as As_2 or As_4 is about ten times greater. Either arsenic vapor species (As_2 or As_4) may be used. Most of Cho's earlier studies utilized Ga together with GaAs as the arsenic source, but Wiegmann,[169] Ilegems,[166] and Cho[165] have also used elemental arsenic. The predominant species effusing from an oven containing elemental arsenic is As_4.

The most extensively investigated III–V solid solution that is grown by MBE is $Al_xGa_{1-x}As$. The sticking coefficients of Al and Ga are unity at the usual substrate temperatures. Therefore, the Ga to Al ratio in the grown layer is the same as the ratio of the Ga to Al flux at the crystal surface. The sticking coefficients of the group V elements on III–V compounds are significantly different from each other. These nonunity sticking coefficients for MBE of III–V solid solutions other than $Al_xGa_{1-x}As$ makes it necessary to empirically determine the sticking coefficient ratios as a function of beam flux for all of the components. These ratios will also be a function of substrate temperature.

A schematic representation[165] of an MBE apparatus used by Cho for growth of $GaAs-Al_xGa_{1-x}As$ heterostructures is given in Fig. 6.6-3. The apparatus contains an ion-pumped vacuum chamber with a substrate mounted on a heating block, several resistively heated pyrolytic BN effusion ovens enclosed in liquid-nitrogen cooled shrouds, and auxiliary diagnostic equipment. The substrate is heated by the Mo heating block. The system is designed to permit the heated substrate or the growing layer to be studied during growth by reflection electron diffraction or analyzed intermittently by Auger spectroscopy. The pumping system is capable of maintaining $10^{-7} - 10^{-10}$ Torr with the effusion ovens cold and $10^{-7} - 10^{-8}$ Torr, which is mostly due to As_4, with the ovens heated. For a typical run, these ovens will contain Ga, Ga plus GaAs, or solid As, Al, and the p- and n-type dopants. The ovens are separated from the substrate with movable shutters.

In a typical run for the growth of a single layer of unintentionally doped GaAs on a GaAs substrate, a carefully polished and etched substrate is placed into intimate thermal contact with the Mo block. The back surface of the substrate is wetted to the Mo heating block with In. After evacuation of the system to about $10^{-9}-10^{-10}$ Torr, the substrate surface is examined by Auger spectroscopy. If necessary, the substrate surface is ion etched to

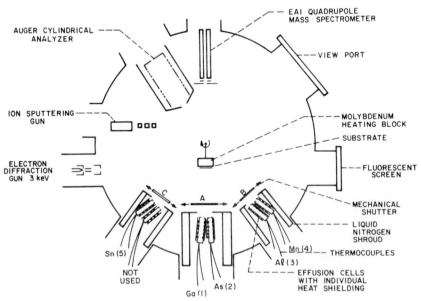

FIG. 6.6-3 Schematic representation of an MBE system for the growth of GaAs–$Al_xGa_{1-x}As$ heterostructures (Ref. 165).

remove surface impurities, primarily carbon, and heated to 500–600°C. During heating, the substrate surface is examined by electron diffraction.

The electron-diffraction pattern and morphology are shown on the left and right, respectively, of Fig. 6.6-4a for a typical {100} surface that was etched and heated sufficiently to remove residual oxides. The electron-diffraction pattern is typical of a microscopically rough (although specular)

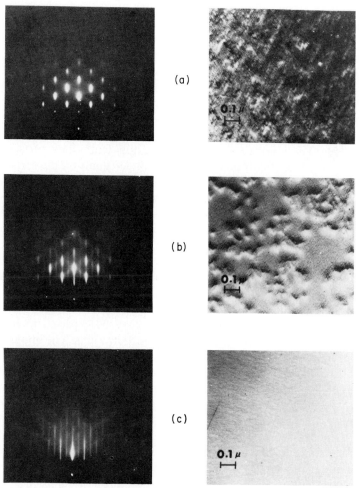

FIG. 6.6-4   Reflection high-energy electron-diffraction patterns (40 keV, [$\bar{1}\bar{1}0$] azimuth) and the corresponding electron photomicrographs (38,400 ×) of Pt–C replica of the same surface. (a) Br$_2$-methanol polish-etched {100} GaAs substrate heated in vacuum to 855°K for 5 min. (b) Deposition of an average thickness of 150 Å of GaAs. (c) Deposition of 1 μm GaAs (Ref. 5).

surface. The appearance is the result of diffraction of the electron beam passing through raised portions of the surface. It is in effect a three-dimensional high-energy electron-diffraction (HEED) pattern. When the shutters are opened to allow beams of the proper intensities of As_2 and Ga to simultaneously strike the surface, the spotted pattern gradually becomes streaked. Figure 6.6-4b shows smoothing of the surface and degeneration of the electron diffraction into a two-dimensional reflection diffraction pattern. Finally, when sufficient epitaxial material has grown, Fig. 6.6-4c shows that the film is microscopically featureless. The electron-diffraction pattern shows not only the two-dimensional overall {100} structure, but also the reconstructed two-dimensional surface as evidenced by additional streaks in the diffraction pattern. The streaked patterns and the observation of two-dimensional surface structures suggest short range smoothness at least on an atomic scale.

A significant observation made by Cho[5,138] was that the reconstructed surface depended upon the As–Ga beam intensity ratio and the substrate temperature. The {100} crystal surface may apparently have surface structure which is either stabilized by Ga atoms or As atoms on the surface. The observation of these patterns, in addition to being of fundamental interest, is useful for epitaxial growth studies. These observations help establish the criteria for smoothness, surface preparation, and stoichiometry. In practice, a sufficiently great As–Ga flux ratio is usually maintained so that the As-stabilized structure is present during growth. This condition is used because excess As evaporates. If the As–Ga flux results in the Ga-stabilized structure, it is difficult to maintain growth without eventually having excess Ga accumulate on the growing surface.

Although specularly reflecting surfaces may be obtained over a wide range of As–Ga flux ratios, the flux ratio may be expected to influence impurity incorporation and native defect concentrations. The impurity and vacancy concentrations may in turn influence the optical and electrical properties of the grown layers. The As–Ga ratio in molecular beams during growth of GaAs influences both the incorporation of Ge as an amphoteric dopant[141] and the incorporation of Mn and C.[170] Germanium- doped GaAs is n-type for the As-stabilized surface and p-type for the Ga-stabilized surface. The Mn acceptor concentration on Ga sites is increased by a larger As–Ga ratio, while the C acceptor concentration on As-sites is decreased.

The impurities used for controlling the electrical characteristics of MBE GaAs and $Al_xGa_{1-x}As$ are quite different from those commonly used in LPE. Those impurity elements with relatively high vapor pressures apparently fail to stick to the surface long enough to be incorporated. Ilegems[166] has pointed out that qualitative insight can be obtained by considering the impurity element partial pressures. The impurity partial pressure in equilibrium with the doped solid is designated P_{eq}. The pressure that corresponds to the impurity flux needed to achieve the impurity concentration in the grown solid during MBE if every incident impurity atom is incorporated is designated P_{min}. These conditions make P_{min} the lowest possible pressure needed to achieve that impurity concentration. Ilegems estimated P_{eq} from the distribution coefficients of the impurity between the solid and liquid at the MBE substrate temperature by extrapolation of phase data from the literature.

The ratio of P_{min}/P_{eq} as a function of the substrate reciprocal temperature is shown in Fig. 6.6-5. The ratio P_{min}/P_{eq} is to first order independent of the impurity concentration. In Fig. 6.6-5, the region where $\log_{10}(P_{min}/P_{eq}) > 0$ is the region where incorporation is arrival rate controlled, while in the region

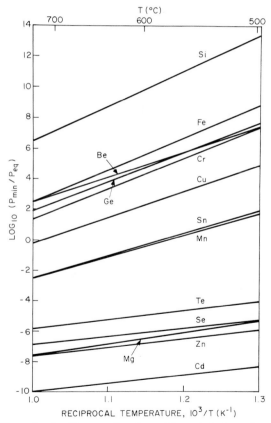

FIG. 6.6-5 The ratio P_{min}/P_{eq} as a function of the substrate reciprocal temperature (Ref. 166).

where $\log_{10}(P_{min}/P_{eq}) < 0$, the incorporation depends primarily upon the equilibrium vapor pressure of the impurity. The impurities in the first category will be expected to be easily incorporated and to be effective dopants for MBE GaAs.

For the above model of the relationship of the partial pressures to impurity incorporation, it was assumed that all impinging species come to thermal equilibrium with the surface but are not strongly chemisorbed to it. Although very crude approximations were frequently necessary in Ilegems'[166] estimation of P_{eq} from the available phase-diagram data, these approximations are probably not very important for comparisons over the 24 orders of magnitude in Fig. 6.6-5. The experimental behavior of a number of impurity elements in GaAs for MBE are summarized in Table 6.6-1.

TABLE 6.6-1 Impurity Incorporation in GaAs by MBE[a]

Element	Donor or acceptor	Maximum carrier concentration (cm^{-3})	Sticking coefficient	Reference
Si	D	$\sim 5 \times 10^{18}$	1	g
Sn[b]	D	$\sim 10^{19}$	1	h
Te	D	$\sim 10^{19}$	0.5–1	i
Ge[c]	D or A	$\sim 5 \times 10^{18}$	1	j
Be	A	$> 10^{19}$	1	k
C[d]	A	—	—	l
Cd	not incorporated		very low	m
Mg	A	10^{16}–10^{17}	$\sim 10^{-5}$	n
Mn[e]	A	$\sim 10^{18}$	—	l
Zn[f]	not incorporated	—	very low	o

[a] At the usual MBE substrate temperature range of 500°–600°C.

[b] Doping profile depends on substrate temperature.

[c] Conductivity type depends on the As to Ga ratio in the beams. For Ga-rich conditions, layer is p-type, while for As-rich conditions, layer is n-type.

[d] Carbon concentration increases with the ratio of As to Ga in the beams.

[e] For As-rich growth conditions. Less Mn is incorporated when the As to Ga beam intensity ratio is decreased.

[f] Zinc has been incorporated with an ionized-Zn beam (see Ref. p).

[g] A. Y. Cho and I. Hayashi, *Metall. Trans.* **2**, 777 (1971).

[h] A. Y. Cho, *J. Appl. Phys.* **46**, 1733 (1975).

[i] J. R. Arthur, *Surface Sci.* **43**, 449 (1974).

[j] A. Y. Cho and I. Hayashi, *J. Appl. Phys.* **42**, 4422 (1971).

[k] M. Ilegems, *J. Appl. Phys.* **48**, 1278 (1977).

[l] M. Ilegems and R. Dingle, *Gallium Arsenide Related Compounds*: 1974 *Symp. Proc.* p. 1. Inst. of Phys., London, 1975.

[m] J. R. Arthur, Private communication.

[n] A. Y. Cho and M. B. Panish, *J. Appl. Phys.* **43**, 5118 (1972).

[o] J. R. Arthur, *Surface Sci.* **38**, 394 (1973).

[p] M. Naganuma and K. Takahashi, *Appl. Phys. Lett.* **27**, 342 (1975).

Comparison of Fig. 6.6-5 with Table 6.6-1 shows that this very qualitative approach is reasonably predictive except for Te. For Te, this approach apparently fails because a stable surface phase containing Te is formed.[171]

As summarized in Table 6.6-1, the usual acceptors such as Zn or Cd are not useful acceptors for MBE. For MBE, Ge is an acceptor only for growth with Ga-stabilized surfaces. Since smoother layers are generally obtained for As-stabilized surfaces, it is not desirable to use Ge as a p-type dopant for heterostructure lasers. Beryllium is the only p-type dopant that gives high hole concentrations.[172] Manganese can give reasonable hole concentrations, but its activation energy of 0.113 eV (see Table 4.3-1) is three times larger than for the shallow acceptors. Although the hole concentration is limited to low values, Mg has been used for DH active layers.[150] However, the photoluminescence intensity of single layers of Mg-doped GaAs is much less than for Ge-doped LPE layers with the same hole concentration. Layers of $Al_xGa_{1-x}As$ may be doped p-type with Mg, Mn, or Be.

There are several good choices for donors in MBE layers. Because the photoluminescent intensities were the best for Sn-doped MBE layers, Sn has been the most extensively used dopant for DH active layers.[7] In fact, the photoluminescent intensities for Sn-doped MBE are as large or larger than comparably doped n-type LPE layers. Tin is also a good donor for n-type MBE $Al_xGa_{1-x}As$ layers. ·

The preparation of GaAs–$Al_xGa_{1-x}As$ DH wafers by MBE that were of sufficiently good quality to permit cw room temperature operation[7] required care in maintaining continuous, noninterrupted growth[147] and a very low contaminant background. The low contaminant background was achieved by allowing Al and/or Mg to coat the walls of the apparatus during growth and by paying scrupulous attention to contaminants that may be present in the effusion ovens. The temperature–time cycles used to grow the DH lasers with the Sn-doped n-type active layer are shown in Fig. 6.6-6.[7] During growth the background pressure is in excess of 2×10^{-7} Torr. The first layer to be grown is a Sn-doped buffer layer and becomes an n-type $Al_xGa_{1-x}As$ layer by opening shutter B. It simplifies the arrangement of effusion cells to use the same donor for the n-type GaAs and $Al_xGa_{1-x}As$ layers. The remaining layers are then grown by opening and closing the shutters and heating the effusion cells to the temperatures indicated in Fig. 6.6-6. The layer thickness varies linearly with growth time, and the growth rate used for this structure is generally 1 μm/h.[7,150,151] Although cw room-temperature operation has been achieved with GaAs–$Al_xGa_{1-x}As$ MBE DH lasers, the threshold current densities are generally about a factor of two higher than for similar LPE devices. This difference appears to be due to the introduction of high concentrations of nonradiative recombination centers in the $Al_xGa_{1-x}As$ layers because of the high reactivity of Al with the residual oxygen.

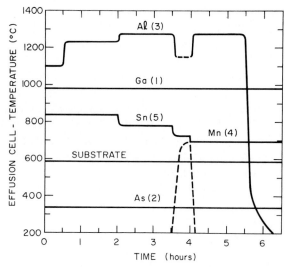

FIG. 6.6-6   Temperature–time cycles used to grow the DH lasers. Solid lines indicate an open shutter, while the dashed line indicates that the shutter is closed. The substrate temperature was 580°C (Ref. 7).

In addition to the usual planar structures, MBE provides a very promising technique for the growth of heterostructures with gradual composition grading rather than the abrupt changes with LPE. The layer thickness control makes MBE very attractive for the growth of waveguides, distributed-feedback devices, and optically integrated circuits. The possibilities for over-growth on a partially processed multilayered structure with MBE is another attractive feature of MBE. Figure 6.6-7 shows the interface between a GaAs wafer with an ion-beam-milled corrugation that was overgrown with a MBE layer of $Al_xGa_{1-x}As$.[153] The growth is coherent and the surface becomes smooth after ~ 1 μm of growth.

Growth of IV–VI Compound Layers and Heterostructures

Unlike the III–V compounds where the equilibrium vapor species consist primarily of molecules of the group V element and atoms of the group III element, the IV–VI compounds can be in equilibrium with a vapor that consists primarily of the binary species $A^{IV}C^{VI}$. In addition, the stoichiometry influences the conductivity and is determined by the flux of group-IV and/or group-VI atoms and molecules. Because of these differences, the MBE growth technique for the IV–VI compounds is somewhat different from the techniques used for the III–V compounds. The early work on the growth of IV–VI MBE epitaxial layers utilized alkali–halide substrates.[173–175]

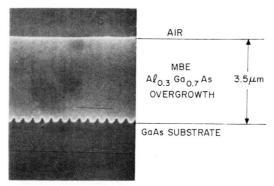

GRATING PERIOD = 0.4 μm

FIG. 6.6-7 Scanning-electron photomicrograph of a cleaved and etched section of an $Al_{0.3}Ga_{0.7}As$ layer (light) grown epitaxially on a GaAs substrate (dark) with an ion-beam milled periodic corrugation (Ref. 153).

The apparatus used by McLane and Sleger[163] to grow

$$N–PbS\,|\,p–PbS_{1-x}Se_x\,|\,P–PbS$$

DH lasers by MBE is shown in Fig. 6.6-8. The properties of these semiconductors and heterostructure lasers were discussed in Section 5.7. As

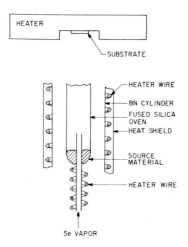

FIG. 6.6-8 Schematic representation of the vacuum deposition system for the MBE of $PbS–PbS_{1-x}Se_x$ DH lasers (Ref. 163).

illustrated in Fig. 6.6-8, the effusion oven that is used to provide the growth components contains the binary or ternary compound as the source material and an additional source of group VI atoms and molecules. With only the binary or ternary source material, the PbS or $PbS_{1-x}Se_x$ layers usually grew n-type even though the starting source material was p-type. To grow p-type layers, the fused-silica reservoir containing Se was used as illustrated in Fig. 6.6-8. Substrate temperatures were $\sim 300°C$ and typical growth rates were $0.5–2$ μm/hr. The laser structures were grown with two source ovens, one containing PbS and the other containing $PbS_{1-x}Se_x$.

Walpole *et al.*[160–162] have prepared a variety of $PbTe–Pb_{1-x}Sn_xTe$ heterostructures by MBE. A description of the DH lasers was given in Section 5.7. This work was extended to the preparation of distributed-feedback $PbTe–Pb_{1-x}Sn_xTe$ DH lasers.[162]

6.7 CHEMICAL-VAPOR DEPOSITION

General Discussion

Chemical-vapor deposition (CVD) is the most widely used technique for the growth of III–V epitaxial layers because it is used for the growth of wafers for visible light-emitting diodes (LED's) of GaP_xAs_{1-x} on GaAs.[176] There are four different CVD techniques used for III–V compounds. The so-called water-vapor transport process is based on the reversible reaction of water vapor with the III–V compound to form the group III element oxide and the group V element vapor.[177] This process is now used primarily for the preparation of high-purity GaP and will not be considered further. The next two CVD processes are based on the same chemistry. In the process called the halide (arsenic or phosphorus trichloride) process,[8] $AsCl_3$ (and/or PCl_3), H_2, and Ga (and/or In) are the initial reactants to grow binary or more complex III–V compounds. In the hydride (arsine and phosphine) process,[9] AsH_3 and PH_3 are used as the sources of arsenic and phosphorus.[9] Gallium (and/or In) is transported via volatile gallium chloride(s) which are produced by passing HCl over the heated Ga. These CVD techniques will be discussed together. In the fourth CVD technique, the decomposition of organometallic compounds is used as a source of group III elements and arsine or other group V hydrides as the source of the group V element.[178–181]

Heterostructure lasers have been prepared by the hydride CVD process[10,11] with $Ga_xIn_{1-x}P$ and $Ga_xIn_{1-y}As$ and by OMD–CVD[11a] with $Al_xGa_{1-x}As$. For DH lasers with $Ga_xIn_{1-x}As$ active layers,[11] the adjacent $Ga_xIn_{1-x}P$ layers lattice match the active layers, but are step graded to the GaAs substrate as discussed in Section 5.6. The growth of $Al_xGa_{1-x}As$ layers of sufficiently high quality to prepare $GaAs–Al_xGa_{1-x}As$ heterostructure lasers by the halide or hydride CVD process has not yet been reported. Johnston and Callahan overcome the problem of Al reacting with the usual fused-silica growth reactor by using high-purity Al_2O_3 ceramic instead and were able to grow good quality AlAs.[182] Growth of high-quality $Al_xGa_{1-x}As$ by this technique is difficult because of its very high reactivity and because the presumed low surface mobility of Al seems to require a high growth temperature. The chemical equilibria require a very high GaCl concentration in the vapor to yield small amounts of Ga in the solid. Just as in LPE, the Ga–Al ratio, now in the vapor, is very high and leads to difficulty in control of composition. These problems are somewhat offset when OMD–CVD is used because the growth conditions are further from equilibrium.

The Halide and Hydride CVD Processes

The most commonly used processes for the epitaxial growth of III–V compounds by open-tube vapor transport are based upon a reaction of the type[183,184]

$$As_4 + 4GaCl + 2H_2 \rightleftarrows 4GaAs + 4HCl, \qquad (6.7\text{-}1)$$

but differ in the way the gaseous components are obtained. The equilibrium constant for the reaction of Eq. (6.7-1) is

$$K(T) = P_{HCl}^4/P_{As_4} \, P_{GaCl}^4 \, P_{H_2}^2, \qquad (6.7\text{-}2)$$

where P is the partial pressure of the subscripted component. The equilibrium constant $K(T)$ is proportional to temperature.

For the halide process the growth apparatus is represented in Fig. 6.7-1. In this process, $AsCl_3$ is used as a source of As and as a reactant with GaAs to transport Ga by the formation of GaCl.[8] Hydrogen is bubbled through $AsCl_3$ which is a liquid above about $-8.5°C$ and boils at about $130°C$. The $AsCl_3$ vapor is thus transported to the heated furnace where the reaction

$$4AsCl_3 + 6H_2 \rightarrow As_4 + 12HCl \qquad (6.7\text{-}3)$$

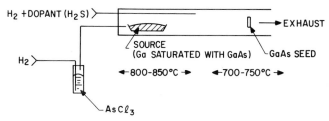

FIG. 6.7-1   Schematic representation of the halide CVD apparatus for the growth of GaAs.

goes essentially to completion. The As_4, HCl, and excess H_2 are then passed over a GaAs source at about $800 \pm 50°C$. Generally, the products of the reaction in Eq. (6.7-3) are passed over Ga, and the Ga becomes saturated with As so that a skin of GaAs forms over the liquid surface. Depending on the flow conditions in the system, the equilibrium of the reaction in Eq. (6.7-1) is more or less established once the Ga has been saturated with As and the GaAs skin formed. Species such as As_2, As, Cl_2, and $GaCl_3$ are present in minor concentrations and do not contribute significantly to the equilibrium. A temperature gradient is established in the reaction tube through which the gaseous components flow. The equilibrium of Eqs. (6.7-1) and (6.7-2) is established at the source in Fig. 6.7-1. The gases flow to the cooler seed region where there is now a thermodynamic driving force to precipitate GaAs. Growth occurs on a GaAs seed placed in this region as illustrated in Fig. 6.7-1.

The other process that utilizes the equilibrium of Eq. (6.7-1) is the hydride (arsine) process[9] in which the group V element is introduced as the hydride and decomposes primarily by the reaction

$$4AsH_3 \rightarrow As_4 + 6H_2. \tag{6.7-4}$$

In this process, the Ga is transported again by its halide

$$2HCl + 2Ga \rightarrow 2GaCl + H_2. \tag{6.7-5}$$

These reactions supply As_4 and GaCl to establish the reaction of Eq. (6.7-1). In the hydride process the partial pressures of the gases are determined by the input flow of HCl and AsH_3. Usually because of rate-limiting steps, Eq. (6.7-4) does not go to completion, so that there is usually some group V hydride present in the growth zone of the furnace. However, the residual hydride also is a source of the group V element contributing to crystal growth. The gas flows are arranged so that the gases mix where the temperature and pressures provide a driving force for the reaction of Eq. (6.7-1) to go to the right and precipitate GaAs on a substrate seed placed in the growth region. The partial pressure ranges for the growth of GaAs are given by Eq. (6.7-2). The stoichiometry of the growing crystal may be modified by varying the ratio P_{As_4}/P_{GaCl}. This ratio modifies the vacancy concentration, which influences impurity incorporation, and provides a degree of freedom not available with LPE. The freedom to vary the P_{As_4}/P_{GaCl} ratio is restricted with the halide process because the ratio is fixed by the reaction of Eq. (6.7-3). Ettenberg et al.[185] prepared wafers for GaAs–$In_{0.5}Ga_{0.5}P$ DH lasers with the hydride process, and obtained improved threshold current densities by decreasing the AsH_3 to HCl ratio, which is proportional to P_{As_4}/P_{GaCl}.

To understand better the processes occurring during CVD by the hydride process, Ban and Ettenberg[184] studied the partial pressures of the reactants and products for the growth of $Ga_xIn_{1-x}P$. These pressures were determined by mass spectrometry. They considered the reactions

$$GaCl + \tfrac{1}{3}PH_3 + \tfrac{1}{6}P_2 + \tfrac{1}{12}P_4 \rightleftarrows GaP + HCl, \tag{6.7-6}$$

and

$$InCl + \tfrac{1}{3}PH_3 + \tfrac{1}{6}P_2 + \tfrac{1}{12}P_4 \rightleftarrows InP + HCl, \tag{6.7-7}$$

which have equilibrium constants of

$$K_2(T) = P_{HCl}a_{GaP}/P_{PH_3}^{1/3}P_{P_2}^{1/6}P_{P_4}^{1/12}P_{GaCl}, \tag{6.7-8}$$

and

$$K_3(T) = P_{HCl}a_{InP}/P_{PH_3}^{1/3}P_{P_2}^{1/6}P_{P_4}^{1/12}P_{InCl}. \tag{6.7-9}$$

In Eqs. (6.7-8) and (6.7-9), a_{GaP} and a_{InP} are the chemical activities of GaP and InP in $Ga_xIn_{1-x}P$. They are obtained from the phase diagrams by the thermodynamic analysis given in Section 6.2. The results of the mass spectrometric studies permitted determination of the equilibrium constants and indicated that it was feasible to consider the system as though it was near equilibrium. With additional thermodynamic information, the partial pressures of the vapor species in equilibrium with $Ga_xIn_{1-x}P$ solid solutions over a range of conditions were predicted. These partial pressures are illustrated in Fig. 6.7-2 at 1000° and 1100°K for a situation in which the group III to group V element ratio in the vapor was unity.

Solid solutions of $Ga_xIn_{1-x}P_yAs_{1-y}$ have been grown by the hydride process with the CVD system shown schematically in Fig. 6.7-3.[186] Both $GaAs–Ga_{0.51}In_{0.49}P$ and $Ga_xIn_{1-x}P–Ga_yIn_{1-y}As$ DH lasers have been prepared with this system.[10,11] It may also be used to grow $Ga_xIn_{1-x}P_yAs_{1-y}$ on InP. The growth process begins with the substrate in the forechamber. The entry value is closed and the forechamber is flushed with H_2. Flows of HCl are established over the Ga and In, and the AsH_3 and PH_3 gases are introduced. The n-type dopant is supplied by H_2S while the p-type dopant is obtained by flowing H_2 over Zn. Composition is determined by the flows of HCl or the group V gases. When the gas flows have been established, the entry valve is opened and the substrate is placed in the preheat zone. A flow of either AsH_3 or PH_3 is passed over the substrate to prevent decomposition. The sample is then moved to the deposition zone and the desired layers grown by controlling the gas flows.

Organometallic Decomposition CVD

Several alkyl compounds of most group III elements are readily available. The compounds containing organic radials that have only one or two carbon atoms are usually moderately volatile liquids at room temperature and

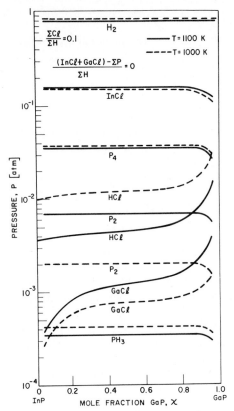

FIG. 6.7-2   The calculated equilibrium partial pressures of gaseous species in equilibrium with $Ga_xIn_{1-x}P$ at 1000° and 1100°K (Ref. 184).

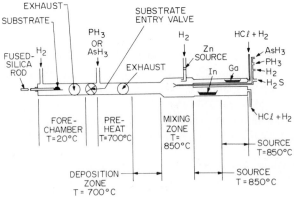

FIG. 6.7-3   Schematic representation of the hydride CVD system for the growth of $Ga_xIn_{1-x}P_yAs_{1-y}$ (Ref. 186).

decompose at several hundred degrees centigrade. The growth of GaAs by the decomposition of trimethyl gallium typifies the process. The trimethyl gallium is usually transported into the reaction chamber as a dilute vapor by bubbling H_2 through it at $0°C$. Arsenic is transported as AsH_3. The reactor is usually a glass chamber with water-cooled walls. The substrate is located on an inductively heated susceptor. For GaAs, epitaxial growth is usually obtained with the substrate in the temperature range $550-700°C$. Epitaxial crystal growth takes place as the result of the decomposition of both the organometallic compound and the hydride. The net reaction is primarily

$$Ga(CH_3)_3 + AsH_3 \xrightarrow{H_2} GaAs + 3CH_4. \qquad (6.7\text{-}10)$$

Details of the mechanism by which this reaction takes place are not known; however, high-quality GaAs and InP epitaxial layers are readily achieved. Doping is generally done by incorporating either organometallics (e.g., $Zn(C_2H_5)_2$) or hydrides (e.g., H_2S) into the reactant gas stream. Since there are no heated walls in the apparatus, the reactants can be present at high supersaturation at the growing surface and the degree of nonequilibrium is probably more representative of MBE than of conventional CVD techniques.

Dupuis et al. have used heterostructures by OMD–CVD for the fabrication of solar cells[187] and heterostructure lasers.[11a,188] Their initial studies with broad area GaAs–$Al_xGa_{1-x}As$ DH lasers suggest that very low thresholds (<1000 A/cm^2) can be achieved. In particular, they reported a threshold current density of 700 A/cm^2 for a DH laser with $d = 0.18$ μm and $x = 0.52$ (Ref. 189). Inspection of Fig. 7.4-9a, b shows that this J_{th} is slightly less than the expected value for this d. If reasonably long life can be demonstrated for these lasers, the OMD–CVD technique will prove an attractive alternative to liquid-phase epitaxy.

6.8 CONCLUDING COMMENTS

An understanding of a particular process for the growth of a heterostructure wafer usually requires information about both the thermodynamic considerations that govern the chemistry of the process and the kinetic considerations that govern the arrival of reactants and their attachment at the growing crystal surface. In this chapter, the thermodynamic considerations, as represented by the phase equilibria and impurity incorporation equilibria for III–V systems, were discussed in detail. Such considerations permit predictions of composition parameters to be used for III–V liquid-phase epitaxy and some of the information needed for interpretation of chemical-vapor deposition processes for the growth of III–V compounds. In addition, a discussion of a kinetic model requiring diffusion-controlled arrival of reactants at the growing LPE interface was presented along with experimental data verifying that model for binary III–V compounds.

The crystal growth techniques for heteroepitaxy by LPE, CVD, and MBE were described. The most commonly used technique for the growth of heterostructure wafers is LPE and it was discussed in detail. Both MBE and CVD may be important for the growth of heterostructure wafers because of their potential for dimensional control over large substrate areas and because they are not as restricted by the liquidus–solidus phase equilibria as is LPE. In addition, MBE permits the growth of structures that are dimensionally quite complex.

REFERENCES

1. H. Nelson, *RCA Rev.* **24**, 603 (1963).
2. J. M. Woodall, H. Rupprecht, and G. D. Pettit, *Solid-State Device Res. Conf.*, Santa Barbara, California (June 1967).
3. H. Rupprecht, J. M. Woodall, and G. D. Pettit, *Appl. Phys. Lett.* **11**, 81 (1967).
4. J. R. Arthur, *J. Appl. Phys.* **39**, 4032 (1968).
5. A. Y. Cho, *J. Vac. Sci. Technol.* **8**, S31 (1971).
6. A. Y. Cho and H. C. Casey, Jr., *J. Appl. Phys.* **45**, 1258 (1974).
7. A. Y. Cho, R. W. Dixon, H. C. Casey, Jr., and R. L. Hartman, *Appl. Phys. Lett.* **28**, 501 (1976).
8. W. F. Finch and E. W. Mehal, *J. Electrochem. Soc.* **111**, 814 (1964).
9. J. J. Tietjen and J. A. Amick, *J. Electrochem. Soc.* **113**, 724 (1966).
10. C. J. Nuese, G. H. Olsen, and M. Ettenberg, *Appl. Phys. Lett.* **29**, 54 (1976).
11. C. J. Nuese, G. H. Olsen, M. Ettenberg, J. J. Gannon, and T. J. Zamerowski, *Appl. Phys. Lett.* **29**, 807 (1976).
11a. R. D. Dupuis and P. D. Dapkus, *Appl. Phys. Lett.* **31**, 466 (1977).
12. M. Ilegems, M. B. Panish, and J. R. Arthur, *J. Chem. Thermodyn.* **6**, 157 (1974).
13. R. A. Swalin, "Thermodynamics of Solids," 2nd ed. Wiley, New York, 1972.
14. E. A. Guggenheim, "Thermodynamics," 5th ed. North–Holland Publ., Amsterdam, 1967.
15. R. A. Swalin, "Thermodynamics of Solids," 2nd ed., p. 125. Wiley, New York, 1972.
16. R. A. Swalin, "Thermodynamics of Solids," 2nd ed., p. 48. Wiley, New York, 1972.
17. O. Kubaschewski, E. LL. Evans, and C. B. Alcock, "Metallurgical Thermochemistry," p. 392. Pergamon, Oxford, 1967.
18. E. A. Guggenheim, "Thermodynamics," 5th ed., p. 197. North–Holland Publ., Amsterdam, 1967.
19. E. A. Guggenheim, "Thermodynamics," 5th ed., p. 192. North–Holland Publ., Amsterdam, 1967.
20. R. A. Swalin, "Thermodynamics of Solids," 2nd ed., p. 127. Wiley, New York, 1972.
21. M. B. Panish and M. Ilegems, "Progress in Solid State Chemistry," (H. Reiss and J. O. McCaldin, eds.), Vol. 7, p. 39. Pergamon, New York, 1972.
22. L. J. Vieland, *Acta Metall.* **11**, 137 (1963).
23. M. B. Panish, *J. Cryst. Growth* **27**, 6 (1974).
24. M. Ilegems and G. L. Pearson, *Gallium Arsenide: 1968 Symp. Proc.* p. 3. Inst. of Phys. and Phys. Soc., London, 1969.
25. A. S. Jordan, *J. Electrochem. Soc.* **119**, 123 (1972).

26. B. Predel and D. W. Stein, *J. Less–Common Met.* **17**, 377 (1969).
27. M. B. Panish and I. Hayashi, "Applied Solid State Science," (R. Wolfe, ed.), Vol. 4, p. 235. Academic Press, New York, 1974.
28. M. B. Panish, unpublished.
29. M. Ilegems and M. B. Panish, *J. Phys. Chem. Solids* **35**, 409 (1974).
30. A. S. Jordan and M. Ilegems, *J. Phys. Chem. Solids* **36**, 329 (1975).
31. R. Sankaran, G. A. Antypas, R. L. Moon, J. S. Escher, and L. W. James, *J. Vac. Sci. Technol.* **13**, 932 (1976).
32. H. C. Casey, Jr. and G. L. Pearson, "Point Defects in Solids" (J. H. Crawford, Jr. and L. M. Slifkin, eds.), vol. 2, p. 163. Plenum Press, New York, 1975.
33. R. A. Swalin, "Thermodynamics of Solids," 2nd ed., p. 107. Wiley, New York, 1972.
34. C. D. Thurmond and M. Kowalchik, *Bell Syst. Tech. J.* **39**, 169 (1960).
35. Y. Furukawa and C. D. Thurmond, *J. Phys. Chem. Solids* **26**, 1535 (1965).
36. M. B. Panish, *J. Less–Common Met.* **10**, 416 (1966).
37. M. B. Panish, *J. Phys. Chem. Solids* **27**, 291 (1966).
38. M. B. Panish, *J. Electrochem. Soc.* **113**, 224 (1966).
39. A. S. Jordan, *Metall. Trans.* **2**, 1965 (1971).
40. M. B. Panish, *J, Appl. Phys.* **44**, 2667 (1973).
41. M. B. Panish, *J. Appl. Phys.* **44**, 2676 (1973).
42. H. Reiss and C. S. Fuller, *J. Met.* **8**, 276 (1956).
43. R. A. Swalin, "Thermodynamics of Solids," 2nd ed., p. 297. Wiley, New York, 1972.
44. F. A. Kröger, "The Chemistry of Imperfect Crystals." Wiley, New York, 1964.
45. W. Van Gool, "Principles of Defect Chemistry of Crystalline Solids." Academic Press, New York, 1966.
46. M. B. Panish and H. C. Casey, Jr., *J. Phys. Chem. Solids* **28**, 1673 (1967).
47. A. S. Jordan, *J. Electrochem. Soc.* **118**, 781 (1971).
48. H. C. Casey, Jr., M. B. Panish, and K. B. Wolfstirn, *J. Phys. Chem. Solids* **32**, 571 (1971).
49. M. B. Panish, *J. Appl. Phys.* **44**, 2659 (1973).
50. F. E. Rosztoczy and K. B. Wolfstirn, *J. Appl. Phys.* **42**, 426 (1971).
51. K.-H. Zschauer and A. Vogel, *Gallium Arsenide: 1970 Symp. Proc.* p. 100. Inst. of Phys., London, 1971.
52. H. C. Casey, Jr., "Atomic Diffusion in Semiconductors" (D. Shaw, ed.), p. 426. Plenum Press, New York, 1973.
53. H. C. Casey, Jr. and M. B. Panish, *J. Cryst. Growth* **13/14**, 818 (1972).
54. A. Many, Y. Goldstein, and N. B. Grover, "Semiconductor Surfaces," p. 165. North-Holland Publ., Amsterdam, 1965.
55. S. M. Sze, "Physics of Semiconductor Devices," p. 363. Wiley, New York, 1969.
56. Y. Nannichi and G. L. Pearson, *Solid-State Electron.* **12**, 341 (1969).
57. R. A. Swalin, "Thermodynamics of Solids," 2nd ed., p. 129. Wiley, New York, 1972.
58. C. J. Hwang and J. R. Brews, *J. Phys. Chem. Solids* **32**, 837 (1971).
59. C. S. Kang and P. E. Greene, *Gallium Arsenide: 1968 Symp. Proc.* p. 18. Inst. of Phys. and Phys. Soc., London, 1969.
60. M. G. Milvidskii and O. V. Pelevin, *Inorg. Mater.* **3**, 1024 (1967) [*Translated from: Izv. Akad. Nauk SSSR, Neorg. Mater.* **3**, 1159 (1967)].
61. P. D. Greene, *Solid State Commun.* **9**, 1299 (1971).
62. L. J. Vieland and I. Kudman, *J. Phys. Chem. Solids* **24**, 437 (1963).
63. G. Schottky, *J. Phys. Chem. Solids* **27**, 1721 (1966).
64. M. S. Abrahams, C. J. Buiocchi, and J. J. Tietjin, *J. Appl. Phys.* **38**, 760 (1967).
65. P. W. Hutchinson and B. D. Bastow, *J. Mater. Sci.* **9**, 1483 (1974).
66. F. E. Rosztoczy, G. A. Antypas, and C. J. Casau, *Gallium Arsenide: 1970 Symp. Proc.* p. 86. Inst. of Phys., London, 1971.

67. M. B. Panish, *J. Electrochem. Soc.* **113**, 861 (1966).
68. K. K. Shih, J. W. Allen, and G. L. Pearson, *J. Phys. Chem. Solids* **29**, 367 (1968).
69. H. C. Casey, Jr., M. B. Panish, and L. L. Chang, *Phys. Rev.* **162**, 660 (1967).
70. F. Ermanis and K. Wolfstirn, *J. Appl. Phys.* **37**, 1963 (1966).
71. D. J. Ashen, P. J. Dean, D. T. J. Hurle, J. B. Mullen, A. M. White, and P. D. Greene, *J. Phys. Chem. Solids* **36**, 1041 (1975).
72. D. R. Ketchow, *J. Electrochem. Soc.* **121**, 1237 (1974).
73. K. L. Ashley and H. A. Strack, *Gallium Arsenide: 1968 Symp. Proc.* p. 123. Inst. of Phys. and Phys. Soc., London, 1969.
74. L. R. Dawson, *J. Appl. Phys.* **48**, 2485 (1977).
75. W. G. Spitzer and M. B. Panish, *J. Appl. Phys.* **40**, 4200 (1969).
76. M. B. Panish and S. Sumski, *J. Appl. Phys.* **41**, 3195 (1970).
77. F. Z. Rosztoczy, *Electrochem. Soc. Fall Meeting, Montreal, Canada* Extended Abstracts (1968).
78. H. C. Casey, Jr. and F. Stern, *J. Appl. Phys.* **47**, 631 (1976).
79. J. K. Kung and W. G. Spitzer, *J. Appl. Phys.* **45**, 2254 (1974).
80. J. K. Kung and W. G. Spitzer, *J. Appl. Phys.* **45**, 4477 (1974).
81. A. J. SpringThorpe, F. D. King, and A. Becke, *J. Electron. Mater.* **4**, 101 (1975).
82. A. V. Novoselova, V. P. Zlomanov, S. G. Karbanov, O. V. Matveyev, and A. M. Gas'kov, "Progress in Solid State Chemistry," (H. Reiss and J. O. McCaldin, eds.), Vol. 7, p. 85. Pergamon, New York, 1972.
83. M. Ilegems and G. L. Pearson, "Annual Review of Materials Science," (R. A. Huggins, R. H. Bube, and R. W. Roberts, eds.), Vol. 5, p. 345. Annual Reviews, Palo Alto, 1975.
84. E. Miller and K. L. Komarek, *Trans. AIME* **236**, 832 (1966).
85. W. Lugscheider, H. Ebel, and G. Langer, *Z. Metallkd.* **56**, 851 (1965).
86. A. S. Jordan, *Metall. Trans.* **1**, 239 (1970).
87. T. C. Harman and I. Melngailis, "Applied Solid State Science," (R. Wolfe, ed.), Vol. 4, p. 1. Academic Press, New York, 1974.
88. R. F. Brebrick and E. Gubner, *J. Chem. Phys.* **36**, 1283 (1962).
89. R. F. Brebrick and A. J. Strauss, *J. Chem. Phys.* **40**, 3230 (1964).
90. J. S. Harris, J. T. Longo, E. R. Gertner, and J. E. Clark, *J. Cryst. Growth* **28**, 334 (1975).
91. T. C. Harman, *J. Nonmet.* **1**, 183 (1973).
92. A. R. Calawa, T. C. Harman, M. Finn, and P. Youtz, *Trans. AIME* **242**, 374 (1968).
93. M. Hansen and K. Anderko, "Constitution of Binary Alloys," McGraw–Hill, New York, 1958.
94. A. J. Strauss and T. C. Harman, *J. Electron. Mater.* **2**, 71 (1973).
95. M. B. Panish, S. Sumski, and I. Hayashi, *Metall. Trans.* **2**, 795 (1971).
96. M. B. Panish, R. T. Lynch, and S. Sumski, *Trans. Metall. Soc. AIME* **245**, 559 (1969).
97. M. Ilegems and M. B. Panish, *J. Cryst. Growth* **20**, 77 (1973).
98. G. B. Stringfellow, *J. Appl. Phys.* **43**, 3455 (1972).
99. G. A. Antypas and L. W. James, *J. Appl. Phys.* **41**, 2165 (1970).
100. J. J. Hsieh, Private communication.
101. J. J. Hsieh, *J. Cryst. Growth* **27**, 49 (1974).
102. D. L. Rode, *J. Cryst. Growth* **20**, 13 (1973).
103. W. A. Tiller, *J. Cryst. Growth* **2**, 69 (1968).
104. M. B. Small and I. Crossley, *J. Cryst. Growth* **27**, 35 (1974).
105. R. L. Moon, *J. Cryst. Growth* **27**, 62 (1974).
106. J. Crank, "The Mathematics of Diffusion," p. 30. Oxford Univ. Press, London and New York, 1956.
107. L. R. Dawson, *J. Cryst. Growth* **27**, 86 (1974).

107a. K.-H. Zschauer, "Festkörper Probleme XV, Advances in Solid State Physics" (H. J. Queisser, ed.) p. 1. Vieweg, Braunschweig, 1975.

107b. K.-H. Zschauer, Private communication.

108. D. L. Rode and R. G. Sobers, *J. Cryst. Growth* **29**, 61 (1975).

109. J. J. Hsieh, J. A. Rossi, and J. P. Donnelly, *Appl. Phys. Lett.* **28**, 709 (1976).

110. F. R. Nash, R. W. Wagner, and R. L. Brown, *J. Appl. Phys.* **47**, 3992 (1976).

111. H. T. Minden, *J. Cryst. Growth* **6**, 228 (1970).

112. I. Crossley and M. B. Small, *J. Cryst. Growth* **19**, 160 (1973).

113. M. B. Panish, *J. Chem. Thermodynam.* **2**, 319 (1970) and unpublished observations.

114. H. C. Casey, Jr., M. B. Panish, W. O. Schlosser, and T. L. Paoli, *J. Appl. Phys.* **45**, 322 (1974).

115. J. Steininger and T. B. Reed, *J. Cryst. Growth* **13/14**, 106 (1972).

116. H. F. Lockwood and M. Ettenberg, *J. Cryst. Growth* **15**, 81 (1972).

117. G. H. B. Thompson and P. A. Kirkby, *J. Cryst. Growth* **27**, 70 (1974).

118. Y. Horikoshi, *Jpn. J. Appl. Phys.* **15**, 887 (1976).

119. Zh. I. Alferov, V. M. Andreyev, S. G. Konnikov, V. R. Larionov, and B. V. Pushny, *Kristallogr. Tech.* **11**, 1013 (1976).

120. F. K. Reinhart and R. A. Logan, *Appl. Phys. Lett.* **25**, 622 (1974).

121. F. K. Reinhart and R. A. Logan, *Appl. Phys. Lett.* **26**, 516 (1975).

121a. J. J. Daniele, D. A. Commack, and P. M. Asbeck, *J. Appl. Phys.* **48**, 914 (1977).

122. B. I. Miller, E. Pinkas, I. Hayashi, and R. J. Capik, *J. Appl. Phys.* **43**, 2817 (1972).

123. R. C. Peters, *Gallium Arsenide Related Compounds: 1972 Symp. Proc.*, p. 55. Inst. of Phys., London, 1973.

124. D. L. Rode, R. W. Wagner, and N. E. Schumaker, *Appl. Phys. Lett.* **30**, 75 (1977).

125. R. H. Saul and D. D. Roccasecca, *J. Appl. Phys.* **44**, 1983 (1973).

126. D. L. Rode, *J. Cryst. Growth* **27**, 313 (1974).

127. R. L. Dawson, Ph.D. Thesis, Univ. Southern California (January 1969).

128. A. U. MacRae and G. W. Gobeli, "Semiconductors and Semimetals" (R. K. Willardson and A. C. Beer, eds.), Vol. 2, p. 115. Academic Press, New York, 1966.

129. F. Jona, *IBM J. Res. Develop.* **9**, 375 (1965).

130. J. E. Rowe, unpublished.

131. D. L. Rode, *Phys. Status Solidi (a)* **32**, 425 (1975).

132. R. A. Logan, Private communication.

133. R. A. Logan and D. L. Rode, Private communication.

134. M. B. Small, A. E. Blakeslee, K. K. Shih, and R. M. Potemski, *J. Cryst. Growth* **30**, 257 (1975).

134a. M. B. Small, J. M. Blum, and R. M. Potemski, *Appl. Phys. Lett.* **30**, 42 (1977).

135. J. R. Arthur and J. J. LePore, *J. Vac. Sci. Tech.* **6**, 545 (1969).

136. J. R. Arthur, U. S. Patent No. 3,615,931 (1971).

137. A. Y. Cho, *J. Appl. Phys.* **41**, 2780 (1970).

138. A. Y. Cho, *J. Appl. Phys.* **42**, 2074 (1971).

139. A. Y. Cho and I. Hayashi, *Solid-State Electron.* **14**, 125 (1971).

140. A. Y. Cho, M. B. Panish, and I. Hayashi, *Gallium Arsenide Related Compounds: 1970 Symp. Proc.*, p. 18. Inst. of Phys., London, 1971.

141. A. Y. Cho and I. Hayashi, *J. Appl. Phys.* **42**, 4422 (1971).

142. A. Y. Cho and I. Hayashi, *Metall. Trans.* **2**, 777 (1971).

143. A. Y. Cho and M. B. Panish, *J. Appl. Phys.* **43**, 5118 (1972).

144. A. Y. Cho and F. K. Reinhart, *J. Appl. Phys.* **45**, 1812 (1974).

145. A. Y. Cho, C. N. Dunn, R. L. Kuvas, and W. E. Schroeder, *Appl. Phys. Lett.* **25**, 224 (1974).

146. A. Y. Cho and D. R. Chen, *Appl. Phys. Lett.* **28**, 30 (1976).
147. A. Y. Cho and F. K. Reinhart, *Appl. Phys. Lett.* **21**, 355 (1972).
148. J. C. Tracy, W. Wiegmann, R. A. Logan, and F. K. Reinhart, *Appl. Phys. Lett.* **22**, 511 (1973).
149. J. L. Merz and A. Y. Cho, *Appl. Phys. Lett.* **28**, 456 (1976).
150. A. Y. Cho and H. C. Casey, Jr., *Appl. Phys. Lett.* **25**, 288 (1974).
151. H. C. Casey, Jr., A. Y. Cho, and P. A. Barnes, *IEEE J. Quantum Electron.* **QE-11**, 467 (1975).
152. H. C. Casey, Jr., S. Somekh, and M. Ilegems, *Appl. Phys. Lett.* **27**, 142 (1975).
153. M. Ilegems, H. C. Casey, Jr., S. Somekh, and M. B. Panish, *J. Cryst. Growth* **31**, 158 (1975).
154. R. Dingle, W. Wiegmann, and C. H. Henry, *Phys. Rev. Lett.* **33**, 827 (1974).
155. R. Dingle, "Festkörper-Probleme XV-Advances in Solid State Physics," p. 21. Pergamon (Vieweg), Oxford, 1975.
156. R. Dingle, A. C. Gossard, and W. Wiegmann, *Phys. Rev. Lett.* **34**, 1327 (1975).
157. R. Ludeke, L. Esaki, and L. L. Chang, *Appl. Phys. Lett.* **24**, 417 (1974).
158. L. L. Chang, L. Esaki, and R. Tsu, *Appl. Phys. Lett.* **24**, 593 (1974).
159. A. C. Gossard, P. M. Petroff, W. Wiegmann, R. Dingle, and A. Savage, *Appl. Phys. Lett.* **29**, 323 (1976).
160. J. N. Walpole, A. R. Calawa, R. W. Ralston, T. C. Harman, and J. P. McVittie, *Appl. Phys. Lett.* **23**, 620 (1973).
161. J. N. Walpole, A. R. Calawa, T. C. Harman, and S. H. Groves, *Appl. Phys. Lett.* **28**, 552 (1976).
162. J. N. Walpole, A. R. Calawa, S. R. Chinn, S. H. Groves, and T. C. Harman, *Appl. Phys. Lett.* **29**, 307 (1976).
163. G. F. McLane and K. J. Sleger, *J. Electron. Mater.* **4**, 465 (1975).
164. H. Preier, M. Bleicher, W. Riedel, and H. Maier, *Appl. Phys. Lett.* **28**, 669 (1976).
165. A. Y. Cho and J. R. Arthur, "Progress in Solid-State Chemistry," (J. O. McCaldin and G. Somorjai, eds.), vol. 10, p. 157. Pergamon Press, New York, 1975.
166. M. Ilegems, Private communication.
167. J. R. Arthur, *J. Phys. Chem. Solids* **28**, 2257 (1967).
168. C. V. Heer, "Statistical Mechanics, Kinetic Theory, and Stochastic Processess," chapter 1. Academic Press, New York, 1972.
169. W. Wiegmann, Private communication.
170. M. Ilegems and R. Dingle, *Gallium Arsenide Related Compounds: 1974 Symp. Proc.* p. 1. Inst. of Phys., London, 1975.
171. J. R. Arthur, *Surf. Sci.* **43**, 449 (1974) and Private communication.
172. M. Ilegems, *J. Appl. Phys.* **48**, 1278 (1977).
173. R. B. Schoolar and J. N. Zemel, *J. Appl. Phys.* **35**, 1848 (1964).
174. E. G. Bylander, *Mater. Sci. Eng.* **1**, 190 (1966).
175. H. Holloway, E. M. Logothetis, and E. Wilkes, *J. Appl. Phys.* **41**, 3543 (1970).
176. R. A. Burmeister, Jr., G. P. Pighini, and P. E. Greene, *Trans. AIME* **245**, 587 (1969).
177. C. J. Frosch, *J. Electrochem. Soc.* **111**, 180 (1964).
178. H. M. Manasevit and W. I. Simpson, *J. Electrochem. Soc.* **116**, 1725 (1969).
179. S. Ito, T. Shinohara, and Y. Seki, *J. Electrochem. Soc.* **120**, 1419 (1973).
180. Y. Seki, K. Tanno, K. Iida, and E. Ichiki, *J. Electrochem. Soc.* **122**, 1108 (1975).
181. Y. Nakayama, S. Ohkawa, H. Hashimoto, and H. Ishikawa, *J. Electrochem. Soc.* **123**, 1227 (1976).
182. W. D. Johnston, Jr. and W. M. Callahan, *Appl. Phys. Lett.* **28**, 150 (1976).
183. A. Boucher and L. Hollan, *J. Electrochem. Soc.* **117**, 932 (1970).

184. V. S. Ban and M. Ettenberg, *J. Phys. Chem. Solids* **34**, 1119 (1973).
185. M. Ettenberg, G. H. Olsen, and C. J. Nuese, *Appl. Phys. Lett.* **29**, 141 (1976).
186. G. H. Olsen and M. Ettenberg, "Crystal Growth: Theory and Techniques" (C. Goodman, ed.), Vol II. Plenum Press, New York, 1978.
187. R. D. Dupuis, P. D. Dapkus, R. D. Yingling, and L. A. Moudy, *Appl. Phys. Lett.* **31**, 201 (1978).
188. R. D. Dupuis, P. D. Dapkus, and G. A. Moudy Tech. Digest, Int Electron Device Meeting, p. 575, Washington, D. C., December 1977.
189. R. D. Dupuis, Private communication.

7.1 INTRODUCTION

An extensive background of the theory that describes heterostructure lasers as well as the epitaxial growth techniques has been presented in the previous chapters. Only structures that confine the injected carriers and guide the radiation in a direction perpendicular to the junction plane (transverse confinement) have been considered. These structures are called broad-area lasers. The most extensively used semiconductor lasers are those that also restrict current along the junction plane (lateral confinement). These lasers have been designated as stripe-geometry lasers. In this chapter, the fabrication and operating characteristics of both broad-area and stripe-geometry heterostructure lasers will be summarized and discussed.

The fabrication of heterostructure lasers utilizes the heteroepitaxial wafers that are prepared by the techniques described in Sections 6.5–6.7. In Section 7.2, the preparation of ohmic contacts and the separation of the wafers into individual device chips are discussed. These techniques are common to both broad-area and stripe-geometry lasers. The techniques for providing current confinement in stripe-geometry lasers are postponed until Section 7.6. Only the general principles of fabrication and a representative example can be given because each laboratory has its own "recipe" which is generally proprietary.

The first broad-area laser to be considered is the single-heterostructure (SH) laser presented in Section 7.3. In terms of device technology, the SH laser served as a link between the homostructure and double-heterostructure (DH) laser. However, the almost immediate development of the lower threshold DH laser prevented extensive quantitative studies of the SH laser. The SH laser has remained an important device because it is a relatively simple structure to prepare, the beam divergence in the direction perpendicular to the junction plane is small, and it produces high-peak power for pulsed excitation.

Numerous properties of DH lasers have been introduced in the previous chapters. The experimental properties such as threshold current density and emission behavior are summarized in Section 7.4. Good agreement is obtained between the room-temperature threshold current density that was calculated without adjustable parameters and the experimental values. The calculation of the gain coefficient for GaAs was given in Chapter 3. A brief discussion of the filamentary nature of the laser emission will be introduced in this section. In all broad-area lasers, the stimulated emission takes place in localized regions, which are called lasing filaments, with a lateral dimension on the order of 10 μm and results in large variations in the optical power intensity across the mirror face.

In Section 7.5, which is the last section on broad-area lasers, the laser properties are considered for the structures that were discussed in Section 2.9 as four- and five-layer heterostructure waveguides. These structures included the large-optical-cavity (LOC) laser, the *Ppn'N* laser, and the symmetric and asymmetric separate-confinement heterostructure (SCH) laser. They are generally intended for high-emission power applications while retaining the low threshold behavior of DH lasers.

The discussion of stripe-geometry lasers begins in Section 7.6 with a description of the various fabrication techniques for lateral current confinement. The most commonly used techniques have been SiO_2 contact masking, proton bombardment to produce high-resistivity regions, or stripes defined by Zn diffusion. The stripe geometry has several beneficial effects in addition to simply reducing the cross-sectional area and hence the operating current. For stripes less than about 10–15 μm wide, single-filament operation as well as emission in the fundamental mode along the junction plane is obtained, and devices selected for well-behaved emission properties permit detailed experimental studies. Most of the examples and discussion of stripe-geometry lasers will be for $Al_{0.08}Ga_{0.92}As–Al_{0.37}Ga_{0.63}As$ DH lasers because a majority of the available experimental data and subsequent analysis is for this structure.

In most stripe-geometry lasers, the current spreading and lateral carrier diffusion in the active layer results in a higher threshold current density than for broad-area lasers. These effects are considered in Section 7.7 where expressions are derived for the carrier distributions along the junction plane. Also, the measurement of the threshold current density is extended from the brief description in Section 3.8 to include differential-voltage measurements. These differential-voltage measurements demonstrate the pinning of the quasi-Fermi levels when threshold is reached and permit determination of the series resistance.

Much of the input power is dissipated as heat in the active region, and therefore device design must consider the quantities that influence the thermal properties of heterostructure lasers. As presented in Section 7.8, the thermal properties of a heterostructure laser may be represented by its mean thermal resistance $\langle R \rangle$. The product of $\langle R \rangle$ and the input power gives the temperature rise of the active region relative to the heat sink. For the dimensions and thermal conductivities of typical $GaAs–Al_xGa_{1-x}As$ stripe-geometry DH lasers, $\langle R \rangle$ is shown to be 20–30°K/W, and a temperature rise of $\sim 5°–10°$K can be expected at room temperature.

The measurement of the gain coefficient in stripe-geometry lasers by the experimental techniques described in Section 7.9 permits comparison with the calculated behavior given in Section 3.8. This experimental measurement of the gain coefficient is necessary for the numerical evaluation of waveguiding along the junction plane that is illustrated in Section 7.10. This waveguiding along the junction plane in stripe-geometry lasers is shown to be primarily due to optical gain. The two-dimensional waveguiding model for stripe-geometry lasers is an extension of the previous analyses in Chapter 2 for waveguiding in the direction perpendicular to the junction plane.

The emission properties of stripe-geometry lasers are summarized in Section 7.11. Many of the properties of the longitudinal, transverse, and lateral modes have been presented in previous chapters. Nonlinearities in the lasing output light intensity with the current above threshold are a serious problem and have been designated "kinks." The properties of kinks and their elimination are discussed in this section. Other emission properties are the relaxation oscillations and the noise resonance of stripe-geometry lasers. These properties influence the possible modulation rates and are discussed briefly in Section 7.11.

In Section 7.12, the experimental properties of distributed-feedback (DFB) lasers are presented. The cw room-temperature properties for a stripe-geometry DFB laser are illustrated for the SCH structure shown in Fig. 2.10-5b. The distributed Bragg reflector (DBR) laser is also illustrated. The integration of the DFB laser with a heterostructure waveguide demonstrates the possibilities for its use in integrated optics.

7.2 DEVICE FABRICATION

Wafer Preparation

The fabrication of discrete devices begins with the heteroepitaxial wafers that are prepared by liquid-phase epitaxy (LPE), chemical-vapor deposition (CVD), or molecular-beam epitaxy (MBE) as described in Chapter 6. The GaAs–Al$_x$Ga$_{1-x}$As heteroepitaxial wafers are most often prepared by LPE, and the surface of a representative LPE wafer is shown in Fig. 7.2-1.[1] Small amounts of the last LPE solution often remain on the surface, either as large drops or as microscopic droplets. The disturbed region in the lower left corner of Fig. 7.2-1 results from this residual solution and must be removed before further processing. The microscopic droplets can readily be removed by anodic oxidation in properly pH-adjusted water.[2] The resulting oxide layer on the sample surface is soluble in HCl, HNO$_3$, and H$_2$SO$_4$ solutions. It is very important to maintain surface cleanliness throughout the fabrication process.

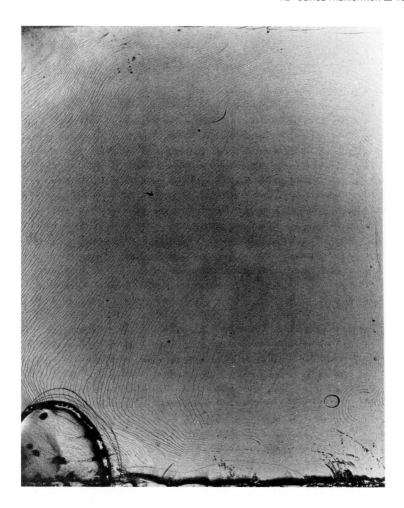

FIG. 7.2-1 Photomicrograph of LPE GaAs–Al$_x$Ga$_{1-x}$As heteroepitaxial wafer. The dimensions are ~1.2 × 1.0 cm (Ref. 1).

The usual procedure for determining the thickness of the various layers grown on the wafer is to cleave off a test bar. It can be etched briefly (~2 min) in 30% H$_2$O$_2$–H$_2$O solution that is brought to a pH of 7.05 with NH$_3$OH solution.[3,4] This solution etches GaAs much faster than Al$_x$Ga$_{1-x}$As and provides slight height differences that facilitate layer thickness measurement either with an optical microscope or a scanning-electron microscope (SEM). Angle lapping to magnify the layer thicknesses, followed by the peroxide etch, permits improved measurement of very thin layers with an optical microscope. Photoluminescence (PL) can be a useful tool for measuring the

$Al_xGa_{1-x}As$ layer composition and in observing the location and detrimental effects of defects in the heteroepitaxial wafer.[5-8] The photon energy of the peak PL intensity occurs very near the direct-energy gap E_g, and the variation of E_g with x given in Fig. 5.3-2 may be used to assign x. If the heteroepitaxial wafer has a top p^+–GaAs layer, as illustrated in Fig. 2.3-1 for a DH laser, the GaAs layer can be removed with the H_2O_2 preferential etch[3,4] for PL measurements.

Contacts

There are several basic guidelines that have been established for providing metallic contacts to heterostructure lasers: (1) avoid alloying the contact to the side with the epitaxial layers because the active layer is only a few microns from the surface; and (2) use an alloyed low-specific-resistance contact to the substrate. Low-resistance contacts to the epitaxial layer may be obtained by using a final epitaxial layer that is sufficiently heavily doped to give a conducting rather than a rectifying Schottky barrier. There are many techniques for obtaining low-specific-resistance contacts to the III–V solid solutions. A useful summary may be found in the review by Rideout.[9]

There are several techniques available for the metallization to heteroepitaxial GaAs–$Al_xGa_{1-x}As$ wafers. A top p^+–GaAs layer, such as illustrated for the DH laser in Fig. 2.3-1, is often used to facilitate ohmic contact. Zinc diffusion with an As-rich source[10] for 20 min at 650°C will ensure a highly conducting p^+ contact when contacted with a thin metallic film. The diffusion depth is $\lesssim 0.2$ μm. In some structures, the top p-type GaAs layer is omitted, and the P–$Al_xGa_{1-x}As$ layer is contacted directly. After diffusion, contact to this layer is obtained by first evaporating or sputtering a thin ~ 500-Å layer of Cr or Ti to facilitate adherence of the subsequent ~ 2000-Å Au or Pt layer. If desired, thicker Au contacts can then be built up by electroplating. Before proceeding to the substrate contact, the wafer is lapped to a thickness of ~ 125 μm to permit cleavage to form the laser mirrors for individual devices. The contact to the n^+–GaAs substrate can be obtained by evaporating and alloying Sn or Au–Ge. The tendency for Sn to ball up during alloying can be reduced by evaporating thin intermediate layers of Pt. The Au–Ge contact has been extensively studied[11-15] because of its use as a contact for GaAs FETs and Gunn oscillators. In Ref. 15, the Au–Ge eutectic alloy (12 wt % Ge) film of 350 Å thickness and a subsequent Au film of 3000 Å thickness were evaporated on n-type GaAs. The contact resistivity was measured for various alloying times and temperatures. By rapid heating and alloying for 3 min at 450°C, a contact resistivity of 10^{-6} Ω-cm² was obtained.[15]

Other III–V solid-solution heterostructure lasers were discussed in Sections 5.4 and 5.5 and the IV–VI solid-solution heterostructure lasers were discussed in Section 5.7. The references in those sections should be consulted for the available descriptions of the fabrication and contacting procedure for those materials.

Device Chips

As described in Section 3.8, the laser cavity is usually formed by the use of parallel reflecting surfaces to form a Fabry–Perot interferometer. These parallel mirrors are readily obtained by cleaving.[16] As illustrated in Fig. 5.2-2, there are {110} natural cleavage planes of GaAs normal to the {100} plane on which the epitaxial layers are grown. The wafer with metallic contacts can be mounted with wax on a thin flexible metal sheet and small indentations scribed near one edge of the wafer with a diamond scriber. Slight flexing will then result in cleavage along {110} planes perpendicular to the surface. This technique ensures perfectly aligned mirrors. For broad-area lasers, the cleaved bars can then be sawed perpendicular to the mirror faces with a diamond or string saw to form the rectangular device chips as illustrated in Fig. 7.2-2. The rough sawed sides and a cavity length-to-width ratio of at least 2.5 appears to prevent excitation of internally circulating modes.[17] Typical dimensions are a width of ~ 125 μm and a length of ~ 350 μm.

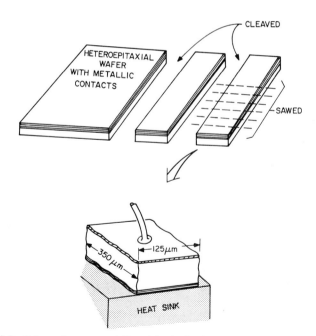

FIG. 7.2-2   Schematic representation of the device fabrication procedure for broad-area lasers.

Devices may be mounted with spring contacts for testing and laboratory measurements with pulse excitation. For cw operation or for use outside the laboratory, the epitaxial layer side is soldered to the Au-plated Cu heat sink with In. The strain introduced by the bonding procedure due to different thermal expansion coefficients of the materials is minimized by the relatively soft In.[18] The other electrical contact is obtained by bonding an Au wire to the metallic layer on the substrate. The mirror faces are sometimes protected by pyrolytically deposited Al_2O_3 layers.[19]

7.3 SINGLE-HETEROSTRUCTURE BROAD-AREA LASERS

Introductory Comments

The application of LPE to the preparation of homostructure lasers resulted in better control over doping and materials and permitted $J_{th}(300°K)$ to be reduced to 26×10^3 A/cm^2.[20] Further reduction in $J_{th}(300°K)$ to about 10×10^3 A/cm^2 was achieved [21-24] with the single-heterostructure (SH) laser illustrated in Figs. 1.2-1b, and 7.3-1. This laser is designated as an n–p–P structure with the notation of the previous chapters and is also called the close-confinement or single-heterojunction laser. Only pulsed operation of SH lasers is possible at room temperature.

Wafers for SH lasers were first prepared by growth of a P–$Al_xGa_{1-x}As$ Zn-doped layer onto a {100} surface of a heavily doped n-type GaAs substrate crystal by LPE.[21,23] The AlAs mole fraction x was usually 0.3–0.5. Either during growth, or by subsequent annealing, sufficient Zn was diffused from the $Al_xGa_{1-x}As$ layer into the GaAs substrate to form the p–n junction a short distance (usually 1–3 μm) from the heterojunction.[21,23,24] Growth temperatures were usually 900°–1000°C in order to attain the Zn diffusion into the substrate. In the diffused SH lasers, the p–n junction is in the substrate wafer, and the resulting lasers can be influenced by the substrate quality. Better control over the properties of SH lasers is achieved when the n- and p-layers are also grown by LPE. Minden and Premo[25] used a multiple LPE technique similar to the processes described in Section 6.5 in order to grow the n-, p-, and P-layers for SH lasers. Germanium is a convenient p-dopant and both Sn and Te have been used as n-type dopants. The incorporation of these dopants into GaAs during LPE was described in Section 6.3.

Threshold Behavior

Although only limited quantitative data are available for the threshold current density of SH lasers, it is clear that J_{th} depends on the thickness of the p-type active layer, the temperature, and the impurity concentration on the n-side of the p–n junction. The $J_{th}(300°K)$ values that have been reported

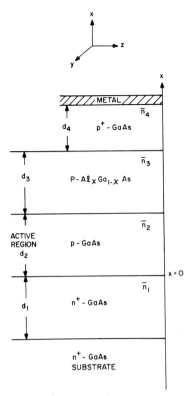

FIG. 7.3-1 Representation of the layers of a GaAs–Al$_x$Ga$_{1-x}$As SH laser.

are for pulse excitation usually with 0.1–0.2 μsec pulses at 100–1000 Hz. For a meaningful comparison of J_{th}, only Fabry–Perot structures without mirror coatings are considered. It is interesting to note that one of the initial studies[22] yielded about the lowest $J_{th}(300°K)$ value, 8.6×10^3 A/cm^2 for a 400-μm cavity, that has been achieved for SH lasers with uncoated mirrors. Unlike the more complex DH and SCH lasers, subsequent work did not result in a significant reduction of this value. The reason for the low $J_{th}(300°K)$ of the diffused SH lasers appears to be the achievement of the optimum active-layer thickness in the initial studies. However, the more complex lasers described in the balance of this chapter had to await improvement in multiple LPE growth techniques. Values of $J_{th}(300°K)$ as low as 6×10^3 A/cm^2 have been obtained by using square, four-mirror, fully internally reflecting SH lasers.[24] Lasers with reflective mirror coatings have given $J_{th}(300°K)$ of 8.5×10^3 A/cm^2 (Ref. 26) and $6.8 \pm 0.4 \times 10^3$ A/cm^2 (Ref. 27).

The variation of $J_{th}(300°K)$ with the p-layer thickness is summarized in Fig. 7.3-2 for GaAs–Al$_x$Ga$_{1-x}$As SH lasers prepared by Zn diffusion from the P–Al$_x$Ga$_{1-x}$As layer. The threshold was determined by the procedure described for Fig. 3.8-10. The threshold current density decreases as the cavity length L is increased[27] so that $J_{th}(300°K)$ should be compared for devices of similar length. The data in this figure from Refs. 24 and 27 are for $L = 400$–500 μm and from Ref. 28 are for $L = 250$ μm. Considerable uncertainty can exist for the p-layer values because this thickness has generally been determined by optical microscope measurement of etched cross sections. The p-layer thickness determined in this manner depends somewhat upon the etching time of the junction stain. Therefore, considerable uncertainty can exist for the p-layer thicknesses in Fig. 7.3-2. The more closely controlled properties of the LPE SH lasers grown by Minden and

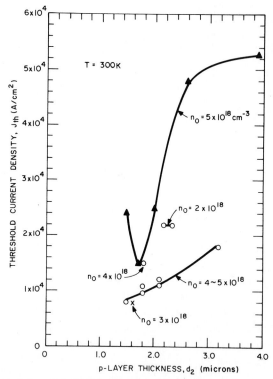

FIG. 7.3-2   Variation of $J_{th}(300°K)$ with p-layer thickness for SH lasers prepared by Zn diffusion from the P–Al$_{0.5}$Ga$_{0.5}$As layer. The data represented by ○ are for $L = 400$–500 μm (Ref. 24), × is for $L = 450$ μm (Ref. 27), and ▲ are for $L = 250$ μm (Ref. 28). Due to the method used to determine the p-layer thickness (see text), there may be significant errors in the d_2 values.

Premo[25] more clearly demonstrated that increasing the carrier concentration of the n^+-layer reduced $J_{th}(300°K)$. However, p-layer thicknesses were not specified, and therefore, their data cannot be used in Fig. 7.3-2.

The variation of J_{th} with temperature for a representative diffused SH laser[24] is shown in Fig. 7.3-3a. The threshold behavior for a homojunction laser is shown for comparison. An exponential variation of J_{th} with T is observed and may be represented by

$$J_{th}(T) = J_0 \exp(T/T_0) \tag{7.3-1}$$

with the empirical parameters J_0 and T_0. The temperature where J_{th} abruptly increases has been labeled T_t. As the p-layer thickness becomes

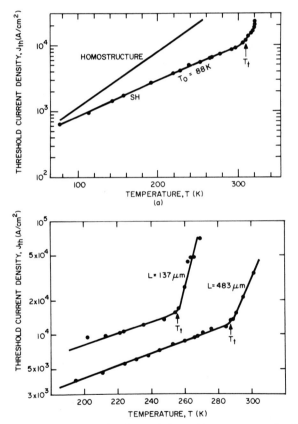

FIG. 7.3-3 Threshold current density variation with temperature for SH laser. The quantity T_t corresponds to the temperature of the abrupt increase in J_{th}. (a) Comparison with homostructure laser. For the SH laser, $d \approx 2$ μm, $n_0 \approx 4 \times 10^{18}$ cm^{-3}, and $L = 500$ μm (Ref. 24). (b) Variation of T_t with L for SH laser with $d \approx 1.7$ μm (Ref. 29).

smaller, T_t moves to a lower temperature.[24] As shown in Fig. 7.3-3b, this transition temperature for a fixed p-layer thickness also depends on the cavity length.[29]

The emission may be shifted to shorter wavelength by sequential growth of an N–$Al_xGa_{1-x}As$ layer and then a P–$Al_yGa_{1-y}As$ layer with $x < y$.[30] Zinc is diffused from the P-layer into the N-layer to give the junction in the N–$Al_xGa_{1-x}As$ layer. The variation of J_{th} with the emission wavelength is shown in Fig. 7.3-4. The threshold current density increases abruptly as the composition of the $Al_xGa_{1-x}As$ layer approaches the composition of the direct–indirect-energy-gap transition (Fig. 4.2-2), and the electrons begin to populate the indirect conduction bands. The relative fraction of the electrons in the direct conduction band as a function of AlAs mole fraction x was given in Fig. 4.6-4.

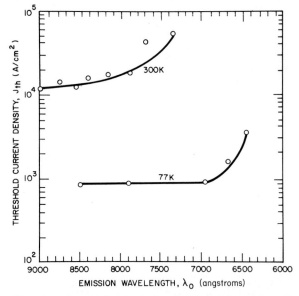

FIG. 7.3-4 Threshold current density J_{th} as a function of the $Al_xGa_{1-x}As$–$Al_yGa_{1-y}As$ SH laser emission wavelength (Ref. 30).

There is insufficient experimental data to permit a detailed analysis of the threshold-current-density behavior for SH lasers. However, the qualitative behavior can be understood. The heterostructure energy-band diagram for the SH represented in Fig. 7.3-1 is shown in Fig. 7.3-5a at zero bias and in Fig. 7.3-5b at high forward bias. This figure was calculated for $n_0 = 4 \times 10^{18}$ cm^{-3}, $p_0 = 1 \times 10^{19}$ cm^{-3}, $x = 0.5$, and $d_2 = 1.5$ μm. It is

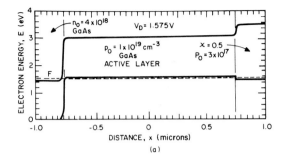

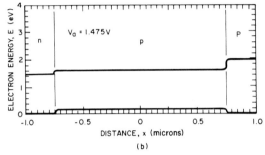

FIG. 7.3-5 Energy-band diagram for GaAs–Al$_{0.5}$Ga$_{0.5}$As *n–p–P* single heterostructure. (a) Zero bias. (b) Forward bias of 1.475 V.

for abrupt changes in impurity concentration as obtained for the LPE SH laser. The equations used for the determination of this energy-band diagram were given in Section 4.3.

The current density J at the *p–n* junction is the sum of the electron current density i_n injected into the *p*-layer and the hole current density i_p injected into the *n*-layer:

$$J(\text{A/cm}^2) = i_n + i_p. \tag{7.3-2}$$

Because of the electron confining *p–P* heterojunction, the expression for i_n will differ from the familiar exponential expression given by Eq. (4.5-35). The solution of the continuity equation was given by Eq. (4.5-30) as

$$n(x) = C_1 \exp(-x/L_n) + C_2 \exp(x/L_n), \tag{7.3-3}$$

where L_n is the electron diffusion length and the thermal equilibrium electron concentration n_{po} has been ignored. At the edge of the space-charge region on the *p*-side, $x = 0$ and $n(0) = n_p$. At $x = d$ for the *p–P* interface, $i_n = 0$ because of the conduction band barrier. These boundary conditions with

Eq. (4.3-50) for i_n give

$$n(x) = n_p \cosh[(d - x)/L_n]/\cosh(d/L_n). \tag{7.3-4}$$

Then at $x = 0$,

$$i_n = qD_n \, dn/dx\big|_{x=0} = -(qD_n n_p/L_n)\tanh(d/L_n), \tag{7.3-5}$$

where D_n is the electron diffusivity.

This expression for i_n may be written in a more useful form by replacing the electron concentration at $x = 0$ in the p-layer, n_p, with the electron concentration of the n-layer, n_n. With the exponential approximation for the Fermi–Dirac integral,

$$n = N_c \exp[F_c - E_c)/kT], \tag{4.3-25}$$

where F_c is the Fermi level and E_c the conduction band edge. From the forward-biased p–n homojunction represented in Fig. 7.3-6,

$$n_p = N_c \exp[(F_{c_p} - E_{c_p})/kT], \tag{7.3-6}$$

and

$$n_n = N_c \exp[(F_{c_n} - E_{c_n})/kT]. \tag{7.3-7}$$

Since $F_{c_n} = F_{c_p}$, these equations may be combined to give

$$n_p = n_n \exp[-q(V_D - V_a)/kT], \tag{7.3-8}$$

where V_D is the built-in potential, V_a the applied bias across the p–n junction, and $q(V_D - V_a) = E_{c_p} - E_{c_n}$. Therefore,

$$i_n = -(qD_n n_n/L_n)\exp[-q(V_D - V_a)/kT]\tanh(d/L_n). \tag{7.3-9}$$

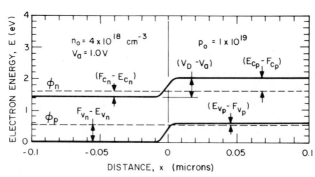

FIG. 7.3-6 Energy band diagram for a GaAs n–p junction with a forward bias of 1 V. The electron and hole quasi-Fermi levels are represented by ϕ_n and ϕ_p, respectively. This figure illustrates the separation of the band edges and the Fermi levels.

In a similar manner, the leakage current i_p may be obtained for the boundary conditions of $p(x) = 0$ at $x \gg L_p$ and $p(x) = p_n$ at $x = 0$, and is

$$i_p = qD_p p_n / L_p, \qquad (7.3\text{-}10)$$

where D_p is the hole diffusivity, p_n the hole concentration on the n-side at $x = 0$, and L_p the hole diffusion length. This current can be written as

$$i_p = (qD_p p_p / L_p) \exp[-q(V_D - V_a)/kT], \qquad (7.3\text{-}11)$$

where p_p is the hole concentration in the p-layer. In Eqs. (7.3-9) and (7.3-11), the diffusivity may be related to the mobility μ as $D = \mu kT/q$. To permit evaluation of these quantities, the mobilities and diffusion lengths[31] for GaAs at room temperature are shown in Fig. 7.3-7. The difficulties in the assignment of L_n and L_p from various experiments were discussed in Section 3.7. These data are for LPE layers. At low temperature, μ becomes larger while L_n and L_p decrease.[32]

These expressions for i_n and i_p are only valid at carrier concentrations where the exponential approximations may be used for the Fermi–Dirac integral. This requirement is approximately $n \lesssim 0.5\,N_c$ and $p \lesssim 0.5\,N_v$.[33] [See also Eqs. (4.3-45) and (4.3-46)] The simple representations in Eqs. (7.3-8) and (7.3-9) do illustrate that n_p approaches n_n as V_a approaches V_D. The high-injection case becomes very complex and requires numerical computer analysis.[34] As V_a approaches V_D, the injected hole concentration in the n-layer also becomes large and gives a significant leakage hole current. Ohmic loss, space-charge neutrality requirements, and the properties of the contacts tend to limit the injected electron concentration to the free electron concentration on the n-side:

$$n_p < n_n. \qquad (7.3\text{-}12)$$

As discussed in Section 4.6, the N–p heterojunction permits $n_p > n_n$ so that "superinjection" is possible in the DH laser.

The electron current density i_n provides the excitation for gain and at threshold equals J_{th} as represented by Eq. (3.8-46), and i_p represents the leakage current density J_L. Therefore, the total current density at threshold may be written as

$$J_{th}(A/cm^2) = J_L + \frac{J_0 d}{\eta} + \frac{d}{\eta \Gamma \beta}\left[\alpha_i + \frac{1}{L}\ln\left(\frac{1}{R}\right)\right], \qquad (7.3\text{-}13)$$

where η is the internal quantum efficiency, Γ the confinement factor, β the gain constant, R the power reflectivity, and J_0 the current where the linear extrapolation of the gain coefficient goes to zero (see Fig. 3.8-7). Equation (7.3-13) together with Fig. 2.6-9 for Γ provide an understanding of the experimental behavior of the threshold current density.

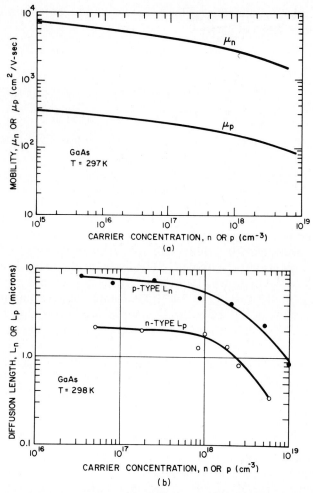

FIG. 7.3-7 (a) Electron and hole mobility as a function of carrier concentration. (b) Minority carrier diffusion length as a function of carrier concentration (Ref. 31).

To describe the behavior of J_{th} with the p-layer thickness, consider the $n_0 = 5 \times 10^{18}$ cm^{-3} data in Fig. 7.3-2 from Ref. 28. At the n–p junction, both the junction current and the refractive index step $\Delta\bar{n}$, which gives Γ, must be considered. With $n_0 = p_0 = 5 \times 10^{18}$ cm^{-3}, $\Delta\bar{n}$ can be estimated from Fig. 2.5-3 to be ~ 0.01. For these values of carrier concentration, L_n in Fig. 7.3-7b is ~ 2 μm, and for $d_3 > 3$ μm, the p–P heterojunction has little influence. For these conditions, $J_{th}(300°K)$ is similar to the homojunction values. As d_2 becomes less than 3 μm, both the carrier and light confinement become better for the SH than for the homostructure laser. The improved optical confinement of the SH laser reduces α_i from $\sim 10^2$ cm^{-1} for the homostructure laser to between 20 and 40 cm^{-1} for SH lasers.[27,35,36] As shown by Eq. (7.3-13), a smaller α_i results in a smaller electron current to reach threshold and thus a smaller V_a and leakage current. For a homostructure, the electron concentration $n(x)$ in the p-layer varies as $\exp(-x/L_n)$, while it decreases more slowly as $\cosh[(d-x)/L_n]/\cosh(d/L_n)$ for the SH. As shown by Figs. 2.6-8 and 2.6-9, the p–P heterojunction aids in confining the light to the p-layer. From Fig. 2.6-9, Γ decreases rapidly as d_2 becomes less than ~ 2 μm. Since the gain coefficient is $g\Gamma$, where g is the uniform-layer gain coefficient, more gain and current are required as Γ becomes smaller. Increased bias to increase i_n also increases the leakage current, and J_{th} becomes larger. At still smaller d_2, lasing can be suppressed when the injected electron concentration approaches the electron concentration of the n-layer or when the waveguide cutoff is reached.

The temperature dependence of J_{th} shown in Fig. 7.3-3 can be expected to be related to the temperature dependence of the nominal current density as shown in Fig. 3.8-8 as well as the larger D_n and the smaller L_n at low temperature. The abrupt increase in current designated by T_t appears to be related to the leakage current J_L. As the cavity is lengthened, less gain is needed to reach threshold, and therefore V_a is smaller, which keeps J_L smaller. Therefore, the leakage current, the temperature dependences of the gain coefficient, D_n, and L_n, and the confinement factor all influence J_{th}. In addition, for the SH laser, the available excitation is limited by the available electron concentration in the n-layer.

Emission Properties

The emission properties of SH lasers are characterized by high-pulsed peak power and small beam divergence. For SH lasers, the emission was observed to be predominately the transverse magnetic (TM) field.[37] Broad-area SH lasers do not emit uniformly along the entire width of the laser facet, but instead they tend to lase in localized regions. These lasing regions are usually referred to as filaments and are discussed more fully in Section 7.4. Longitudinal modes similar to those illustrated in Fig. 3.8-12d are observed and have a spacing given by Eq. (3.8-11).

Gill[26] reported the emission for a SH laser that was Zn diffused into the $n_0 \approx 4 \times 10^{18}$ cm^{-3} substrate to give $d_2 \approx 2$ μm. The device was 180 by 300 μm and had a reflective film on one facet. The $J_{th}(300°$K) was 8.5×10^3 A/cm^2, and the differential quantum efficiency η_D was 0.53. At a current of 20 A (37×10^3 A/cm^2), the output power from one mirror was 11 W, and the external quantum efficiency was 0.40. The maximum emission power is limited by catastrophic facet damage as described in Section 8.2.

For SH lasers with all layers prepared by LPE, Minden and Premo[25] showed that high electron concentrations in the n-layer permitted high emission power.

Because the refractive index step is small at the p–n junction, the fundamental mode is expected even for large active layer thicknesses. The fundamental mode was observed for a p-layer thickness d_2 of 2.5 μm, while for $d_2 = 5.0$ μm, the emission was the second-order mode.[37] With the wide thickness of the active layer and small refractive index step, small beam divergences (see Section 2.7) in the direction perpendicular to the junction plane $\Theta_\perp$ are expected. For SH lasers with $d_2 = 2.0$ μm, $\Theta_\perp$ between $\sim 14°$ and $20°$ were observed.[38] By using an anti-reflection coated facet in conjunction with a diffraction grating, the lasing linewidth was limited to 0.4 Å.[39] The emission properties of SH lasers are summarized in Table 7.3-1.

TABLE 7.3-1   Summary of SH Laser Emission Properties at 300°K with Pulse Excitation[a]

$J_{th}(300°K)^b$	8.5×10^3 A/cm^2
Peak power from one mirror[b]	11 W at 20 A
Differential quantum efficiency	$\sim 50\%$
$\Theta_\perp$	~ 14–$20°$
$\Theta_\parallel$	$\sim 10°$
Emission polarization	TM

[a] See text for literature references.
[b] Reflective coating on one mirror, active-layer thickness ~ 2.0 μm, and 180×300-μm broad-area device.

Time Delays and Internal Q-Switching

When a current pulse of sufficient amplitude to give stimulated emission is applied to a SH laser, two distinct modes of response are observed.[40] In one, there is a delay of a few nanoseconds[29] before the stimulated emission is observed as illustrated in Fig. 7.3-8a. This short delay is related to the carrier lifetime[41] and is observed for homojunction as well as all types of heterostructure lasers. In the other mode of response, stimulated emission only occurs at the end of the pulse even if the pulse width or amplitude is varied as illustrated in Fig. 7.3-8b–d. This effect occurs only above a transition temperature T_t and has been called internal Q-switching.[42] It occurs for both homojunction[42] and SH lasers.[29] This transition temperature is also the temperature where J_{th} in Fig. 7.3-3b abruptly increases. As discussed previously, it seems reasonable to suggest that the transition temperature T_t is also related to J_L. However, the relationship between this

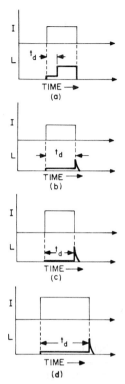

FIG. 7.3-8 Schematic representation of the time response of the SH laser output L for the pulse excitation current I. (a) Normal lasing after a short time delay t_d. (b), (c), and (d) Long time delay which is equal to the length of the excitation pulse and lasing occurs only after the end of the pulse even if the pulse amplitude (c) or length (d) is changed (Ref. 40).

increase in J_L and the observed long-time delay and internal Q-switching is not clearly established or understood. In addition to the long time delays and internal Q-switching, a response designated H-pulsing has been reported for SH lasers.[43] In this case, short light pulses are superimposed on the beginning and end of a steady laser emission at particular temperatures and currents.

The temperature and current region for internal Q-switching for a Zn-diffused SH laser is shown in Fig. 7.3-9. Normal lasing behavior is observed up to the transition temperature T_t. Above this temperature, there is a current and temperature range where internal Q-switching is observed as shown by the shaded region in Fig. 7.3-9. Numerous papers have been published on internal Q-switching in SH lasers, and a critical review was given by Ripper and Rossi.[40] Extensive references to the publications on this subject can be found in that review. Most of the explanations[40] of the

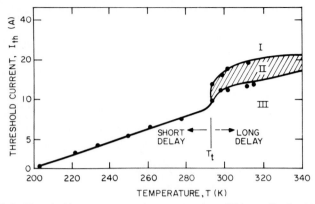

FIG. 7.3-9 Threshold current versus temperature for a SH laser. Region I is the normal lasing region, Region II is the internal Q-switching region (shaded), and Region III is the spontaneous emission region (Ref. 29).

long time delay and internal Q-switching require assumptions such as a particular trapping behavior or nonthermalized carrier distributions. These explanations have not been substantiated. More recently, Nunes *et al.*[44] have proposed a model based on the effects of the injected carriers, the temperature distribution, and gain guiding on the ability of the laser cavity to confine the radiation. This explanation appears quite promising.

7.4 DOUBLE-HETEROSTRUCTURE BROAD-AREA LASERS

Introductory Comments

The GaAs–Al$_x$Ga$_{1-x}$As or Al$_x$Ga$_{1-x}$As–Al$_y$Ga$_{1-y}$As DH laser has been the most extensively studied semiconductor laser, and at the present time its technology is the most advanced. It was the first injection laser to be operated continuously at room temperature[45,46] and above.[47] As discussed in Chapter 8 for these DH lasers, extrapolated room-temperature lifetimes at power levels useful for optical communications are in excess of 10^5 hr.[48] Although stripe-geometry DH lasers are used in most applications, it is instructive to first consider those properties primarily influenced by the parallel layer structure without any kind of lateral restriction. Those properties are most readily investigated with broad-area lasers. For these lasers, data are usually given for pulsed operation with pulse widths of 50–200 μsec and low duty cycles, and only limited data are available for cw operation. This section of Chapter 7 is devoted to the experimental threshold current density behavior and emission properties of GaAs–Al$_x$Ga$_{1-x}$As DH broad-area lasers.

The preceding chapters have given considerable analysis of the broad-area DH laser. The DH layer structure is $N–p–P$ or $N–n–P$ as illustrated in Figs. 1.4-2, 2.3-1, and 2.3-2. Waveguiding in both asymmetric and symmetric DH lasers was considered and numerical values of the confinement factors were given in Chapter 2. Expressions for the threshold current density were derived in Section 3.8. The energy-band diagrams for the DH were presented in Section 4.3, and numerical examples are shown for forward bias in Figs. 4.3-16 and 4.3-17. Carrier confinement in this GaAs–Al$_x$Ga$_{1-x}$As structure was considered in Section 4.6, where it was shown that the carriers were generally well confined. The multiple-layer LPE growth was described in Section 6.5, and the devices are usually fabricated by techniques similar to those presented in Section 7.2.

Threshold Current Dependence at Room Temperature

As would be expected from the discussion of Chapters 2, 3, 4, and 6, the threshold current density and transverse mode behavior of the GaAs–Al$_x$Ga$_{1-x}$As DH laser is dependent primarily upon the dimensions of the structure and upon the refractive index step at the heterojunction interface. Many of the properties of DH lasers can be illustrated with the measurements of Pinkas et al.[49] made on devices fabricated from highly uniform wafers. The threshold current density $J_{th}(300°K)$ as a function of active-layer thickness for DH lasers with identical length and doping are shown in Fig. 7.4-1.

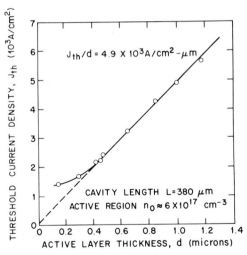

FIG. 7.4-1 Threshold current density at 300°K versus active-layer thickness for DH lasers with n-type GaAs active layers (Ref. 49).

The active layers are n-type GaAs, and the $Al_xGa_{1-x}As$ layers have $x = 0.25$. The measurement of the threshold current was illustrated in Fig. 3.8-10, and the techniques for measuring the active-layer thicknesses were discussed in Section 7.2. The normalized threshold current density J_{th}/d was found to be 4.9×10^3 A/cm²-μm. Additional $J_{th}(300°K)$ data will be presented and discussed later in this part of Section 7.4.

By measuring J_{th} as a function of cavity length, several laser parameters may be numerically evaluated. Equation (3.8-33) for the differential quantum efficiency may be written as

$$1/\eta_D = (1/\eta_{stim})[1 + \alpha_i L/\ln(1/R)], \qquad (7.4\text{-}1)$$

where η_{stim} is the internal quantum efficiency at threshold and α_i the total internal loss. Therefore, $1/\eta_D$ has been plotted in Fig. 7.4-2 as a function of L to permit assignment of $1/\eta_{stim}$ and α_i by Eq. (7.4-1).[49] The intercept at $L = 0$ gives $\eta_{stim} = 0.65$, and solving for α_i at any value of L gives $\alpha_i = 12$ cm^{-1}. These are representative values for DH lasers. The data in Fig. 7.4-2 also emphasizes that η_D decreases as the cavity is lengthened. For example, η_D goes from 0.53 for $L = 225$ μm to 0.29 for $L = 990$ μm.[49]

Until recently it was not understood why η_{stim} did not approach 1.0 because of the lifetime shortening due to stimulated emission and the saturation of nonradiative processes at high excitation levels. Experiments by Henshall[49a] have resolved this dilemma. For sawn-cavity broad-area lasers, he obtained η_{stim} of 0.67, but for proton isolated lasers (see Section 7.6) η_{stim} was 0.90 and $\alpha_i = 12.9$ cm^{-1}. The stripe widths used by Henshall were wide enough to eliminate effects of stripe width on J_{th}. Henshall attributed the difference between η_{stim} for the sawn-cavity broad-area and the proton

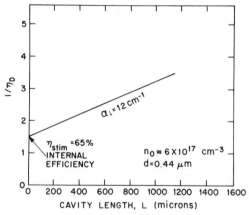

FIG. 7.4-2 Reciprocal of the external differential quantum efficiency versus cavity length for DH lasers at 300°K (Ref. 49).

isolated DH lasers to the presence of internally circulating modes in the sawn-cavity lasers.

The conditions where higher-order transverse modes are obtained were discussed by Yonezu *et al.*[50] The transverse mode order may readily be identified from the far-field emission patterns as illustrated in Fig. 7.4-3. As the active layer thickness d becomes small, the higher-order modes are cut off. At values of d where higher-order modes are permitted, the mode gain is influenced by the mode confinement factor Γ_m that was given in Fig. 2.5-14 and the mode reflectance loss $\ln(1/R_m)$ that was illustrated in Fig. 2.8-2. Threshold will be reached by the mode that first satisfies the threshold relation given by Eq. (3.8-42) as

$$g\Gamma_m = \alpha_i + (1/L)\ln(1/R_m). \tag{7.4-2}$$

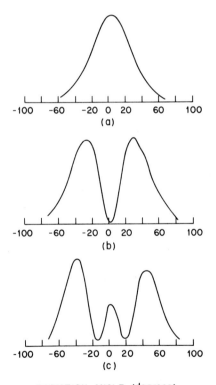

RADIATION ANGLE (degrees)

FIG. 7.4-3 Far-field patterns in the direction perpendicular to the junction plane for $x = 0.43$. (a) Fundamental mode, $d = 0.35\ \mu$m, (b) First-order mode, $d = 0.62\ \mu$m, and (c) Second-order mode, $d = 1.35\ \mu$m (Ref. 50).

At $x = 0.3$ for a symmetric DH laser, the first-order $m = 1$ mode is possible at $d = 0.38$ μm, but the $m = 1$ mode is not observed until $d > 0.7$ μm.[51] The $m = 2$ mode is observed for $d > 1.0$ μm.[51] As x gets larger, the higher-order modes occur at smaller d. Only $J_{th}(300°K)$ for the fundamental mode will be considered in detail.

Most of the experimental studies of DH lasers are for the important case of lasers with d small enough to permit only the fundamental mode. Dyment et al.[52] prepared broad-area DH lasers with $0.1 < d < 0.2$ and obtained the 300°K threshold current density dependence shown in Fig. 7.4-4. Threshold data were also obtained for DH lasers with phosphorus added to the $Al_xGa_{1-x}As$ layers.[52] In that case, J_{th} was lower by about 20%, but the reason for the decreased J_{th} is not understood and will not be considered. The data of Figs. 7.4-1 and 7.4-4 demonstrate that for $d < 0.2$ μm J_{th} continues to decrease with d, but no longer linearly.

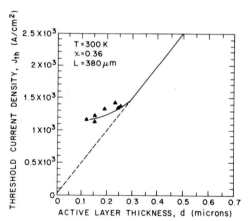

FIG. 7.4-4 Variation of threshold current density with active-layer thickness for GaAs–$Al_xGa_{1-x}As$ DH lasers in the region 0.1–0.25 μm (Ref. 52).

The influence of the $Al_xGa_{1-x}As$ layer composition is illustrated in Fig. 7.4-5 for the data from Ettenberg[53] and Kressel and Ettenberg.[54] The active layers were doped with Sn to give $n_0 \approx 5 \times 10^{17}$ cm^{-3}. For $d > 0.2$ μm, this data is consistent with the data in Figs. 7.4-1 and 7.4-4, and x has little influence on J_{th}. Although the data are scattered at $d \approx 0.1$ μm, J_{th} does decrease for larger x. For the $x = 0.25 \pm 0.05$ data at $d = 0.1$ μm, the J_{th} from Ref. 54 appears somewhat larger than the results from Fig. 7.4-1 at $d < 0.2$ μm and from Ref. 52 as shown by the arrow and open circle. For the $x = 0.50 \pm 0.05$ data at $d \approx 0.1$ μm, the J_{th} values are in good agreement with other results for $x \approx 0.40$.[55] However, for $d = 0.05$ μm, the abrupt increase suggests that this point labeled with the question mark may not

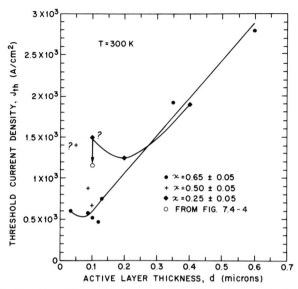

FIG. 7.4-5   Variation of threshold current density with active-layer thickness for GaAs–$Al_xGa_{1-x}As$ DH lasers with the indicated $Al_xGa_{1-x}As$ layer compositions (Ref. 54).

be a representative J_{th}. The data for $x = 0.65 \pm 0.05$ at $d \leq 0.1$ μm are well behaved. For such thin active layers with $d < 0.1$ μm, considerable scatter is expected and scattering loss due to interface roughness can greatly increase J_{th}.[56]

Another effect of x on $J_{th}(300°K)$ was presented in Section 4.6. Rode[57] showed that $J_{th}(300°K)$ increased for $x < 0.25$. In Fig. 4.6-7, it was shown that this increase in $J_{th}(300°K)$ for $x < 0.25$ was due to the leakage current at the p–P or n–P heterojunction. A detailed discussion of the leakage current in GaAs–$Al_xGa_{1-x}As$ DH lasers due to unconfined carriers was given in Section 4.6.

A critical examination of the preceding threshold current density behavior permits giving a representative summary for GaAs–$Al_xGa_{1-x}As$ broad-area DH lasers. These lasers showed that J_{th} was the same for uncompensated n- or p-type active layers as long as the free-carrier concentration was $\sim 1 \times 10^{18}$ cm^{-3} or less. For $d \gtrsim 0.2$ μm, these lasers are characterized by a normalized threshold current density J_{th}/d of about 5.0×10^3 A/cm^2-μm for $L = 400$–500 μm. The one exception is the closely compensated active layer. For $d > 0.2$ μm, Pinkas et al.[49] showed that J_{th}/d for lasers with closely compensated active layers was 3.9×10^3 A/cm^2-μm. A similar result was obtained by Selway and Goodwin[58] and by Hayashi et al.[59] when their J_{th} for shorter cavities are corrected to $L = 500$ μm. However, as d was decreased to about 0.2 μm, J_{th} was essentially the same as for lasers with uncompensated

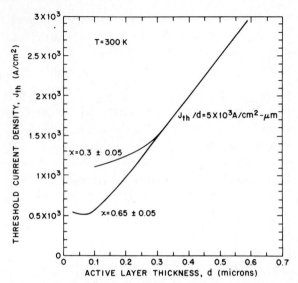

FIG. 7.4-6 Variation of threshold current density with active-layer thickness for GaAs–Al$_x$Ga$_{1-x}$As DH lasers with cavity length $L = 500$ μm. These curves were obtained from a critical assessment of the available experimental data.

active layers. To summarize the J_{th} versus d behavior for broad-area DH lasers with uncompensated active layers, representative values obtained from a critical assessment of the J_{th} data given in Refs. 49, 50, 52, and 54 are given in Fig. 7.4-6 for $x = 0.3 \pm 0.05$ and $x = 0.65 \pm 0.05$. All values have been adjusted to a cavity length of 500 μm. For example, a J_{th} for $L = 400$ μm would be decreased by $\sim 5\%$ for $L = 500$ μm.

Comparison of Experimental and Theoretical Threshold Current Density

The threshold current density dependence on active-layer thickness and composition can be understood from the variation of the required gain coefficient g_{max} with d and x. These gain coefficient values can then be related to J_{th} with Stern's[60] calculated g_{max} dependence on J_{nom} given in Fig. 3.8-7. The calculated g_{max} dependence on J_{nom} is not expected to be significantly different for n- and p-type active layers that are not heavily doped. The gain coefficient at threshold from Eq. (7.4-2) for $m = 0$ may be written as

$$g_{max} = (1/\Gamma)[\alpha_i + (1/L)\ln(1/R)]. \tag{7.4-3}$$

And from Eq. (3.8-25),

$$\alpha_i = \Gamma\alpha_{fc} + (1 - \Gamma)\alpha_{fc,x} + \alpha_s + \alpha_c, \tag{7.4-4}$$

where α_{fc} is the free-carrier loss in the active layer, $\alpha_{fc,x}$ the free-carrier loss in the adjacent Al$_x$Ga$_{1-x}$As layers, α_s the scattering loss, and α_c the coupling loss. For the low J_{th} devices represented in Fig. 7.4-6, α_c is expected to be negligible, and for this discussion, α_s is neglected. From Fig. 3.8-9, $\alpha_{fc} \approx$ 10 cm^{-1}, and for the usual carrier concentrations in the N- and P-layers, $\alpha_{fc,x}$ may also be taken as ~ 10 cm^{-1} to give $\Gamma\alpha_{fc} + (1 - \Gamma)\alpha_{fc,x} \approx 10$ cm^{-1}. These approximations are in reasonable agreement with the experimental data that are generally obtained. The right side of Eq. (7.4-3) has been plotted in Fig. 7.4-7a with $\ln(1/R)$ taken from Fig. 2.8-2, $\alpha_i = 10$ cm^{-1}, and Γ taken from Figs. 2.5-13a,b. The Al$_x$Ga$_{1-x}$As layer composition has been taken as $x = 0.3$ and 0.6. The cavity length is 500 μm. The difference between the two curves results mostly from the difference in Γ for the two values of x. The variation of g_{max} with J_{nom} in Fig. 3.8-7 is reproduced in Fig. 7.4-7b. It should be recalled that the gain-coefficient spectrum shifts with excitation, and that g_{max} is the maximum gain coefficient at a given excitation. Figure 7.4-7 summarizes the gain-coefficient behavior necessary for discussion of the experimental J_{th} dependence on d and x.

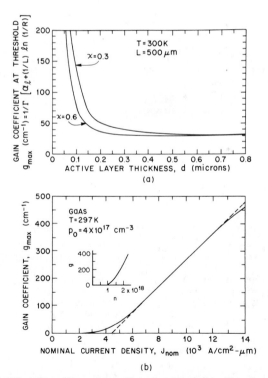

FIG. 7.4-7 (a) Variation of the gain coefficient at threshold with active-layer thickness. (b) Variation of the gain coefficient with the nominal current density. The dashed line represents a linear dependence. The insert shows the relationship between the gain coefficient and the injected electron concentration (Ref. 60).

Figure 7.4-7a shows that at 300°K in the absence of scattering or coupling losses, g_{max} at threshold varies from ~ 200 cm^{-1} near 0.05 μm to ~ 30 cm^{-1} for $d \gtrsim 0.5$ μm. The gain coefficient over this same range of g_{max} is shown in Fig. 7.4-7b to be superlinear at low g_{max} and then varies linearly with J_{nom} for $50 \lesssim g_{max} \lesssim 400$ cm^{-1}. In either case, the zero of g_{max} is offset from $J_{nom} = 0$. For the low gain region, the g_{max} given in Fig. 7.4-7b may be written as

$$g_{max} = 4.7 \times 10^{-6}(J_{nom} - 2 \times 10^3)^2, \tag{7.4-5}$$

and for the higher gain linear region,

$$g_{max} = 5.0 \times 10^{-2}(J_{nom} - 4.5 \times 10^3). \tag{7.4-6}$$

The values of g_{max} calculated from Eqs. (7.4-5) and (7.4-6) are compared in Table 7.4-1. This comparison shows that these equations give approximately the same values for $g_{max} > 75$ cm^{-1}.

The threshold current density was related to J_{nom} by Eq. (3.8-18) as

$$J_{th}(A/cm^2) = J_{nom}d/\eta, \tag{7.4-7}$$

with d in microns for J_{nom} defined for an active-layer thickness of 1 μm. The expression for J_{th} with the gain coefficient represented by Eq. (7.4-5) and g_{max} at 300°K taken as Eq. (7.4-3) becomes

$$J_{th}(A/cm^2) = \frac{2 \times 10^3}{\eta} d + \frac{d}{\eta}\left\{\frac{1}{4.7 \times 10^{-6}\Gamma}\left[\alpha_i + \frac{1}{L}\ln\left(\frac{1}{R}\right)\right]\right\}^{1/2}. \tag{7.4-8}$$

A somewhat different expression results if Eq. (3.8-19), which ignores the J_{nom} zero-offset, is used to relate g_{max} to J_{nom}. Although either representation gives essentially the same numerical result, Eq. (7.4-8) more closely represents the dependence of the gain coefficient on current. In a similar manner for

TABLE 7.4-1 Comparison of g_{max} Calculated from a Linear and Squared Current Dependence

J_{nom} $(10^3$ A/cm^2-μm)	g_{max}(cm^{-1}) $= 4.7 \times 10^{-6}(J_{nom} - 2 \times 10^3)^2$	g_{max}(cm^{-1}) $= 5.0 \times 10^{-2}(J_{nom} - 4.5 \times 10^3)$
2	—	—
3	5	—
4	19	—
5	42	25
6	75	75
7	118	125
8	170	175
9	230	225
10	300	275

g_{max} at 300°K represented by Eq. (7.4-6),

$$J_{th}(A/cm^2) = \frac{4.5 \times 10^3}{\eta} d + \frac{20d}{\eta\Gamma}\left[\alpha_i + \frac{1}{L}\ln\left(\frac{1}{R}\right)\right]. \qquad (7.4-9)$$

This equation is for a linear dependence of the gain coefficient on current which would correspond to $b = 1$ in Eq. (3.8-19), where the J_{nom} zero-offset is ignored. However, in this case, different numerical results are obtained. Therefore, Eq. (7.4-9), which correctly includes the current offset shown in Fig. 7.4-7b, must be used.

Comparison of the experimental and theoretical behavior requires consideration of both the gain coefficient and threshold current density. The experimental gain coefficient obtained from Eq. (7.4-3) for different cavity lengths can be plotted as a function of $J_{th}(300°K)/d$ to permit comparison with g_{max} calculated from Eq. (7 4-5) with Eq. (7.4-7) to relate $J_{th}(300°K)$ to J_{nom}. The case to be considered here is for $d \gtrsim 0.4$ μm so that g_{max} is small and in the superlinear region. Then, the variation of the experimental $J_{th}(300°K)$ with d that was summarized in Fig. 7.4-6 will be compared with the theoretical $J_{th}(300°K)$ represented by Eq. (7.4-9). Active layers as thin as 0.05 μm are considered. For thin active layers, g_{max} is large, and $J_{th}(300°K)$ may be represented by the linear relation of Eq. (7.4-9).

For $d \gtrsim 0.4$ μm, $\Gamma \approx 1$, and Eq. (7.4-3) may be used to obtain g_{max} at threshold for a given cavity length.[49] By selecting a range of cavity lengths, a range of g_{max} versus $J_{th}(300°K)$ may be obtained. In this manner, g_{max} for $\alpha_i = 12$ cm^{-1} and $\ln(1/R) = 1.1$ have been plotted in Fig. 7.4-8 as a function of the normalized threshold current $J_{th}(300°K)/d$. This figure illustrates the effect of the active-layer doping on the gain coefficient. It shows that the gain coefficient for compensated layers is larger at low $J_{th}(300°K)/d$, but effects of doping become insignificant at $g_{max} \gtrsim 100$ cm^{-1}. The g_{max} calculated from the current-squared expression of Eq. (7.4-5) is also shown, and it agrees very closely with the experimental g_{max} for the uncompensated active layers.

For d sufficiently large that $\Gamma \approx 1$ and $\alpha_i + (1/L)\ln(1/R) \approx 30$ cm^{-1}, $J_{th}(300°K)$ from Eq. (7.4-8) gives $J_{th}(300°K)/d = 4.5 \times 10^3$ A/cm^2-μm, and Eq. (7.4-9) gives $J_{th}(300°K)/d = 5.1 \times 10^3$ A/cm^2-μm when η is taken as unity. The experimental $J_{th}(300°K)/d$ is 4.9–5.0 $\times 10^3$ A/cm^2-μm. It should be noted that g_{max} in Figs. 3.8-7 and 7.4-8 was calculated from first principles without any adjustable parameters.

The calculated $J_{th}(300°K)$ is compared to the experimental J_{th} of Fig.7.4-6 in Fig. 7.4-9. Values of R and $\ln(1/R)$ are taken from Figs. 2.8-1 and 2.8-2, and $\ln(1/R)$ varies from 1.25 to 0.85 over the range of d and x considered in Fig. 7.4-9. The values for Γ are taken from Fig. 2.5-13a, b. The loss has been taken as $\alpha_{fc} = \alpha_{fc,x} = 10$ cm^{-1}, and $L = 500$ μm. In Fig. 7.4-9a, Eq. (7.4-8),

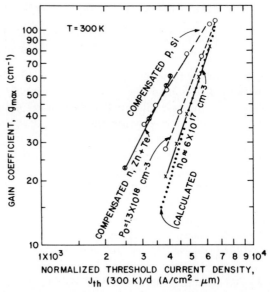

FIG. 7.4-8 Dependence of the gain coefficient for DH lasers on the normalized threshold current density $J_{th}(300°K)/d$ for differently doped active layers (Ref. 49). The theoretical g_{max} calculated from Eq. (7.4-5) is shown by the dotted line.

representing the current squared variation of the gain coefficient, has been used with $\eta = 0.9$ in order to obtain agreement between the calculated and experimental J_{th} at $d = 0.5$ μm. The calculated and experimental J_{th} for $x = 0.6$ are in very good agreement; however, for $x = 0.3$ and $d \lesssim 0.2$ μm the calculated J_{th} is less than the experimental J_{th}. This difference is ~ 300 A/cm^2 at $d = 0.1$ μm. In Fig. 7.4-9b, Eq. (7.4-9), representing the linear variation of the gain coefficient with current, has been plotted with $\eta = 1$. Again the fit for $x = 0.6$ is very good, while for $x = 0.3$ the calculated and experimental J_{th}^* differ by ~ 400 A/cm^2 at $d = 0.1$ μm. Other choices of parameters do not improve the fit for $x = 0.3$ at small d. Expressions for J_{th} based on Eq. (3.8-19) may be curve fit at larger d ($d > 0.5$) with various choices of the power dependence parameter b. These representations of J_{th} also do not improve the fit at small d for $x = 0.3$. Since Eqs. (7.4-8) and (7.4-9) each give almost the same numerical results, it is most convenient to use the linear expression given by Eq. (7.4-9) for calculation of $J_{th}(300°K)$. These curves for the J_{th} variation with d that were calculated from first principles provide a useful guide to the expected minimum J_{th} for a given x and d. In fact, the recent low value $J_{th}(300°K)$ results of Dupuis et al.[60a] for the GaAs–Al$_x$Ga$_{1-x}$As DH lasers prepared by organometallic decomposition CVD are in good agreement with the calculated curves given in Fig. 7.4-9b. For example, at $x = 0.52$ and $d = 0.05$ μm, $J_{th}(300°K)$ was 630 A/cm^2, and at the same x but

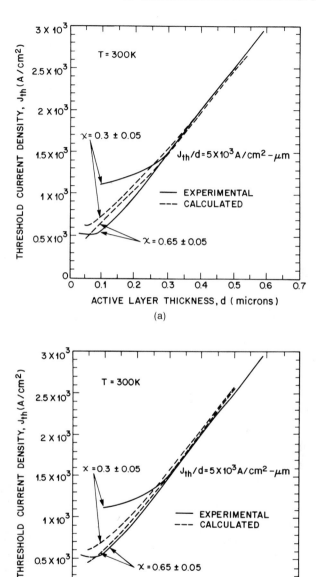

FIG. 7.4-9 Comparison of the experimental and calculated J_{th}. (a) Calculated curve from Eq. (7.4-8) for $g_{max} = \beta(J_{th} - J_0)^2$. (b) Calculated curve from Eq. (7.4-9) for $g_{max} = \beta(J_{th} - J_0)$.

with $d = 0.18$ μm, $J_{th}(300°K)$ was 940 A/cm^2. At $x = 0.38$ and $d = 0.16$ μm, $J_{th}(300°K)$ was 1×10^3 A/cm^2.

Before considering the excess current for $d < 0.2$ and $x = 0.3$, it is useful to plot each term of Eq. (7.4-9) for $x = 0.3$ and 0.6 as a function of d. The first term [see Eqs. (7.4-6) and (7.4-7)], $4.5 \times 10^3 d/\eta$, represents the excitation necessary for band-to-band absorption to be reduced to zero and varies directly with d as shown in Fig. 7.4-10 for $\eta = 1.0$. The second term, $(20d/\eta\Gamma)[\alpha_i + (1/L)\ln(1/R)]$, represents the additional gain coefficient that is necessary to overcome the losses. Since most of the variation of this term is due to Γ for $\alpha_i = 10$ cm^{-1} and $(1/L)\ln(1/R) = 20$ cm^{-1}, the second term may be written as $600d/\Gamma$ for $\eta = 1.0$. This term has also been plotted in Fig. 7.4-10 for $x = 0.3$ and 0.6 to illustrate that Γ (see Fig. 2.5-13) for a given x varies approximately as d, and then the $600d/\Gamma$ term and hence J_{th} are relatively independent of Γ.

The excess current for $d < 0.2$ and $x = 0.3$ may now be discussed by considering the $(20d/\Gamma)[\alpha_i + (1/L)\ln(1/R)]$ term. From the analysis for leakage current due to unconfined carriers[60b] given in Section 4.6, the calculated leakage current for $x = 0.3$ is less than 100 A/cm^2 for the expected injected electron concentration [see Fig. 7.4-7b)] of $\sim 2 \times 10^{18}$ cm^{-3}. Most DH lasers have Al$_x$Ga$_{1-x}$As layers that are sufficiently thick to prevent

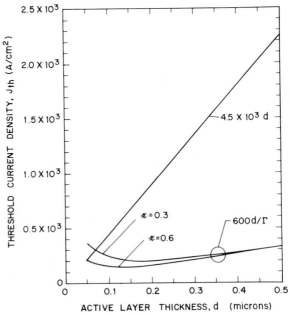

FIG. 7.4-10 Illustration of the influence of Γ on J_{th} calculated from each term of Eq. (7.4-9) with Γ from Fig. 2.5-13.

significant coupling losses α_c. The results of an investigation of scattering loss by Thompson et al.[60c] showed that losses of 12 cm^{-1} result for a roughness amplitude of only 0.01 μm. Since the scattering loss becomes larger as d is decreased,[56] it appears that effects of α_s at small d may account for the difference in the experimental and calculated J_{th} at $d = 0.1$ and $x = 0.3$. A scattering loss of ~ 30 cm^{-1} can double the $(20d/\Gamma)[\alpha_i + (1/L)\ln(1/R)]$ term from 240 A/cm^2 to 480 A/cm^2 to give $J_{th} = 930$ A/cm^2. As α_s becomes significant, the loss $(1/\Gamma)[\alpha_i + (1/L)\ln(1/R)]$ increases and a larger n is required. When $n = 3 \times 10^{18}$ cm^{-3}, the leakage current becomes ~ 100 A/cm^2 and grows rapidly for $n > 3 \times 10^{18}$ cm^{-3}. Since α_s also increases with the refractive index step, the absence of a significant scattering loss for $x = 0.6$ suggests a more planar heterojunction interface for $x = 0.6$ than $x = 0.3$. However, since Γ at $x = 0.6$ is larger than for $x = 0.3$ and α_s enters J_{th} as α_s/Γ, the effect for the same α_s would be larger for $x = 0.3$ than $x = 0.6$. Also, at $x = 0.6$, the injected electron concentration could become large before any significant leakage current occurs. It appears that for small d and x near 0.3, scattering can increase the loss, which increases the necessary injected electron concentration to levels where carrier leakage currents also become significant. Nash et al.[56] related the observed J_{th} variations for a given d and x to the scattering loss.

Threshold Current Density Temperature Dependence

The temperature dependence of J_{th} for a DH laser in which carriers are completely confined is expected to depend almost entirely on the temperature dependence of the gain coefficient. The variation with temperature of the refractive index steps, mirror reflectivities, free-carrier losses, scattering losses, and coupling losses is expected to have a much smaller effect. The experimental dependence of $J_{th}(T)$ is illustrated with the early measurements by Hayashi et al.[59] and Panish et al.[61] with GaAs–Al$_x$Ga$_{1-x}$As ($x = 0.2$–0.4) DH lasers that had Si-doped (compensated) active layers with $0.5 \leq d \leq 2.0$ μm. These data are the only measurements of $J_{th}(T)$ over an extensive temperature range at room temperature and below that have been reported for DH lasers. The temperature dependence of J_{th} is illustrated for $d = 0.5$, 1.0, and 2.0 μm in Fig. 7.4-11. The temperature variation of J_{th} may be represented by Eq. (7.3-1) for T_0 between 120° and 165°K. For comparison, a calculated $J_{nom}(T)$ is also shown. It was obtained with the GHLBT–SME model for the gain coefficient (see Sections 3.7 and 3.8) and is the $N_A = 13 \times 10^{18}$, $N_D = 10 \times 10^{18}$ cm^{-3} curve given in Fig. 3.8-8. This comparison confirms that the experimental variation of J_{th} from approximately 100° to 300°K is in fact due primarily to the variation of the gain coefficient.

At room temperature and above, the current due to incomplete carrier confinement can also affect $J_{th}(T)$. As shown in Fig. 4.6-6, the electron leakage

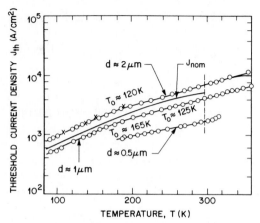

FIG. 7.4-11   Threshold current density versus temperature for DH lasers (Ref. 59). The calculated J_{nom} is from Fig. 3.8-8.

current depends on x, the temperature, and electron concentration. Since the greatest dependence is upon x, it is possible to compare $J_{th}(T)$ for DH lasers prepared by different workers even though there are differences in geometry and doping. The changes in J_{th} between 10° and 65°C obtained by Goodwin et al.[62] and between 22° and 70°C obtained by Kressel and Ettenberg[54] are shown in Fig. 7.4-12. For some of these lasers there is a small amount of Al in the active layer so that the composition parameter is Δx rather than x. The J_{th} values are for pulse excitation. Part of the scatter in this data probably results from the use of lasers with different doping, L, and d. For the lasers with the highest Δx, almost all of the increase in J_{th} over the approximately 50°C temperature range results from the temperature dependence of the gain coefficient. The increase in J_{th} due to g_{max} is approximately 30%. The remainder of the increase for the other lasers in Fig. 7.4-12 can be ascribed to electron leakage. These comparisons of the temperature dependence of J_{th} on x above room temperature are particularly important because they cover a range of active region temperatures that is useful for cw degradation studies as well as possible cw operating temperatures.

Influence of $Al_xGa_{1-x}As$ Layer Thickness on Threshold Current Density

In the discussion of the $GaAs–Al_xGa_{1-x}As$ DH lasers presented in the previous parts of this section, it has been assumed that the N- and P-layers that bound the active layer were sufficiently thick to terminate the optical fields. As shown in Fig. 2.3-1, these N- and P-layers are bounded by the n^+ substrate and usually a p^+ contact layer. If the N- or P-layer becomes too thin, the optical fields begin to penetrate into the adjacent n^+- or p^+-layers.

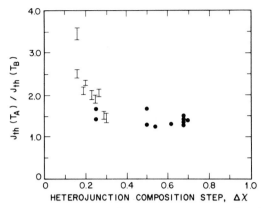

FIG. 7.4-12   The ratio $J_{th}(T)$ at two different temperatures as a function of composition difference Δx between the active layer and the bounding $Al_xGa_{1-x}As$ layers. I: A = 65°C, B = 10°C (Ref. 62). ●: A = 70°C, B = 22°C (Ref. 54).

Optical energy is then lost to these layers. This additional loss is the previously designated coupling loss and results in an increase in J_{th} and a reduction in η_D. Both experimental studies[63] and theoretical analysis[64,65] of this problem have been reported. The influence of the $Al_xGa_{1-x}As$ layer thickness on the threshold current density is illustrated by the comparison of the analysis by Streifer *et al.*[65] with the experimental results of Casey and Panish.[63]

The DH lasers used for the experimental measurements had N–$Al_{0.3}Ga_{0.7}As$ layers with a thickness in excess of 3 μm. The GaAs active layer was Si-doped and had a thickness d_2 of not more than 0.15 μm or less than 0.10 μm, with a typical value of 0.12 μm. The thickness of the P–$Al_{0.3}Ga_{0.7}As$ layer d_3 was varied between 0.25 and 2.3 μm. The P–$Al_{0.3}Ga_{0.7}As$ layer was bounded by the p^+–GaAs contact layer. As shown in Fig. 7.4-13a, J_{th} abruptly increases for $d_3 < 0.8$ μm, while in part (b) η_D abruptly decreases. From consideration of the optical intensity distribution,[63] a useful guideline for the $Al_xGa_{1-x}As$ layer thickness to terminate the optical fields for d_2 near 0.1 μm was found to be

$$d_3(\mu m) \approx 0.24/x, \qquad (7.4\text{-}10)$$

or for d_2 near 0.2 μm,

$$d_3(\mu m) \approx 0.18/x. \qquad (7.4\text{-}11)$$

In their analysis, Streifer *et al.*[65] considered the flow of optical power through the thin $Al_xGa_{1-x}As$ layer into an adjacent GaAs layer. The calculated J_{th} followed the data given in Fig. 7.4-13a. They also showed that for thick active layers, the coupling loss was dependent on the mode order

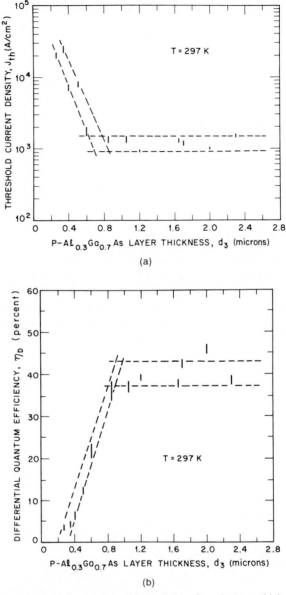

(a)

(b)

FIG. 7.4-13   Variation of J_{th} and η_D with the P–$Al_{0.3}Ga_{0.7}As$ layer thickness. The range of J_{th} or η_D observed for several devices from the same wafer is represented by the length of the short vertical lines. The dashed line represents the approximate boundaries of the data. (a) Threshold current density; (b) Differential quantum efficiency (Ref. 63).

and could be used to retain the fundamental mode when the first-order mode normally would dominate. This analysis led to a broad-area DH laser with so-called leaky-wave coupling through a 0.1 μm N–$Al_{0.24}Ga_{0.76}As$ layer to the substrate.[66] The leaky-wave coupling provided a highly collimated output beam through the substrate at the cleaved mirror with an approximately 2° beam divergence perpendicular to the junction plane. The peak pulsed power at $2J_{th}$ was 1.5 W from one facet with approximately one-third of the power in the collimated beam. These characteristics were obtained at an increase of J_{th} of approximately 30% when compared to otherwise similar DH lasers with N- or P-layers sufficiently thick to terminate the optical fields.

$Al_yGa_{1-y}As$ Active Layers

As with SH lasers, the emission may be shifted to shorter wavelength by adding Al to the active layer to give $Al_xGa_{1-x}As|Al_yGa_{1-y}As|Al_xGa_{1-x}As$ DH lasers. These DH lasers are of particular interest because an important application of the DH laser with an $Al_yGa_{1-y}As$ active layer is for optical-fiber (lightwave) communication systems. A representative optical-loss spectrum for the optical fibers available in quantity for lightwave communication systems is shown in Fig. 7.4-14.[67] The loss peaks between 0.85 and 1.0 μm are due to OH-ion absorption. The optical-loss spectrum for an optical fiber produced in the laboratory with low OH-ion concentration was shown in Fig. 5.1-1. Emission in the low-loss 0.85-μm-wavelength region may be obtained with $0.05 \lesssim y \lesssim 0.1$ and $0.3 \lesssim x \lesssim 0.4$. Practical DH lasers for lightwave communication applications are stripe-geometry rather than

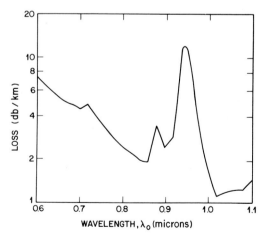

FIG. 7.4-14   Loss spectrum for an optical fiber with a SiO_2 core and B_2O_3–SiO_2 cladding (Ref. 67).

broad-area lasers. However, the $Al_xGa_{1-x}As$ active layer DH lasers will be briefly described here because the carrier confinement at the heterojunctions rather than the lateral confinement along the junction plane influences the laser behavior as Al is added to the active layer.

The lasing wavelength may be decreased further by simultaneously increasing x and y until y approaches the direct–indirect crossover composition near 0.4. Miller *et al.*[68] first reported visible cw operation with emission at wavelengths as short as 0.773 μm with $y = 0.21$ for active layer thickness of 0.4–0.6 μm. Itoh *et al.*[69] used larger values of x and obtained lasing wavelengths of 0.761 μm for cw excitation and 0.668 μm for pulsed excitation. More recently Kressel and Hawrylo[70] reported data for DH lasers with $x = 0.6$ and y varied to give emission wavelengths as short as 0.70 μm for pulsed excitation. The active-layer thicknesses were between 0.08 and 0.15 μm, and the P–$Al_{0.6}Ga_{0.4}As$ layers were doped with Zn. Comparative experiments using Ge and Zn for the acceptor in the P–$Al_{0.6}Ga_{0.4}As$ layer showed that it was more difficult to achieve highly conductive layers with Ge than with Zn.[70]

A summary of J_{th} versus the emission wavelength is shown in Fig. 7.4-15 for the data of Miller *et al.*,[68] Itoh *et al.*,[69] Kressel and Hawrylo,[70] Ettenburg,[53] and Alferov *et al.*[71] Much of the difference in J_{th} obtained by the various authors at a particular wavelength is due to the differences in active layer thickness. The abrupt increase in J_{th} near 0.77 μm in Fig. 7.4-15

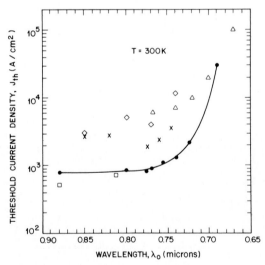

FIG. 7.4-15 Threshold current density versus emission wavelength for Al_xGa_{1-x}-$As|Al_yGa_{1-y}As|Al_xGa_{1-x}As$ DH lasers (Ref. 70). ×—Ref. 68, △—Ref. 69, ●—Ref. 70, ◇—Ref. 71, and ☐—Ref. 53.

is due to the thermal excitation of injected carriers into the indirect conduction bands. Those carriers do not contribute to stimulated emission. The distribution of electrons between the direct and indirect conduction bands was discussed in Section 4.6.

Emission Properties

Many of the emission properties of GaAs–Al$_x$Ga$_{1-x}$As DH lasers were discussed in detail in the preceding chapters. In Section 2.7, the far-field pattern was related to the optical-field confinement due to the refractive index steps at the heterojunctions. An example of the far-field emission both perpendicular and parallel to the junction plane was shown in Fig. 2.7-4. The full angle at the half-power points (FAHP) for the emission perpendicular to the junction plane as a function of active layer thickness for x between 0.1 and 0.6 was given in Fig. 2.7-5. Variation of the emission spectra with current, both below and above J_{th}, was illustrated in Fig. 3.8-12. In lasers with lightly doped active layers, two peaks have been observed in the spontaneous spectra. However, for lightly doped n-type active layers ($n_0 \approx 2 \times 10^{16}$ cm^{-3}), Kressel et al.[72] have shown that the lower energy peak is spurious and results from selective internal absorption of spontaneous radiation in the GaAs substrate.

A family of longitudinal modes is illustrated in Fig. 7.4-16. Polarization is predominately TE. Generally, for broad-area DH lasers at $J > J_{th}$, the mode

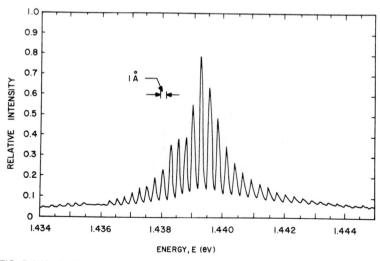

FIG. 7.4-16 Lasing spectrum of a single transverse-mode DH laser with multiple longitudinal modes.

spectrum suggests the presence of several mode families which are presumably the result of the filamentary lasing described below. As the current is increased, more filaments reach threshold and the minima between the discrete lines begin to fill in. The longitudinal mode spacing was given by Eq. (3.8-11). The lasing envelope occurs at a few meV below the energy gap for high purity GaAs and has about the same temperature dependence as the energy gap.[73] The variation of the optical output as a function of the laser current was illustrated in Fig. 3.8-10.

The near-field emission of a broad-area GaAs–$Al_xGa_{1-x}As$ DH laser is shown in Fig. 7.4-17a. Part (b) shows the variation of the emission intensity

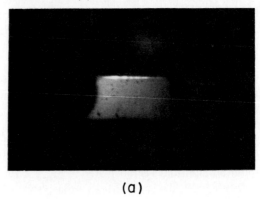

(a)

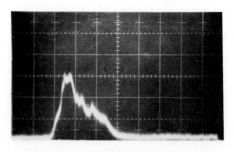

(b)

FIG. 7.4-17   Near-field emission at 297°K of a GaAs–$Al_xGa_{1-x}As$ DH laser to illustrate the filamentary emission. (a) Emission observed with an infrared image converter. The width of the mirror facet is 165 μm. (b) Single line scan of the near-field intensity as measured with a Si-target vidicon.

as measured by a single-line scan with a Si-target vidicon. The distinct and localized regions of stimulated emission are referred to as filaments. Visual observation of the onset of the filaments through an infrared image-converter microscope is a very convenient technique for observing the threshold of broad-area lasers. As the current is increased, the number of lasing filaments increases. Each filament appears to have its own threshold, and lasers with high differential efficiency have the most uniform near-field emission. The effect of near-field uniformity on catastrophic failure of heterostructure lasers is discussed in Section 8.2. The filament formation has been attributed to a localized increase in the refractive index due to a depletion of the injected carrier concentration,[74] and a refractive index step due to differences between the quasi-Fermi levels of lasing and nonlasing regions.[75] Presently no general agreement on the origin of filaments has been obtained. The lateral optical confinement of an individual filament due to gain guiding in stripe-geometry lasers is considered in Section 7.10.

A summary of the emission properties of GaAs–$Al_xGa_{1-x}As$ DH lasers is given in Table 7.4-2. The emission properties have a strong depencence on the active layer thickness and the composition of the bounding $Al_xGa_{1-x}As$ layers. High peak power for pulse excitation was considered by Kirkby and Thompson.[76] The maximum output power for pulsed operation is limited by catastropic degradation of the mirror facet and is discussed in Section 8.2. The maximum power for cw operation is generally limited by heating. The parameters that influence the power efficiency at high power levels have been investigated by Whiteaway and Thompson.[76a]

TABLE 7.4-2 Summary of Typical GaAs–$Al_xGa_{1-x}As$ DH
Laser Emission Properties at 300°K[a,b]

Pulse excitation	
$J_{th}(300°K)^b$	$0.6–1.5 \times 10^3$ A/cm²
Peak power from one mirror	2–5 W
η_D	$\sim 40–50\%$
$\Theta_\perp{}^c$	$\sim 20–40°$
$\Theta_\parallel$	$\sim 10°$
Emission polarization	TE
cw Operation	
Maximum power from one mirror[d]	0.39 W at ~ 3 A

[a] Broad-area laser (~ 100 μm wide and ~ 400 μm long) with $d \leq 0.2$ μm.

[b] See Fig. 7.4-6 for J_{th} versus d with $x = 0.3$ and 0.6.

[c] See Fig. 2.7-5 for $\Theta_\perp$ versus d for x between 0.1 and 0.6.

[d] N. Chinone, R. Ito, and O. Nakada, *J. Appl. Phys.* **47**, 785 (1976). This device was an 80-μm-wide mesa-stripe laser with a 300-μm cavity length.

Other Properties

Often, the initial measurement of an injection laser is the forward bias current–voltage (I–V) characteristic. An I–V characteristic for a representative broad-area GaAs–Al$_{0.3}$Ga$_{0.7}$As DH laser is shown in Fig. 7.4-18. The voltage at 1 mA is generally near 1.1–1.2 V. If the forward bias current at a given voltage significantly exceeds the values shown here, the device generally has excess current paths and a high J_{th}. The reverse breakdown depends on the impurity concentrations and generally is greater than 6 V. The semilogarithmic I–V plot shows that the current varies as $\exp(qV/2kT)$ for many decades. At higher currents near threshold, heating influences the I–V measurements, but it appears that I continues to vary as $\exp(qV/2kT)$. The models for I–V behavior were presented in Section 4.5. It has been shown by Henry et al.[76b] that the $\exp(qV/2kT)$ current in GaAs–Al$_x$Ga$_{1-x}$As heterojunctions is due to surface recombination. The expected current dependence as $\exp(qV/kT)$ for a diffusion current is not observed. The development of a

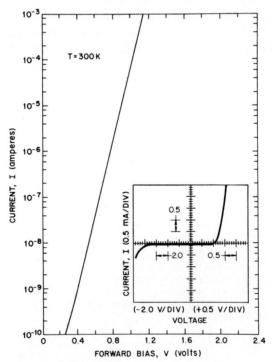

FIG. 7.4-18 Current–voltage characteristic for a broad-area GaAs–Al$_{0.3}$Ga$_{0.7}$As DH laser. The cross-sectional area is 6.0×10^{-4} cm^2.

theoretical model that describes the experimental I–V behavior of GaAs–$Al_xGa_{1-x}As$ heterojunctions would be useful.

There are a number of topics pertaining to broad-area GaAs–$Al_xGa_{1-x}As$ DH lasers that have not been presented here in order to keep this presentation reasonably brief. These topics include, for example, discussions of the power per cavity mode[77,78] and the flexural and longitudinal vibrations that occur during pulse excitation.[79] Modifications to the usual DH laser have been made, such as an additional junction to give N–p–n–P lasers that switch rapidly.[80,81] Also, properly designed broad-area DH lasers can be used as phase[82] or intensity modulators.[83] It should be noted that by eliminating one mirror, the DH laser becomes a super-radiant light-emitting diode (LED) with a higher radiance and smaller beam divergence than for other LED configurations.[84]

7.5 SEPARATE-CONFINEMENT BROAD-AREA LASERS

Introductory Comments

Waveguiding in four- and five-layer heterostructures has been discussed in Section 2.9. Carrier confinement by heterojunctions was illustrated in Section 4.6. With the background provided by these two sections, the basic concepts of separate-confinement heterostructure (SCH) lasers may readily be illustrated. The notation that uses lowercase n or p for the smallest energy-gap semiconductors and uppercase N or P for the larger energy-gap semiconductors is conveniently subscripted to give n_x, N_y, or P_z, where x, y, z are the AlAs mole fraction of the solid solution. As with the SH and DH lasers, SCH lasers can be fabricated as either broad-area or stripe-geometry lasers. In this section, the discussion will be restricted to those properties primarily influenced by carrier and optical confinement perpendicular to the junction plane. Further application of the SCH laser to distributed-feedback structures will be presented in Section 7.12.

Consideration of the carrier and optical confinement properties of hetero-junctions illustrates how these properties may be exploited further by using multiple-layer structures. For an asymmetric N_xpP_y heterostructure with $x > y$, the energy band diagram is schematically represented in Fig. 7.5-1a at high forward bias. Although the injected electron concentration in the p-active layer was shown in Fig. 4.6-1 to decrease exponentially with energy in the conduction band, the level of the injected electrons is schematically represented by the dashed line. In this example, the barrier at the p–P_y interface is too small to adequately confine the injected electrons and gives a disffusive electron leakage current as illustrated in Figs. 4.6-6 and 4.6-7. An additional heterojunction is added to give a $N_xpP_yP_x$ structure as shown

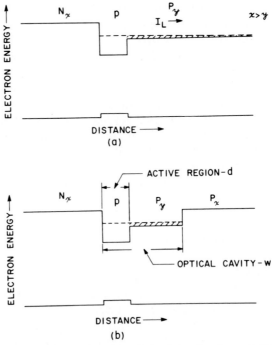

FIG. 7.5-1 Schematic representation of the heterojunction energy band diagram. (a) For the N_xpP_y structure, the unconfined electrons are indicated by the cross-hatched regions and contribute the leakage current I_L. (b) For the $N_xpP_yP_x$ structure, the leakage current is prevented by the P_y–P_x heterojunction.

in Fig. 7.5-1b. Although the electrons are still not totally confined at the p–P_y interface, the P_y–P_x interface does provide confinement and prevents a diffusive leakage current. Almost all the carriers are confined to the active layer even for $y \approx 0.1$. Thus, the carriers are adequately confined to the active layer by the small conduction band step at the p–P_y interface, while the optical field is largely confined on the p-side by the refractive index step at the P_y–P_x interface as illustrated in Fig. 2.9-2. This behavior has led to the development of several types of heterostructures in which most of the injected carriers are confined to a region significantly narrower than the waveguide. All of these structures may be classified as separate-confinement heterostructure (SCH) lasers.

There are two convenient subclassifications of the SCH lasers, symmetric and asymmetric, as well as several analogous lasers having a p–n homojunction or a p–n heterojunction within the waveguide. The LOC lasers,[85–88] which have a p–n junction within the waveguide, are frequently designated as $NnpP$ structures[89,90] and were illustrated in Fig. 2.9-4. When a small amount of Al is added to the n region of an $NnpP$ laser, the resulting structure has a p–n heterojunction in the waveguide and is usually referred to as a $Nn'pP$ laser.[91–93] The symmetric SCH lasers are $N_x N_y pP_y P_x$ or $N_x N_y nP_y P_x$ with $x > y$.[55,94–96] In the symmetric case, the N_y-layer thickness is the same as the thickness of the P_y-layer thickness, and this structure was illustrated in Fig. 2.9-1. The asymmetric SCH lasers are $N_x N_y nP_z P_u$ or $N_x N_y pP_z P_u$ with $x > y$ and $z < u$.[97,98] Some layers may be omitted, and there is no restriction on the thickness of the N_y or P_z layers. For all the above structures, the p- or n-active region was written as containing no Al, but it can contain Al and frequently does. Fabrication procedures for SCH lasers are the same as previously described in Section 7.2.

Large-Optical Cavity Laser

The large-optical cavity (LOC) laser was first introduced in the $NnpP$ form by Lockwood et al.[85] Most of the junction current is the injection of electrons into the p-layer which is the active region. The p–P heterojunction provides both carrier and optical confinement. The n–N heterojunction provides optical confinement and prevents the optical field from spreading as it does in the SH laser (see Fig. 2.6-8). Thus, the optical cavity width w is the sum of the n- and p-layer thicknesses. Also, the n–N heterojunction prevents a hole leakage current. The small refractive index step due to doping at the p–n junction also influences the optical field as discussed in Section 2.9 for the $Nn'pP$ laser. The carrier and optical field confinement properties of the heterojunctions permit moderately low threshold current densities even with rather large optical cavity thickness. The variation of $J_{th}(300°K)$ and η_D with the n-layer thickness d_n is shown in Fig. 7.5-2. Unfortunately, there is insufficient information on the refractive index profile of these lasers to permit meaningful calculations of the optical fields as was done for the $Nn'pP$ structure in Section 2.9.

Experimentally, $NnpP$ lasers with composition, doping, and dimensional parameters similar to the lasers used for Fig. 7.5-2 emit radiation with TE polarization and higher-order transverse modes. The dominant mode ranged from $m = 3$ to $m = 6$ with $0.3 \leq d \leq 0.5$ μm and $2.8 \leq w \leq 4$ μm.[88] These lasers with large-optical cavities have higher power output before catastrophic mirror damage than most DH lasers because the optical power is not so highly confined in the active layer. Pulsed power outputs of 0.6 W from one mirror for 2.5 A were reported.[87]

The $Nn'pP$ form of the LOC laser described in Section 2.9 was suggested[91,92] for the attainment of several desired properties. These properties are operation in the fundamental transverse mode while maintaining a relatively low J_{th}, a high-power catastrophic damage limit, and a relatively

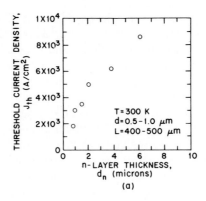

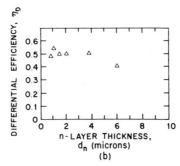

FIG. 7.5-2 Properties of LOC lasers with active-layer thickness between 0.5 and 1.0 μm as a function of the *n*-layer thickness d_n. (a) Threshold current density. (b) Differential quantum efficiency (Ref. 86).

narrow beam divergence.[91-93] Unfortunately, there is little experimental data for lasers with this structure. Figures 2.9-6 and 2.9-7 illustrate how selection of the active-layer and optical-cavity thickness can be used to obtain fundamental transverse mode emission. Detailed studies that follow the suggestions in Ref. 93 would be helpful.

Symmetric SCH Laser

The slab waveguide for the symmetric SCH laser was illustrated in Fig. 2.9-1. This laser structure was suggested by Hayashi[96] and by Thompson and Kirkby[97] in order to obtain lasers with low $J_{th}(300°K)$ while maintaining the fundamental transverse mode and a moderate beam divergence. A scanning-electron photomicrograph of the cross section of a symmetric SCH laser was given in Fig. 6.5-9 together with the energy gap and refractive index profile.

The previous expressions for J_{th} that were derived in Section 7.4 for the DH laser can also be used for the SCH laser. Equation (7.4-9), which represents a linear dependence of the gain coefficient on current, can be used for J_{th} with α_i given by

$$\alpha_i = \Gamma\alpha_{fc} + \Gamma_y\alpha_{fc,y} + \Gamma_x\alpha_{fc,x} + \alpha_s + \alpha_c, \qquad (7.5\text{-}1)$$

where Γ_y is the fraction of the optical field in the N_y and P_y layers, and Γ_x is the fraction of the optical field in the N_x and P_x layers. For this calculation of J_{th}, the scattering loss α_s and coupling loss α_c are neglected, and α_i is taken as 10 cm^{-1}. In the absence of calculated values of the facet reflectivity for SCH lasers, the value from DH lasers of $\ln(1/R) \approx 1.0$ that was given in Fig. 2.8-2 will be used. For $L = 500$ μm, $[\alpha_i + (1/L)\ln(1/R)]$ in Eq. (7.4-9) becomes 30 cm^{-1}. The value of $\eta = 0.77$ obtained in Ref. 55 gives J_{th} in Eq. (7.4-9) as

$$J_{th}(\text{A/cm}^2) = 5.8 \times 10^3 d + 780d/\Gamma. \qquad (7.5\text{-}2)$$

The J_{th} calculated from Eq. (7.5-2) with Γ from Fig. 2.9-3 for $w = 0.5$ and 1.0 μm with $x = 0.3$ and $y = 0.1$ is shown in Fig. 7.5-3. Experimental values of J_{th} from Refs. 55 and 95 with $L \approx 500$ μm are also shown. The values of x and y as well as the layer thicknesses and cavity lengths and widths are tabulated in Refs. 55 and 95. Typical values are $y = 0.1$–0.12, $x = 0.30$–0.40 with w between 0.8 and 1.5 μm. Agreement is remarkable between the

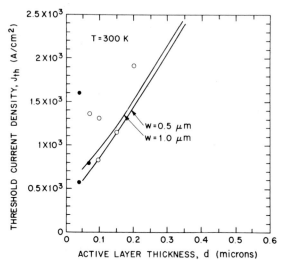

FIG. 7.5-3 Comparison of the calculated and experimental J_{th} for symmetric SCH lasers. The calculated J_{th} is from Eq. (7.5-2) with Γ from Fig. 2.9-3 for $x = 0.3$ and $y = 0.1$. The experimental data given by ○ are from Ref. 55 and by ● are from Ref. 95.

lowest experimental J_{th} values and J_{th} calculated from Eq. (7.5-2). This agreement demonstrates the absence of leakage current due to unconfined carriers at the N_y–p or p–P_y interfaces. For a DH laser with $x = 0.1$, it is shown in Fig. 4.6-7 that the leakage current would be $\sim 2 \times 10^4$ A/cm^2. It seems likely that the low threshold lasers of Fig. 7.5-3 are ones with negligible excess currents through junction defects or negligible scattering losses due to layer nonplanarity. The higher-than-predicted J_{th} that is observed for some lasers must be related to poorer quality with respect to one or both of these properties.

The lasers from Ref. 55 were characterized by more uniform near-field emission then generally observed for DH lasers. This emission uniformity results in η_D values that are 0.50 to 0.60 for the shorter cavities. Plots of $1/\eta_D$ versus L, as in Fig. 7.4-2, gave α_i between 10 and 19 cm^{-1} and the internal quantum efficiency η as 0.77.[55] As pointed out in Section 7.4, η obtained in this manner is probably somewhat low. However, the difference in the calculated $J_{th}(300°$K$)$ with $\eta = 0.77$ or Henshall's[49a] value of 0.90 is not significant for the purposes of this discussion. Comparison of the experimental beam divergence $\Theta_\perp$ with the calculated $\Theta_\perp$ versus d curves in Fig. 2.7-5 shows that $\Theta_\perp$ for symmetric SCH lasers is characteristic of the optical cavity width w rather than the active layer thickness. Since the active layer is the thin center layer, the fundamental mode is retained for optical cavity thicknesses that would give higher order modes for DH lasers.

Only limited data are available for the cw or pulsed output powers of symmetric SCH lasers. The pulse excitation output power from one mirror and the total external quantum efficiency for a symmetric SCH laser are shown in Fig. 7.5-4. For this device, $d = 0.1$ μm, and $w = 1.56$ μm, the area is 508×143 μm^2, and J_{th} was 1.3×10^3 A/cm^{2}.[55] The pulse width was 0.2 μsec and the repetition rate was ~ 100 Hz. No mirror damage was observed for an emission of 3.6 W for a single mirror, and this emission was limited by the current available from the pulse generator rather than by catastrophic mirror damage.

Asymmetric SCH Lasers

For the five-layer structure, $N_x N_y p_z P_u P_v$ or $N_x N_y n_z P_u P_v$, that is based on the Al–Ga–As system, neither the compositions nor the dimensions of any of the layers need be the same. However, the AlAs mole fractions in each layer generally are related as $x > y > z < u < v$ in order to obtain separate optical and carrier confinement. The only detailed study of the five-layer asymmetric SCH laser is the study of the structure described by Thompson et al.,[98] and this structure is illustrated in Fig. 7.5-5. In these asymmetric SCH lasers, $x \approx 0.28$, $y \approx x - 0.02$ with a thickness $b \approx 0.80$–1.40 μm, $z = 0.05$ with an active-layer thickness $d \approx 0.05$–0.15 μm, $u \approx 0.30$

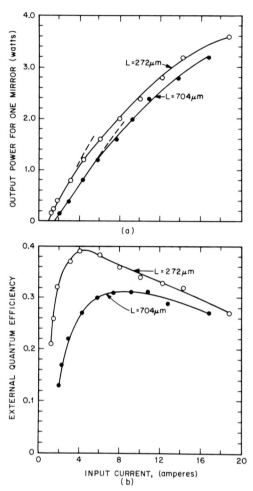

FIG. 7.5-4 Pulsed output properties for symmetric SCH lasers with a cavity width of 165 μm and the indicated lengths. (a) Output power from one mirror. (b) External quantum efficiency (Ref. 55).

and the thickness $c \approx d$, and $v \approx 0.45$. With one mirror coated to give $R = 0.8$, these lasers are distinguished by J_{th} near 600–700 A/cm². Also, a small temperature sensitivity of J_{th} above 300°K is obtained.

The terminology used by Thompson *et al.*[98] differs somewhat from that used here. They designated the SCH lasers as localized-gain-region (LGR) lasers and expressed a total effective waveguide thickness S_{eff} as

$$S_{eff} = \int_{-\infty}^{\infty} |\mathscr{E}_y|^2 \, dx / |\mathscr{E}_y|_{max}^2, \qquad (7.5\text{-}3)$$

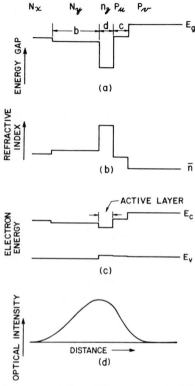

FIG. 7.5-5 Schematic representation of the asymmetric SCH laser. (a) Energy gap. (b) Refractive index. (c) Heterojunction energy-band diagram. (d) Optical intensity distribution.

where $\mathscr{E}_y$ is the optical electric field and $|\mathscr{E}_y|^2_{\max}$ the maximum intensity. A coupling constant k (to the optical field) for the active layer is given as

$$k = \int_{-d/2}^{d/2} |\mathscr{E}_y|^2 \, dx / |\mathscr{E}_y|^2_{\max} d, \qquad (7.5\text{-}4)$$

where the integral is taken over the active layer, and generally has a value near unity.[98] The ratio of Eq. (7.5-4) to Eq. (7.5-3) gives

$$k/S_{\text{eff}} = (1/d)\left(\int_{-d/2}^{d/2} |\mathscr{E}_y|^2 \, dx \right) \Big/ \left(\int_{-\infty}^{\infty} |\mathscr{E}_y|^2 \, dx \right), \qquad (7.5\text{-}5)$$

which from the previous definition of Γ gives

$$k/S_{\text{eff}} = \Gamma/d. \qquad (7.5\text{-}6)$$

The effective waveguide width S_{eff} relates the actual intensity distribution to an equivalent distribution of $|\mathscr{E}_y|^2_{\max}$ over a distance S_{eff}.

The solution of the wave equations for the asymmetric five-layer wave-guide follows the procedures used in Section 2.9 for the symmetric SCH laser. However, the asymmetric case required solution of an 8×8 matrix rather than the 4×4 matrix. Thompson et al.[98] therefore obtained estimates for the optical field in the five-layered structure of Fig. 7.5-5 by computing the behavior of the field in the simpler four-layer $N_x N_y p_x P_v$ structure. The insertion of the P_a layer to form the five-layer structure was considered to give approximately the same optical field for selected layer thickness ratios. They summarized the results of these computations as S_{eff} and k. The computed optical distribution in the four-layer structure was also used to derive $\Theta_\perp$. Values of $\Theta_\perp$ were calculated from Eq. (2.7-28) as the Fourier transform of the optical field distributions. The obliquity factor was neglected because $\Theta_\perp$ is small for these lasers. This calculation was summarized by plotting S_{eff} versus $\Theta_\perp$ as shown in Fig. 7.5-6. Three different thicknesses of b were considered as shown in the insert, and d is the independent variable.

The relationship between S_{eff} and $\Theta_\perp$ is also plotted in Fig. 7.5-6 for the fundamental mode of the DH laser. This curve will be used in Section 8.2 for the discussion of catastrophic mirror damage. For the DH laser there are two curves. Curve 1 corresponds to large values of d with a one-half sinusoidal period of $\mathscr{E}_y$ within the active layer. Curve 2 corresponds to small values of d with an exponential $\mathscr{E}_y$ entirely outside the active layer.

The dimensions and performance properties of the asymmetric five-layer structure by Thompson et al.[98] are given in Table 7.5-1. For these lasers, one mirror face had a reflective coating consisting of a half-wavelength-thick layer of Al_2O_3 plus a layer of Al to give $R = 0.8$ for that mirror. For $L = 500 \ \mu m$, one coated mirror reduces the end losses from $\sim 20 \ cm^{-1}$ to ~ 13

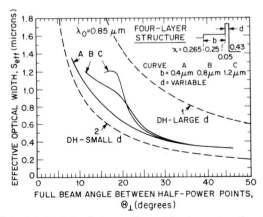

FIG. 7.5-6 Calculated relation between $\Theta_\perp$ and S_{eff} for various four-layer asymmetric SCH lasers and three-layer DH lasers. The active-layer width d is the independent variable (Ref. 98).

TABLE 7.5-1 Asymmetric Five-Layer SCH Lasers[a]

Wafer	x	y $b(\mu m)$	z $d(\mu m)$	u $c(\mu m)$	v	Avg. $J_{th}(300°K)$ (A/cm²) $L = 530\ \mu m$	$L = 300\ \mu m$	Avg. η_D for $L = 530\ \mu m$	Avg. η_D for $L = 300\ \mu m$	$\Theta_\perp$ (deg)	$\dfrac{J_{th}(338°K)}{J_{th}(283°K)}$	S_{eff} (μm)	k	Γ	Exp. J_{th} (A/cm²)	Cal. J_{th} (A/cm²)
KW 27	0.295	0.28 (1.40)	0.05 (0.09)	0.31 (0.10)	0.46	500	660	0.26	0.34	19–37	—	—	—	—	—	—
28	0.285	0.27 (0.81)	0.05 (0.08)	0.30 (0.10)	0.45	630	930	0.25	0.35	15–25	1.4	—	—	—	—	—
29	0.275	0.26 (0.83)	0.05 (0.13)	0.29 (0.17)	0.44	660	890	0.26	0.29	40	1.5	0.36	0.95	0.34	660	980
30	0.265	0.25 (1.70)	0.05 (0.08)	0.28 (0.15)	0.43	690	920	0.27	0.34	30	1.9	0.40	0.95	0.19	690	715
42	0.295	0.28 (1.10)	0.05 (0.13)	0.31 (0.10)	0.46	610	780	0.33	0.38	40	1.5	0.35	0.98	0.36	610	970
43	0.285	0.27 (0.75)	0.05 (0.07)	0.30 (0.05)	0.45	610	820	0.30	0.38	18–28	1.5	—	—	—	—	—
44	0.275	0.26 (0.88)	0.05 (0.09)	0.29 (~0.03)	0.44	710	830	0.31	0.40	12–30	1.5	—	—	—	—	—
46	0.255	0.24 (0.80)	0.05 (0.08)	0.27 (~0.04)	0.42	920	1050	0.24	0.40	12–21	1.4	—	—	—	—	—
49	0.305	0.29 (0.60)	0.05 (0.07)	0.32 (~0.06)	0.47	970	1080	0.33	0.43	17	—	0.73	0.98	0.09	970	870
52	0.305	0.29 (0.74)	0.05 (0.08)	0.32 (0.15)	0.47	750	920	0.29	0.36	47	1.6	0.35	0.98	0.22	750	680
53	0.295	0.28 (0.69)	0.05 (0.08)	0.31 (0.05)	0.46	640	860	0.30	0.42	34	1.6	0.38	0.98	0.21	640	690
54	0.285	0.27 (1.0)	0.05 (0.08)	0.30 (0.08)	0.45	650	810	0.32	0.41	34	1.5	0.39	0.98	0.20	650	700

[a] One mirror of each laser is coated so that $R = 0.8$. All data from Ref. 98 except for last three columns

cm^{-1}. Values of J_{th} and η_D in Table 7.5-1 were obtained with procedures similar to those described in Section 3.8. The ratio of $J_{th}(338°K)/J_{th}(283°K)$ in Table 7.5-1 shows that the asymmetric SCH lasers have a temperature dependence of J_{th} similar to the DH laser temperature dependence shown in Fig. 7.4-12 for $\Delta x > 0.3$. However, $\Theta_\perp$ is similar to DH lasers with $\Delta x < 0.3$ which have a large temperature dependence of J_{th}. In Table 7.5-1, values of S_{eff} and k are given only for those wafers which Thompson et al.[98] reported unique values of $\Theta_\perp$, and hence S_{eff}. The confinement factor is obtained from Eq. (7.5-6) as kd/S_{eff}.

In Ref. 98, the plots of $1/\eta_D$ versus L that are used to determine η tend to have a significant range of scatter, and it is difficult to judge the accuracy of the resulting values. Therefore, the same η of 0.77 as used for the symmetric SCH lasers has been used here, and Eq. (7.4-9) becomes

$$J_{th}(A/cm^2) = 5.8 \times 10^3 d + 600d/\Gamma. \tag{7.5-7}$$

In Eq. (7.5-7), α_i has been taken as $10\ cm^{-1}$, and $(1/2L)\ln(1/R_1 R_2)$ as $13\ cm^{-1}$ for $L = 500\ \mu m$, $R_1 = 0.32$, and $R_2 = 0.8$. The J_{th} values calculated from Eq. (7.5-7) are given in the last column of Table 7.5-1 and are compared to the experimental J_{th} values for $L = 530\ \mu m$.

Thompson et al.[98] found that the experimental J_{th} data could be fitted with the empirical relation

$$J_{th}(A/cm^2) = 4.0 \times 10^3 d + (28d/\Gamma)[\alpha_i + (1/2L)\ln(1/R_1 R_2)]. \tag{7.5-8}$$

Since $[\alpha_i + (1/2L)\ln(1/R_1 R_2)]$ is $\sim 23\ cm^{-1}$, the second term becomes $644d/\Gamma$ as compared to $600d/\Gamma$ for the theoretical expression in Eq. (7.5-7). The first terms in Eqs. (7.5-7) and (7.5-8) differ by a larger amount. It is interesting to note that the derived J_{th} expression in Eq. (7.5-7) and the empirical J_{th} expression in Eq. (7.5-8) are of identical form and have similar numerical values.

7.6 STRIPE-GEOMETRY LASER FABRICATION

Introductory Comments

The broad-area lasers of Sections 7.3–7.5 illustrate the features of confinement of light and carriers by slab structures. However, most heterostructure lasers intended for use outside the laboratory are stripe-geometry lasers that also restrict current along the junction plane. Stripe widths are typically 5–30 μm. This lateral confinement serves several purposes: (1) reduction of the cross-sectional area which also reduces the operating current; (2) single filament operation and fundamental mode emission along the junction plane for stripe widths $S \lesssim 15\ \mu m$; and (3) improved degradation by removing most of the junction perimeter from the surface. However, it is shown in Section 7.8 that the temperature rise of the active region of a stripe-geometry DH laser does not significantly differ from that of a broad-area DH laser.

Furnanage and Wilson[99] first suggested the use of an active region in the shape of a long, narrow rectangle in order to control the modes along the junction plane. Dyment[100] made contact to 50-μm-wide stripes etched in a SiO_2 layer in order to obtain Hermite–Gaussian-mode patterns in homo-structure GaAs lasers. Dyment and D'Asaro[101] reduced the SiO_2 stripe width to 12.5 μm and obtained cw operation of homostructure GaAs lasers up to 200°K. These homostructure lasers with 12.5-μm-wide stripes were also used to study the Gaussian-mode patterns.[102] Dyment et al.[47] introduced the use of proton-bombardment-induced high-resistivity layers to define active regions of stripe-geometry GaAs–$Al_xGa_{1-x}As$ DH lasers. Planar-stripe lasers were prepared by Yonezu et al.[103] by the diffusion of Zn through stripe windows in the SiO_2 film. The Zn diffusion is through the top n–GaAs layer into the P–$Al_xGa_{1-x}As$ layer. There are several modifications of these techniques that are also used, but the oxide stripe, proton-bombarded stripe, and the planar stripe are the most extensively used stripe-geometry lasers.

Although any of the broad-area lasers presented in Sections 7.3–7.5 can be fabricated as stripe-geometry lasers, most of the work on stripe-geometry lasers has been with DH lasers. The fabrication procedures presented in Section 7.2 are extended in this section to the techniques used for the preparation of GaAs–$Al_xGa_{1-x}As$ stripe-geometry lasers. A description of the various stripe-geometry lasers is also given. The most commonly used techniques will be briefly summarized. There are numerous stripe-geometry structures, and more can be expected.

Contact Stripe

In the contact stripe-geometry laser, contact to the p–GaAs top layer of a DH laser is limited by an insulating layer as illustrated in Fig. 7.6-1. The barrier is usually SiO_2 (Ref. 104), but Si_3N_4 (Ref. 105) has also been used. Layers of SiO_2 may be deposited on GaAs by the reaction of silane (0.5%) in nitrogen with oxygen at ~ 350°C. Sputtered SiO_2 may also be used. For contact stripes, the insulating layer is usually 1500–3000 Å thick. The stripe is opened in the oxide by standard photolithographic procedures by etching with buffered $HF(7-NH_4F:1-HF)$. The contacting procedures then follow the metallization techniques described in Section 7.2.

Proton-Bombardment Isolation

The irradiation of a semiconductor with energetic particles such as protons creates lattice defects as they dissipate their energy. These damaged

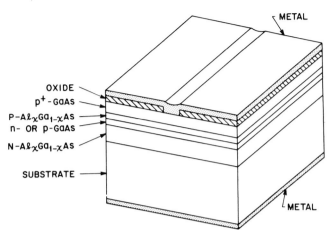

FIG. 7.6-1   Stripe-geometry DH laser with four heteroepitaxial layers on the n^+–GaAs substrate. The oxide layer isolates all but the stripe contact. The rectangular bar is typically 380 μm long, 250 μm wide, and 120 μm thick. The drawing is not to scale in order to show the various layers (Ref. 104).

regions can have high resistivity.[106] Foyt *et al.*[107] used proton bombardment for isolating GaAs junction devices. Stripe-geometry lasers are readily prepared by masking with a tungsten wire as shown in Fig. 7.6-2 or by masking with an evaporated metallic stripe.[104] The proton bombardment introduces a high resistivity layer outside the stripe, and therefore confines the lateral flow of the current. An array of wires placed over the wafer for bombardment provides a simple batch-processing technique. Contact is obtained by a metallization of the entire bombarded surface.

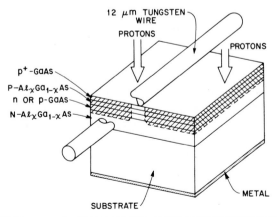

FIG. 7.6-2   Stripe-geometry DH laser fabricated by proton bombardment (Ref. 104).

The effect of 300-keV proton bombardment and subsequent annealing on the optical absorption and electrical resistivity of p-type GaAs was studied by Dyment et al.[108] Proton bombardment also greatly increases the resistivity of $Al_xGa_{1-x}As$.[109] Dyment et al.[108] showed that the resistivity increase is accompanied by optical loss. However, the optical loss can be reduced to its unbombarded value by selected annealing temperatures and times, while retaining sufficient resistivity for current confinement. Proton bombardment at 300 keV with a dose of 3×10^{15} cm^{-2} produces a high resistivity layer 3-μm deep. The isolation depth is 1 μm per 100 keV of proton energy.[107] Annealing at 450°C for 15 min returns the optical absorption to its unbombarded value, while the final resistivity is 100 times its unbombarded value. Therefore, a 10^{-2} Ω-cm p-layer before bombardment becomes 1 Ω-cm after bombardment and annealing. Care must be taken in the subsequent processing not to anneal out the remaining damage that would return the layer to its unbombarded resistivity.

Oxygen-ion implantation has also been used for stripe formation in DH lasers.[110] Because of the heavier ion, energies greater than 1 MeV are required. The damage due to implantation may readily be annealed out, but the layer is semi-insulating due to the implanted oxygen.[111] It is not clear whether any significant differences in laser operating or degradation behavior exist for stripe-geometry devices prepared by these two techniques.

Planar Stripe

The planar-stripe laser described by Yonezu et al.[103] is shown in Fig. 7.6-3a. Note that the top layer is n-type GaAs. To prepare this structure, a SiO_2 film is sputtered onto that surface and stripe windows of the desired width are opened in the SiO_2 by masking and etching. A reproducible diffusion source[10] is used at 730°C to diffuse Zn through the windows to a depth sufficient to reach the $P-Al_xGa_{1-x}As$ layer. The SiO_2 film is removed, and metal contacts are evaporated onto the top surface. The p^+-n and $n-P$ junction provide current confinement to the stripe region.

Yonezu et al.[112] extended the Zn diffusion into the active layer or $N-Al_xGa_{1-x}As$ layer as shown in Fig. 7.6-3b. With this structure, they observed improved linearity of the light output and a stable single transverse mode along the junction plane. The nonlinearities in the light–current curves that are frequently observed in stripe-geometry lasers are designated as "kinks" and are discussed in Section 7.11. A structure similar to the planar stripe laser of Ref. 112 was also reported by Tabusagawa et al.[113]

Aiki et al.[114,114a] found that planar-stripe lasers grown on channeled substrates as shown in Fig. 7.6-3c also eliminated kinks. This structure has many good operating characteristics such as single longitudinal mode emission and absence from relaxation oscillations.[114a] The heteroepitaxial

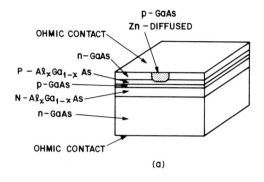

(a)

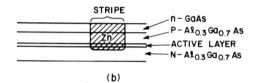

(b)

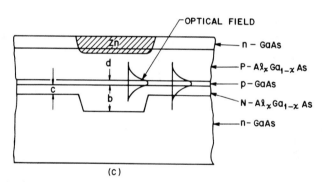

(c)

FIG. 7.6-3 (a) Conventional planar-stripe laser (Ref. 103). (b) Schematic representation of cross section for new planar-stripe laser (Ref. 112). (c) Channeled substrate planar-stripe geometry laser. The active-layer thickness $d \approx 0.1\ \mu m$, while $c \approx 0.4\ \mu m$ and $b \approx 1.4\ \mu m$ (Ref. 114).

layers for this device were grown on a n–GaAs substrate with an etched channel $\sim 1\ \mu m$ deep and 5 to 20 μm wide. The active layer thickness d is $\sim 0.1\ \mu m$, and the N–Al$_x$Ga$_{1-x}$As layer thickness outside the channel is $\sim 0.4\ \mu m$. In this structure, the tail of the evanescent wave reaches the lossy substrate in the region outside the channel and therefore provides improved confinement to the channel region. This structure is called the channeled-substrate planar (CSP) laser. A detailed discussion of the CSP laser has been given by Aiki *et al.*[114a]

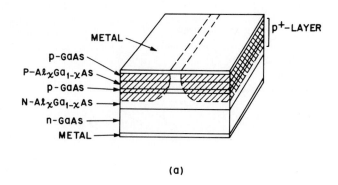

(a)

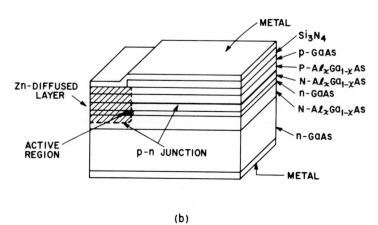

(b)

FIG. 7.6-4 (a) Junction stripe-geometry laser (Ref. 115). (b) Transverse-junction stripe-geometry laser (Ref. 116).

A Zn-diffused structure called the junction-stripe geometry laser[115] is shown in Fig. 7.6-4a. The stripe region was masked by a Si_3N_4 film, and Zn was diffused at 650°C into the N-$Al_xGa_{1-x}As$ layer. The Si_3N_4 film is removed for contact metallization. Similar current confinement is obtained in the transverse-junction-stripe (TJS) geometry laser[116,117] shown in Fig. 7.6-4b. Since the injection in this case is from the n–GaAs layer into the Zn-diffused p–GaAs, this device is a very thin homojunction laser. The conditions that influence injection currents into the other layers will be discussed in Section 7.7.

Mesa Stripe

The cross-sectional area of the broad-area laser has also been reduced by the use of the mesa-stripe-geometry DH laser shown in Fig. 7.6-5a.[118] These lasers are made by masking the stripe photolithographically and

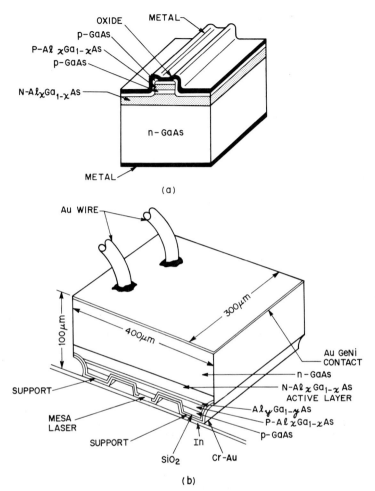

FIG. 7.6-5 (a) Mesa-stripe-geometry DH laser. The width of the stripe region is 10–40 μm and the cavity lengths are 200–600 μm (Ref. 118). (b) Heat-sinking and mounting of mesa-stripe-geometry laser (Ref. 119).

etching with $4-H_2SO_4:1-H_2O_2:1-H_2O$. Phosphosilicate glass (PSG) was used as the etching mask, and the layers were etched into the $N-Al_xGa_{1-x}As$ layer. After removing the PSG etch mask, PSG is redeposited and reetched as the mask for metallization. For heat sinking, adjacent electrically inactive mesas are used as shown in Fig. 7.6-5b for mechanical support.[119]

Buried Heterostructure

For buried-heterostructure (BH) lasers, the active region is completely surrounded by $Al_xGa_{1-x}As$ as shown in Fig. 7.6-6.[120] The mesa etching is

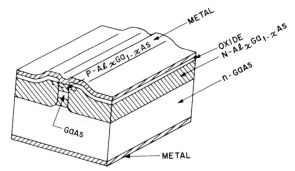

FIG. 7.6-6 Buried-heterostructure laser. The GaAs active region is completely surrounded by $Al_xGa_{1-x}As$ (Ref. 120).

deep enough to reach the n–GaAs. An etch of $1-H_3PO_4 : 1-H_2O_2 : 3-CH_3OH$ was used because it has the same etch rate for GaAs and $Al_xGa_{1-x}As$.[120] The shape of the mesa is dependent on the crystallographic direction, and the $\langle 01\bar{1} \rangle$ direction was selected. It is very difficult to get LPE growth on an air-exposed $Al_xGa_{1-x}As$ surface with $x > 0.05$. However, LPE growth is readily obtained on the exposed sides of mesa-etched $Al_xGa_{1-x}As$. A shallow Zn diffusion is used in order to restrict the current flow. The BH laser is characterized by an active region as small as 1 μm square. With such small active regions, the threshold current is as small as 15 mA, and a nearly symmetrical far-field pattern is obtained.[120] The active layer width and thickness must be $\lesssim 1$ μm to prevent higher order modes.

Strip-Buried Heterostructure

With the buried heterostructure, the large change in the refractive index along the junction plane limits fundamental mode operation to stripe widths of ≤ 1 μm. In the strip-buried heterostructure (SBH) laser,[120a] the introduction of a N–$Al_{0.1}Ga_{0.9}As$ layer as shown in Fig. 7.6-7 converts the channel waveguide in a BH laser to a strip-loaded waveguide. The optical mode is no longer confined to the thin p–GaAs active region, but spreads mostly into the N–$Al_{0.1}Ga_{0.9}As$ low-loss waveguide and thereby results in a reduction of the effective refractive index along the junction plane. Therefore, the SBH laser retains the two-dimensional carrier confinement as with the BH laser, while permiting the light to spread out along the junction plane. The reduced light confinement permits stable fundamental mode operation for a strip width as wide as 5 μm, and there are no light–current nonlinearities. Studies of cw lasers have also shown single longitudinal mode emission and the absence of relaxation oscillations.[120b] The spreading of the light into the N–$Al_{0.1}Ga_{0.9}As$ layer also permits higher pulsed output power. Details of the

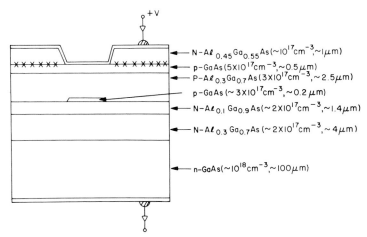

FIG. 7.6-7 Schematic representation of the strip-buried heterostructure laser. The active region is the p–GaAs between the P–Al$_{0.3}$Ga$_{0.7}$As and N–Al$_{0.1}$Ga$_{0.9}$As layers. Lateral current confinement is provided by the reverse-biased p–N heterojunction marked by X–X (Ref. 120a).

heterepitaxial growth as well as the device preparation and operating properties were given by Tsang et al.[120a]

Junction-Isolated Stripes

Burnham et al.[121] introduced lateral-current confinement by a p–N junction at the substrate N–Al$_x$Ga$_{1-x}$As interface as shown in Fig. 7.6-8a. The stripes on the substrate surface were masked with Si$_3$N$_4$, and Zn was diffused into the substrate from a Zn$_3$As$_2$ source at 700°C for 10 min. The Si$_3$N$_4$ is removed and the heteroepitaxial layers are grown. Another junction isolation technique was demonstrated by Itoh et al.[122] By growing a top Al$_x$Ga$_{1-x}$As layer with $0.4 < x < 0.6$ and etching a stripe to permit contacting the p–GaAs layer, lateral current confinement is provided by the N–p junction as shown in Fig. 7.6-8b. Tsang and Logan[123] combined reverse-biased p–N junctions at the substrate and top surface as shown in Fig. 7.6-8c. In this case, a p–GaAs layer was first grown by LPE and the channel etched, and then the heteroepitaxial layers were grown. The structure was found to have linear light–current curves.[123]

Junction isolation has been extended to heteroepitaxial growth in channels to give a semicircular GaAs active region that is surrounded by Al$_x$Ga$_{1-x}$As.[124] Burnham and Scifres called their device the etched-buried heterostructure laser.[124] Kirkby and Thompson[125] prepared the channeled-substrate buried-heterostructure laser shown in Fig. 7.6-9a. The active region

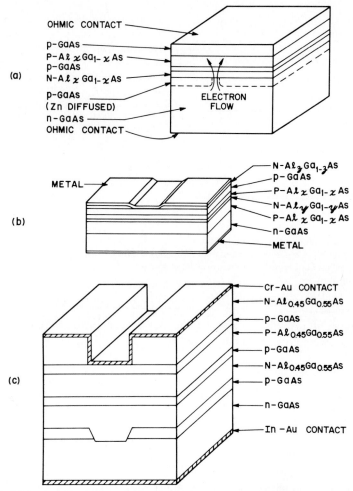

(a)

OHMIC CONTACT
p-GaAs
P-Al $_x$ Ga$_{1-x}$ As
p-GaAs
N-Al $_x$ Ga$_{1-x}$ As
p-GaAs
(Zn DIFFUSED)
n-GaAs
OHMIC CONTACT

ELECTRON FLOW

(b)

METAL

N-Al $_z$ Ga$_{1-z}$ As
p-GaAs
P-Al $_x$ Ga$_{1-x}$ As
N-Al $_y$ Ga$_{1-y}$ As
P-Al $_x$ Ga$_{1-x}$ As
n-GaAs
METAL

(c)

Cr-Au CONTACT
N-Al$_{0.45}$Ga$_{0.55}$As
p-GaAs
P-Al$_{0.45}$Ga$_{0.55}$As
p-GaAs
N-Al$_{0.45}$Ga$_{0.55}$As
p-GaAs
n-GaAs
In-Au CONTACT

FIG. 7.6-8   Junction-isolated stripe-geometry lasers. (a) Striped-substrate laser (Ref. 121). (b) Heteroisolation-stripe laser (Ref. 122). (c) Double-lateral current-confinement laser (Ref. 123).

of the 10- and 20-μm-wide stripes are parabolic in cross section, taper to zero at the edges, and are completely embedded in Al$_x$Ga$_{1-x}$As.

A stripe-geometry laser with current confinement obtained by growth of a polycrystalline insulating layer is shown in Fig. 7.6-9b.[126] This structure was grown by molecular-beam epitaxy. In the window of the SiO$_2$, the P–Al$_{0.35}$Ga$_{0.65}$As grows single crystal, while on the SiO$_2$ film the Al$_{0.35}$Ga$_{0.65}$As grows as a polycrystalline-insulating layer.

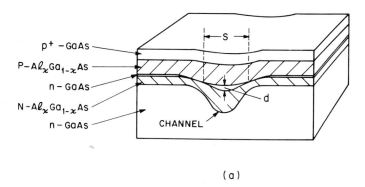

(a)

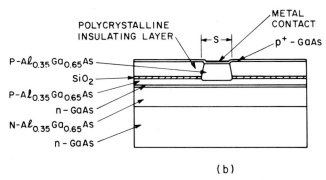

(b)

FIG. 7.6-9 (a) Channeled-substrate laser with stripe width S and active-layer thickness d (Ref. 125). (b) Embedded stripe-geometry laser grown by MBE (Ref. 126).

7.7. THRESHOLD CURRENT OF STRIPE-GEOMETRY LASERS

Current Spreading and Lateral Carrier Diffusion

In broad-area lasers, the current flow is one dimensional and the current density in the active region is the external current divided by the cross-sectional area. In structures such as the contact-stripe laser, the current flow through the p- and/or P-layers is by a majority carrier drift current which spreads laterally as illustrated in Fig. 7.7-1. Because of spreading, the current flows through an area in the active region that is larger than the stripe-contact area. Within the active layer, there is a lateral diffusive current of minority carriers due to recombination which also broadens the current distribution. These two effects greatly influence the threshold current behavior and the emission properties of stripe-geometry lasers. In this part of Section 7.7, the current-spreading expressions given by Yonezu et al.[103] will be used to extend the active-layer carrier-diffusion model of Hakki[127] to

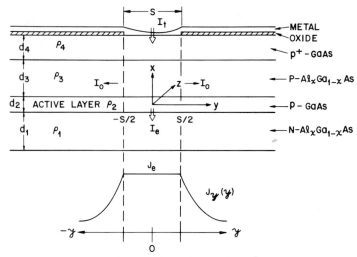

FIG. 7.7-1   Schematic representation of current spreading in a contact stripe-geometry laser. The total current is I_t, the current through the active region under the stripe is I_e with a current density of J_e. The lateral spreading current is I_0, and the distribution of current density across the junction at y is $J_y(y)$ (Ref. 103).

include both current spreading and lateral carrier diffusion. An approximate representation of the current spreading that was suggested by Tsang[128] will be used to obtain an expression for the carrier distribution in the active layer. This expression can be used for structures such as stripe-contact lasers where both current spreading and lateral carrier diffusion must be considered or for proton-bombarded stripe-geometry lasers where only lateral carrier diffusion is important.

A model for current spreading in stripe-geometry lasers has been presented.[103,104,129–130a] In Fig. 7.7-1, the total current I_t is shown to be the sum of the uniform current under the stripe I_e and the spreading current I_0 flowing in the $\pm y$ direction:

$$I_t = I_e + 2I_0. \tag{7.7-1}$$

In Appendix A of Ref. 103, it was shown that the current density across the junction at $y > |S/2|$ is

$$J_y(y) = I_0/l_0 L[1 + (|y| - S/2)/l_0]^2, \tag{7.7-2}$$

where

$$l_0 = 2L/\beta \rho_s I_0. \tag{7.7-3}$$

In Eq. (7.7-3), β is the exponential junction parameter q/nkT, L the cavity length, and ρ_s the composite sheet resistivity given by

$$1/\rho_s = 1/(\rho_4/d_4) + 1/(\rho_3/d_3). \tag{7.7-4}$$

It was also shown by Yonezu et al.[103] that

$$J_e = \beta\rho_s I_0^2/2L^2 = I_0/l_0 L, \tag{7.7-5}$$

and

$$I_0 = \frac{[1 + (S\beta\rho_s/2L)I_t]^{1/2} - 1}{S\beta\rho_s/2L}. \tag{7.7-6}$$

With Eq. (7.7-4), it can be shown that the layer with the smallest ρ/d determines ρ_s and will be the layer that dominates the spreading. For a given structure, the current spreading will also have a current dependence as expressed by Eqs. (7.7-2), (7.7-3), and (7.7-6), and the fraction of the total current under the stripe increases with current.

To combine the current spreading with lateral diffusion in the active layer in a form that permits analytical solution for the carrier concentration profile, Tsang[128] suggested representing $J_y(y)$ by an exponential that gives the same total lateral current I_0. For $|y| > S/2$,

$$J_y(y) = M \exp[-a(|y| - S/2)]. \tag{7.7-7}$$

Equation (7.7-2) at the stripe edge gives $J_y(S/2) = I_0/l_0 L$ so that $M = I_0/l_0 L$. The total lateral current I_0 is

$$I_0 = \int_0^L \int_{S/2}^\infty \frac{I_0}{l_0 L} \exp\left[-a\left(|y| - \frac{S}{2}\right)\right] dy \, dz, \tag{7.7-8}$$

and gives

$$a = 1/l_0. \tag{7.7-9}$$

Therefore, the approximate $J_y(y)$ for $|y| \geq S/2$ becomes

$$J_y(y) = (I_0/l_0 L) \exp[-(|y| - S/2)/l_0]. \tag{7.7-10}$$

This representation of $J_y(y)$ shows that $1/l_0$, which is $\beta\rho_s I_0/2L$, is a decay constant, and therefore the current spreading increases rapidly for small ρ_s.

The carrier concentration profile due to lateral diffusion may be found from the continuity equation for electrons given in Eq. (4.5-26). Within the stripe, the generation rate $g(y)$ is (J_e/qd). For the diffusive current given by Eq. (4.3-50), the electron concentration in the p-type active region at steady state for $-S/2 < y < S/2$ is governed by

$$\frac{d^2n}{dy^2} - \frac{n}{L_n^2} = -\left(\frac{J_e}{qD_nd}\right) \equiv -G, \qquad (7.7\text{-}11)$$

where L_n is the electron diffusion length and D_n the electron diffusivity. The carrier lifetime τ_n is related to these quantities by $L_n = (D_n\tau_n)^{1/2}$. Solution of Eq. (7.7-11) gives

$$n(y) = A\exp(-y/L_n) + B\exp(y/L_n) + GL_n^2. \qquad (7.7\text{-}12)$$

For the symmetric case with $n(-y) = n(y)$, $A = B$, and

$$n(y) = 2A\cosh(y/L_n) + GL_n^2. \qquad (7.7\text{-}13)$$

Outside the stripe for $|y| > S/2$, $g(y) = J_y(y)/qd$. With the exponential representation of Eq. (7.7-10) for $J_y(y)$, the solution of Eq. (7.7-11) is

$$n(y) = C\exp\left(\frac{-(|y| - S/2)}{L_n}\right)$$
$$+ \left(\frac{l_0^2 L_n^2}{l_0^2 - L_n^2}\right)\left(\frac{I_0}{ql_0LD_nd}\right)\exp\left(\frac{-(|y| - S/2)}{l_0}\right). \qquad (7.7\text{-}14)$$

The constants A in Eq. (7.7-13) and C in Eq. (7.7-14) are determined from the requirement that $n(y)$ and the lateral current must be continuous at $|S/2|$. For the diffusive current to be continuous, dn/dy at $|S/2|$ must be continuous. Equating $n(y)$ and dn/dy from Eqs. (7.7-13) and (7.7-14) at $|y| = S/2$ gives A and C. For $-S/2 < y < S/2$,

$$n(y) = \left(\frac{I_e\tau_n}{qSLd}\right)\left[1 - \cosh\left(\frac{y}{L_n}\right)\exp\left(\frac{-S}{2L_n}\right)\right]$$
$$+ \left(\frac{1}{l_0 + L_n}\right)\left(\frac{I_0\tau_n}{qLd}\right)\cosh\left(\frac{y}{L_n}\right)\exp\left(\frac{-S}{2L_n}\right), \qquad (7.7\text{-}15)$$

and for $|y| > S/2$

$$n(y) = \left[\frac{I_e\tau_n/qSLd}{1 + \coth(S/2L_n)} - \left(\frac{1}{l_0^2 - L_n^2}\right)\left(\frac{I_0\tau_n}{qLd}\right)\left(\frac{l_0 + L_n\coth(S/2L_n)}{1 + \coth(S/2L_n)}\right)\right]$$
$$\times \exp\left[\frac{-(|y| - S/2)}{L_n}\right] + l_0\left(\frac{1}{l_0^2 - L_n^2}\right)\left(\frac{I_0\tau_n}{qLd}\right)$$
$$\times \exp\left[\frac{-(|y| - S/2)}{l_0}\right]. \qquad (7.7\text{-}16)$$

Equations (7.7-15) and (7.7-16) may be written in a reduced form by replacing I_0 by $J_e l_0 L$. However, the present form emphasizes that for proton-bombarded stripe-geometry lasers the spreading current I_0 goes to zero, and $n(y)$ becomes the expressions given by Hakki[127] for lateral diffusion without spreading. Hakki also included a different L_n for $|y| < S/2$ and $|y| > S/2$ to allow for effects on L_n when the protons penetrate the active layer. In the other limit of current spreading but no lateral diffusion, $n(y)$ becomes the previous $J_y(y)(\tau_n/qd)$ with $J_y(y)$ given by the expression in Eq. (7.7-10). The relation between carrier concentration and current density, $n = J\tau_n/qd$, is derived in Eq. (7.7-27).

The effects of current spreading and lateral diffusion are illustrated in Figs. 7.7-2 and 7.7-3. For the geometry shown in Fig. 7.7-1 with $d_4 = 1$ μm,

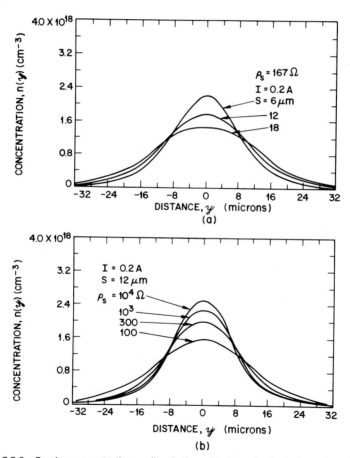

FIG. 7.7-2 Carrier concentration profiles in the active layer for the indicated conditions. The device parameters are specified in the text. (a) Variation with stripe width. (b) Variation with spreading resistance.

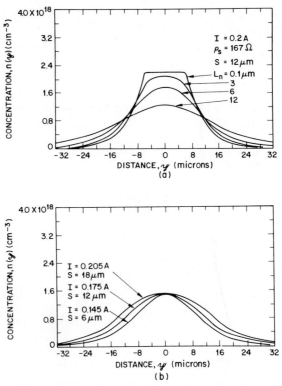

FIG. 7.7-3   Carrier concentration profiles in the active layer for the indicated conditions. The device parameters are specified in the text. (a) Variation with diffusion length. (b) Values of current necessary to retain $n(0) = 1.5 \times 10^{18}$ cm^{-3} as the stripe width is varied.

$\rho_4 = 2 \times 10^{-2}$ Ω-cm, $d_3 = 1$ μm, and $\rho_3 = 1 \times 10^{-1}$ Ω-cm, Eq. (7.7-4) gives ρ_s as 167 Ω. In the next part of this section, n in q/nkT is found to be ~2. The active layer thickness is taken as 0.2 μm and the cavity length is 380 μm. Figure 7.7-2a shows the variation of $n(y)$ for $I = 0.2$ A for the above parameters and $S = 18$, 12, and 6 μm. In Fig. 7.7-2b, the variation of $n(y)$ for $S = 12$ μm, and $\rho_s = 100$, 300, 1×10^3, and 1×10^4 Ω is shown. The carrier profiles for $\rho_s \gtrsim 1 \times 10^3$ Ω are not significantly influenced by current spreading. The variation of $n(y)$ with L_n is shown in Fig. 7.7-3a for the indicated parameters. For $L_n = 0.1$ μm, $n(y)$ is dominated by current spreading. To maintain a constant carrier concentration at $y = 0$ as the stripe width is increased, it is necessary to increase the current. The variation of $n(y)$ and the total current I necessary to maintain $n(0) = 1.5 \times 10^{18}$ cm^{-3} is given for several different stripe widths S in Fig. 7.7-3b.

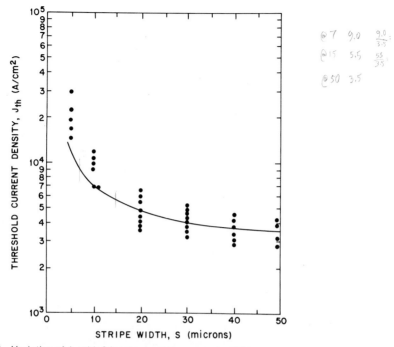

FIG. 7.7-4   Variation of J_{th} with S for planar-stripe geometry DH lasers at room temperature. The experimental data are from Ref. 103. The solid curve is calculated from Eq. (7.7-15) and demonstrates that the variation of J_{th} with S is due largely to lateral carrier diffusion.

The variation of the threshold current density with stripe width for planar-stripe GaAs–Al$_x$Ga$_{1-x}$As DH lasers is shown in Fig. 7.7-4.[103] Because of current confinement in the top n-layer of this structure, the only current spreading is in the P-layer. For the lasers in Ref. 103, $\rho_3 = 0.2$ Ω-cm, and $d_3 = 2$ μm to give $\rho_s = 1 \times 10^3$ Ω, and therefore current spreading will not be very significant. The DH lasers in Fig. 7.7-4 were reported to have active layer thicknesses of 0.7 μm and cavity lengths of 300 μm. The threshold current density for broad-area lasers was 3.3×10^3 A/cm^2. With this J_{th} used to give $n(0)$ as $J_{th}\tau_n/qd$, the current necessary to retain this $n(0)$ constant as S is varied may be found from Eq. (7.7-15) with L_n taken as 6 μm. This current when divided by $S \times L$ gives the variation of J_{th} with S shown by the solid line in Fig. 7.7-4. For proton-bombarded stripe-geometry lasers, J_{th} varies with S in a similar manner, and J_{th} at 12 μm is typically twice as large as for otherwise comparable broad-area lasers. The influence of stripe width on J_{th} for contact-stripe GaAs–Al$_x$Ga$_{1-x}$As DH lasers was investigated by

Ladany.[130a] The study of the variation of J_{th} with stripe width was extended to InP–Ga$_x$In$_{1-x}$P$_y$As$_{1-y}$ DH lasers by Hsieh and Shen.[130b] They investigated contact-stripe, proton-bombarded, and two types of buried heterostructures. For these DH lasers, J_{th} increased most rapidly as the stripe width was decreased for the oxide-defined contact stripe.

In addition to the effects of current spreading and lateral carrier diffusion in the active layer, J_{th} can be influenced by optical mode loss. This loss is due to absorption in both the active region and the surrounding Al$_x$Ga$_{1-x}$As layers and diffraction losses due to the optical field spreading outside the active region both transverse and along the junction plane. Tsang[128] considered the relative importance of current spreading, lateral carrier diffusion, and optical mode loss on the stripe-width dependence of J_{th}. The influence of optical mode loss is not as important as current spreading and lateral carrier diffusion in the active layer and for this reason can generally be neglected.[128]

Derivative Measurements of the Current–Voltage Characteristic

Derivative techniques can be very useful in the characterization of heterostructure lasers, and this technique has been considered in several studies.[131–135] These measurements permit the direct determination of the series resistance, the exponential junction parameter $\beta = q/nkT$, and the laser threshold current. The junction voltage is also shown to saturate at the onset of lasing. The relationships for the expressions that describe the various parameters may be derived by considering an ideal p–n junction with a series resistance R_s.[131,132,136] The current–voltage behavior is represented by

$$I = I_s[\exp \beta(V - IR_s) - 1]. \qquad (7.7\text{-}17)$$

By neglecting the term -1 and assuming the parameters are current independent, differentiation of Eq. (7.7-17) gives[131,132,136]

$$dV/dI = 1/I\beta + R_s \qquad (7.7\text{-}18)$$

and

$$d^2V/dI^2 = -1/I^2\beta. \qquad (7.7\text{-}19)$$

The more convenient forms of Eqs. (7.7-18) and (7.7-19) are

$$I\,dV/dI = 1/\beta + IR_s, \qquad (7.7\text{-}20)$$

and

$$I^2\,d^2V/dI^2 = -\frac{1}{\beta}. \qquad (7.7\text{-}21)$$

Since β may be obtained as the $I = 0$ intercept with the first derivative, all the desired parameters may be evaluated by plotting $I(dV/dI)$.

The experimental derivative measurements[131,133] use a sinusoidally modulated driving current and measure the voltage response. The voltage at the signal frequency is related to the first derivative, and the second harmonic voltage is related to the second derivative.[131,133,134] The strongly peaked second derivative is a particularly convenient measure of laser threshold.[131] An example of $I(dV/dI)$ and the light output L versus I for a proton-bombarded stripe geometry DH laser is shown in Fig. 7.7-5. Calibration curves with 1.0 and 4.3 ohm resistances are also shown. The $I = 0$ intercept gives $\beta = 15$ V^{-1}, and for currents below threshold, the linear region gives $R_s = 1.78 \, \Omega$.[133]

At threshold, the L versus I curve abruptly increases and $I(dV/dI)$ decreases. This behavior is due to the saturation of the junction voltage at threshold.[132] There has been some controversy as to whether saturation of the spontaneous emission and hence voltage, occur at threshold.[137,138] Most measurements suggest saturation. For an ideal semiconductor laser, the gain coefficient remains constant above threshold so that the electron and hole quasi-Fermi levels become "pinned" and the additional injected carriers contribute to the stimulated emission. Since the junction voltage V_j is related to the quasi-Fermi level separation as $F_n - F_p = qV_j$, the I–V relation above threshold becomes

$$V = IR_s + (V_j)_{th}. \tag{7.7-22}$$

Therefore, dV/dI becomes a constant equal to the series resistance at currents above threshold. The abrupt decrease of $I(dV/dI)$ near threshold represents its change from $1/\beta + IR_s$ below threshold to IR_s above threshold.

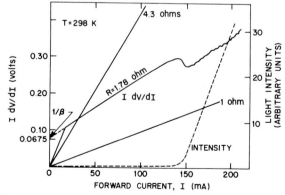

FIG. 7.7-5 Plot of $I(dV/dI)$ and light output L versus laser current I (Ref. 133).

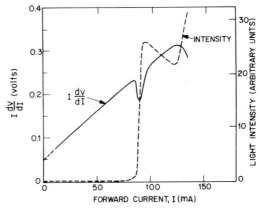

FIG. 7.7-6   Experimental variation of $I(dV/dI)$ and light output with current for a proton-bombarded stripe-geometry DH in which the voltage is not saturated above threshold. Note the nonlinear current dependence of the lasing output occurs simultaneously with loss of voltage saturation (Ref. 132).

Although the behavior shown in Fig. 7.7-5 was presented as a typical example,[133] not all lasers show complete voltage saturation over that large a range. An example of incomplete saturation together with a nonlinear variation of the light–current curve,[132] which is the so-called "kink," is shown in Fig. 7.7-6. The loss of voltage saturation accompanies the nonlinear $L–I$ curve.

The lasing threshold in a semiconductor laser has usually been assigned from the knee in the $L–I$ curve or the extrapolation of the $L–I$ curve to zero light as illustrated in Fig. 3.8-10. Because it is difficult to determine the cross-sectional area to within 5 to 10%, precise I_t has not been sought in the evaluation of threshold current density. However, by measurement of the noise fluctuations in the emitted light intensity, Paoli[135] has been able to relate the threshold for amplitude-stabilized oscillation to the first and second derivatives of the current–voltage characteristic. Near J_{th}, as the stimulated emission becomes significant, the intensity noise reaches a maximum at the threshold for regenerative oscillation. A comparison of $I(dV/dI)$ versus I and the relative noise power are shown in Fig. 7.7-7. This comparison shows that the onset of stabilization occurs at a current somewhat above the current where the voltage is fully saturated.

Time Delay

As previously mentioned in Section 7.3, the initial short time delay (nanoseconds) between the application of a current pulse and the observation of stimulated emission is related to the minority carrier lifetime τ_n or τ_p. This

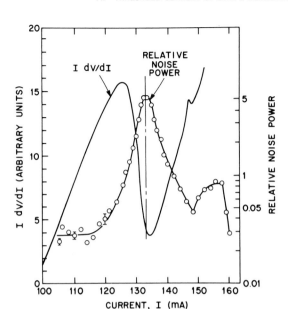

FIG. 7.7-7 Comparison of the first voltage derivative and the relative intensity fluctuations in a 10-kHz interval centered at 50 MHz near the laser threshold. Note that quieting expected for an amplitude-stabilized oscillator occurs at a current slightly below the relative minimum in the first derivative curve (Ref. 135).

initial short time delay is observed for all homostructure and heterostructure lasers and is the only time delay observed for DH lasers. In this part of Section 7.7, this initial short time delay t_d will be related to τ_n for p-type active layers. Knowledge of the carrier lifetime permits evaluation of the injected carrier concentration from the current density. The basic relationships for the representation of t_d were given by Konnerth and Lanza[41] for GaAs homostructure lasers. These concepts have been extended to heterostructure lasers by several authors.[139–142]

The time variation of the injected electron concentration in the p-type active region is given by the continuity equation, which for one-dimension was given by Eq. (4.5-26). For the time-delay model, the current is assumed to be uniform across the active layer so that the $\partial i_n/\partial x$ term is zero. It is convenient to take the junction current, when divided by the area and active layer thickness, as a uniform generation rate $g(x)$. With these assumptions and the injected electron concentration n much greater than the thermal equilibrium value n_0, Eq. (4.5-26) becomes

$$dn/dt = I/qAd - n/\tau \qquad (7.7\text{-}23)$$

with τ_n written as τ. A similar equation may be written for holes in n-type active layers. The solution of this equation for $n(0) = 0$ is

$$n(t) = (\tau I/qAd)[1 - \exp(-t/\tau)], \qquad (7.7\text{-}24)$$

or

$$t = \tau \ln\left[\frac{I}{I - qn(t)Ad/\tau}\right]. \qquad (7.7\text{-}25)$$

When $n(t)$ reaches the threshold value, $n(t) = n_{th}$ and

$$I_{th} = qn_{th}Ad/\tau, \qquad (7.7\text{-}26)$$

or

$$n_{th} = J_{th}\tau/qd. \qquad (7.7\text{-}27)$$

The expression given by Eq. (7.7-27) is frequently used to relate J_{th} to the injected carrier concentration. Since $t = t_d$ at $n(t) = n_{th}$, substitution of Eq. (7.7-26) into Eq. (7.7-25) gives[41]

$$t_d = \tau \ln[I/(I - I_{th})]. \qquad (7.7\text{-}28)$$

Hwang and Dyment[141] measured t_d for a group of proton-bombarded stripe-geometry DH lasers with Ge acceptor concentrations N_A in the active layer from 2×10^{17} to 3×10^{19} cm^{-3}. Their results are shown in Fig. 7.7-8 and give a decreasing t_d as N_A becomes larger. The lifetime derived from time-delay measurements is generally $3 \pm 2 \times 10^{-9}$ sec. This lifetime is related to the radiative τ_r and nonradiative τ_{nr} lifetime by Eq. (3.7-6). However, both the radiative and nonradiative lifetimes may be influenced by the high level of injection. Namizaki et al.[142] found that τ varied as $J_{th}^{-1/2}$. The internal quantum efficiency η is the radiative recombination rate, $R_r = \Delta n/\tau_r$, divided by the total recombination rate, $R = \Delta n/\tau$, or

$$\eta = \tau_{nr}/(\tau_{nr} + \tau_r). \qquad (7.7\text{-}29)$$

Therefore, with $\eta \geq 0.5$, $\tau_{nr} \geq \tau_r$.

Values of n_{th} may be obtained from Eq. (7.7-27) with J_{th}, d, and the τ determined from the time-delay measurements. For typical cases, $n_{th} \approx 2 \pm 0.5 \times 10^{18}$ cm^{-3}. At this high electron concentration, the requirement for electrical neutrality, as expressed by Eq. (3.7-9), results in hole injection. For example with $(N_A^- - N_D^+) = 2.5 \times 10^{17}$ cm^{-3} and $n_{th} = 2 \times 10^{18}$ cm^{-3}, p is increased from its thermal equilibrium value of $\sim 2.5 \times 10^{17}$ cm^{-3} to 2.25×10^{18} cm^{-3}.

Dyment et al.[139] demonstrated that the time delays can be reduced by prebiasing the laser to a current near threshold. If the laser is prebiased to

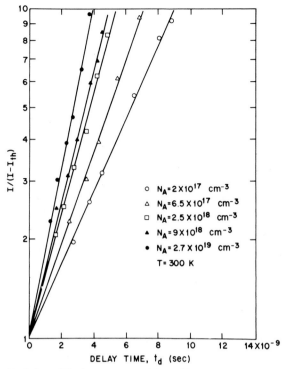

FIG. 7.7-8 Variation of the laser turn-on delay with current above threshold for active layers with the indicated Ge acceptor concentrations (Ref. 141).

$I_0 < I_{th}$, solution of Eq. (7.7-23) with the initial condition $n(0) = I_0\tau/Aqd$ gives[139]

$$\tau_d = \tau \ln[(I - I_0)/(I - I_{th})]. \tag{7.7-30}$$

In their example, prebiasing reduced t_d from 5×10^{-9} sec to 0.7×10^{-9} sec.

Transverse-Stripe Shunting Current

The analysis of the current flow in the stripe-geometry lasers was concerned with lateral confinement. However, for the junction-stripe (JS) laser and the transverse-junction-stripe (TJS) laser that were illustrated in Fig. 7.6-4, it is important to consider the shunting current.[117,143] Only the TJS laser will be considered,[117] but a similar analysis applies to the JS laser. The problem in the TJS laser is the relative amount of current that crosses the p–n junction in the active region to the shunting current of the P–N junction marked by the heavy line in Fig. 7.6-4b. There are two properties of this structure that influence the shunting current.

The first of these properties is the ratio of the current densities through the $p–n$ and $P–N$ junctions. From arguments that are similar to the derivation of Eq. (4.5-38) for a heterojunction, the ratio of the injection current density through the $p–n$ junction i_n to the injection current density through the $P–N$ junction i_N will be

$$i_n/i_N \approx \exp[\Delta E_g/kT], \qquad (7.7\text{-}31)$$

where ΔE_g is the difference in energy gaps of the GaAs for the $p–n$ junction and the $Al_xGa_{1-x}As$ for the $P–N$ junction. Equation (7.7-31) is for the same voltage across each junction. The area of the $p–n$ junction is $d \times L$, and the area of the $P–N$ junction is $W \times L$. Therefore, the current ratio $I_n/I_N \approx (d/W)\exp(\Delta E_g/kT)$ is reduced from the ratio of the current densities by d/W.

The second property that leads to significant shunting current is the difference in voltage across the $p–n$ and $P–N$ junctions. The junction voltage V_j is the applied voltage V less the series resistance voltage drop: $V_j = V - I_j R_j$. Because the p-layer of the active region is so thin, R_j for the $p–n$ junction is much greater than for the $P–N$ junction, and V_j for the $p–n$ junction will be less than for the $P–N$ junction. This effect further reduces the i_n/i_N ratio. Experimentally, the TJS laser was found to have a large temperature dependence of J_{th} which was attributed to the temperature dependence of the shunting current.[117]

The effects of the shunting $P–N$ junction were eliminated by Susaki et al.[144] by adding an additional n-layer as shown in Fig. 7.7-9. The $P–n$ junction is reverse biased and eliminates the shunting current. This structure gave a temperature dependence of J_{th} between $-40°$ and $100°C$ that was almost identical to the dependence of a conventional broad-area DH laser.[144] Threshold currents for this new structure are 30–40 mA for cw operation at room temperature. Single longitudinal-mode emission as well as a fundamental transverse mode are obtained for currents up to twice threshold.[144]

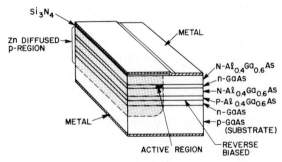

FIG. 7.7-9 Transverse-junction stripe-geometry laser with n-layer added to provide reverse biased $P–n$ junction in order to eliminate shunt currents (Ref. 144).

7.8 THERMAL PROPERTIES OF STRIPE-GEOMETRY LASERS

Steady-State Thermal Resistance

The thermal behavior for a particular device configuration is represented by its mean thermal resistance $\langle R \rangle$. The thermal resistance of the active layer is given by the mean temperature rise of the active layer relative to the heat sink divided by the heat generation rate in the active layer. Therefore, $\langle R \rangle$ influences device operation through its effect upon the active-region temperature, and an increase in temperature increases J_{th} because of the basic temperature dependence of the threshold as presented in Section 7.4. Higher temperature also decreases the operating life of the device as discussed in Chapter 8.

Joyce and Dixon[145] considered the uniform generation of heat in a plane-stripe source which is in a rectangular layered structure. The stripe-geometry DH laser bonded to the heat sink is schematically represented in Fig. 7.8-1. Nominal layer parameters are also given. The heat flow is two

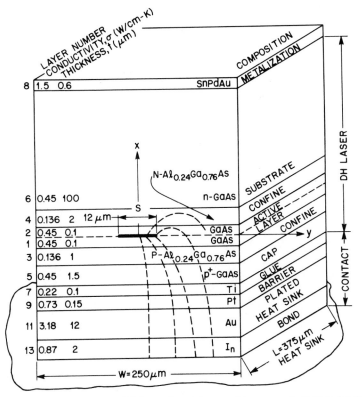

FIG. 7.8-1   Stripe-geometry DH laser dimensions and layer conductivities for the calculation of the thermal resistance (Ref. 145).

dimensional in the x–y plane as shown by the dashed lines, and the thermal resistance will depend on the stripe width S, the cavity length L, and also the layer thickness t and thermal conductivity σ of each layer. The thermal conductivity depends on the composition and is shown for $Al_xGa_{1-x}As$ in Fig. 7.8-2 as the thermal resistivity $\rho = 1/\sigma$.[146] The thermal conductivities for several other III–V binary compounds and ternary solid solutions have been summarized by Maycock.[147]

The temperature $T(x, y)$ within a layer is obtained from a solution of Laplace's equation.[145,148] The thermal resistance along the stripe is given by

$$R(y) = T_1(0, y)/P, \tag{7.8-1}$$

where P is the heat generation rate in the active layer and $T_1(0, y)$ the temperature along the stripe. The evaluation of $T_1(0, y)$ and hence $R(y)$ requires a series summation as described in Ref. 145. Only the results of numerical examples will be considered here. As discussed by Yonezu et al.,[149] the heat generation rate is the device current–applied voltage product less the optical output. At threshold, the external quantum efficiency is $\sim 5\%$, and the optical output power can be ignored. At $J > J_{th}$, the external efficiency may be ~ 20–40%, and therefore the optical output power must be taken into account. For the experimental internal efficiency of ~ 0.6–0.9, there is high conversion of the current to stimulated emission. It is difficult to determine where this emission is absorbed and how it influences the device temperature. These uncertainties do not influence the value of $\langle R \rangle$, but they can influence the value of T calculated from $\langle R \rangle P$.

The mean thermal resistance $\langle R \rangle$ is

$$\langle R \rangle = \frac{1}{S} \int_{-S/2}^{S/2} R(y)\, dy. \tag{7.8-2}$$

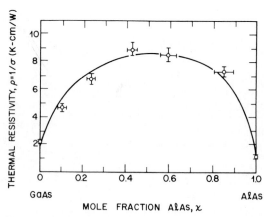

FIG. 7.8-2 Thermal resistivity as a function of the AlAs mole fraction (Ref. 146).

In Fig. 7.8-1, the heat source is embedded in the vertical center of the active layer. This approximation to the uniform vertical distribution in the active layer has negligible influence on the results. With the dimensions and conductivities given in Fig. 7.8-1,[145]

$$\langle R \rangle = 20.6°\text{K/W} \tag{7.8-3}$$

within the active layer. For operation at 0.2 A and 1.6 V, the mean active-layer temperature rise ΔT is $0.2 \times 1.6 \times 20.6 = 6.6°\text{K}$, when the optical output is ignored.

Joyce and Dixon[145] also considered the effect of factor-of-two variations in several dimensions about the nominal values given in Fig. 7.8-1. Their results are shown in Fig. 7.8-3. With ΔT taken as $\langle R \rangle IV$, the current will vary as L for a constant current density, and $\langle R \rangle$ will vary as $1/L$ as shown in the figure. It is also shown that doubling S to 24 μm reduces $\langle R \rangle$ from 20.6 to 12.7°K/W, while halving S to 6 μm raises $\langle R \rangle$ to 31.9°K/W. At $S = 4$ μm, $\langle R \rangle = 39.8°\text{K/W}$; at $S = 3$ μm, $\langle R \rangle = 45.9°\text{K/W}$; and at $S = 2$ μm, $\langle R \rangle = 54.4°\text{K/W}$. As illustrated in Fig. 7.7-4, J_{th} also increases as the stripe width is narrowed. However, the product $\langle R \rangle \times J_{th} \times S \times L$ varies slowly with S until J_{th} becomes very large for $S < 10$ μm.

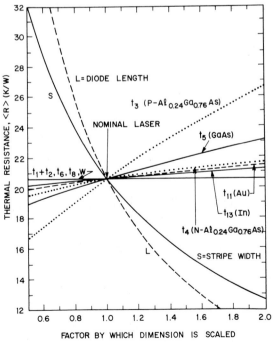

FIG. 7.8-3 Thermal resistance of the stripe-geometry DH laser of Fig. 7.8-1 as a function of factor-of-two changes in characteristic dimensions (Ref. 145).

A factor of ± 2 in the thickness of the P–$Al_{0.24}Ga_{0.76}As$ layer (layer 3) changes $\langle R \rangle$ by 6.1 to 3.9°K/W. Elimination of the p^+–GaAs layer (layer 5) reduces $\langle R \rangle$ by 3.2°K/W. Factors of two in any other dimensions account for less than ± 1.2°K/W. The "heat spreader" layer (layer 11) is added on the assumption that the thermal resistance of the In bond would be reduced. This reduction would occur because the heat first spreads over a large area in the highly conductive Au layer before reaching the less conductive In. The calculated results show that the Au layer is actually unnecessary for thermal considerations. Also, about 40% of the temperature drop between the center of the active region and the heat sink occurs within the active region.

Because the thermal conductivity[104,150] of type II diamond is 20 W/cm-°K as compared to 4.0 W/cm-°K for pure Cu,[151] it would appear helpful to use a diamond heat sink. However, determination of $\langle R \rangle$ for diamond on a Cu stud gives an additional 7.3°K/W, while the addition to $\langle R \rangle$ for the Cu heat sink would be 10.1°K/W. At a power of 0.25 W the active-region temperatures of two lasers of the type shown in Fig. 7.8-1 would differ by only 1°K if one were mounted on diamond and the other on copper. This provides little justification for the diamond. Yonezu et al.[149] also considered mounting on a Si heat sink to more closely match the thermal expansion of GaAs. With a Si heat sink, it is possible to use "hard" bonding methods with higher melting temperatures than for the "soft" In without introducing excessive bonding strain.[149] The thermal resistance is increased, however, as compared to a Cu heat sink.

Mounting in the junction-up configuration with the substrate on the heat sink was also considered.[145] For this case of junction-up mounting, the thermal resistance $\langle R \rangle$ is raised from 20.6 to 82.9°K/W. The substrate becomes a dominant part of the resistance, and the heteroepitaxial layer thicknesses make little difference. In this case, the heat spreader (layer 1) is helpful, and with a 12-μm-thick spreader on the laser of Fig. 7.8-1, $\langle R \rangle = 49.6$°K/W.

The thermal resistance based on one-dimensional heat flow straight down from the stripe gives $\langle R \rangle = 39.2$°K/W for $S = 12$ μm as compared to 20.6°K/W for two-dimensional heat flow. For a 250-μm-wide broad-area laser with the same layer parameters, $\langle R \rangle = 39.2(12/250) = 1.9$°K/W. However, the current is much larger, and a numerical example shows the predicted mean active region temperature rise is about the same for the broad-area and stripe-geometry DH laser. From Fig. 7.7-4, $J_{th} = 8 \times 10^3$ A/cm^2 for $S = 10$ μm, and $J_{th} = 4 \times 10^3$ A/cm^2 for $S = 50$ μm. For the stripe-geometry laser, $\Delta T = 20.6 \times 8 \times 10^3 \times 10 \times 10^{-4} \times 380 \times 10^{-4} \times 1.6 = 10.0$°K, and with the same J_{th} for $S = 250$ μm as for $S = 50$ μm, $\Delta T = 1.9 \times 4 \times 10^3 \times 250 \times 10^{-4} \times 380 \times 10^{-4} \times 1.6 = 11.6$°K for the broad-area DH laser. For further examples and discussion of the steady-state thermal resistance of stripe-geometry DH lasers, Ref. 145 should be consulted. It should be noted that the thermal properties for the other stripe-geometry lasers presented in Section 7.6 may differ from the proton-bombarded case considered here.

Paoli[152] measured the thermal resistance of stripe-geometry DH lasers by determining the exact wavelength of a single Fabry–Perot mode. This measurement is based on the temperature dependence of the refractive index [Eq. (2.3-1)]. In this technique, the decrease in heat-sink temperature required to maintain an individual Fabry–Perot mode at a preselected wavelength is measured as the operational duty cycle is increased at constant current from near 0 to 100%. For two 13-μm-wide stripe-geometry DH lasers mounted p-side down on Cu, $\langle R \rangle$ values of 22 and 58°K/W were obtained. Since the layer thicknesses and compositions were not specified for these lasers, it is not possible to directly compare these experimental $\langle R \rangle$ values with the $\langle R \rangle$ of 20.6°K/W for the structure of Fig. 7.8-1. However, it is interesting to note that the lower experimental $\langle R \rangle$ value is near the calculated value.

Kobayashi and Iwane[152a] extended the numerical analysis of the thermal properties of GaAs–Al$_x$Ga$_{1-x}$As DH lasers to the three-dimensional case. This analysis permitted investigation of the influence of solder voids on the temperature distribution in the active region. They found that solder voids must be less than 4 μm × 4 μm to prevent local heating from exceeding 10% of the uniform temperature rise. The local heating due to solder voids probably explains why it was possible in the initial work with DH lasers to obtain cw operation more readily with stripe-geometry lasers than with broad-area lasers. The broad-area lasers increased the chances for significant solder voids. Kobayashi and Iwane[152a] also gave experimental temperature distributions along the stripe active region and suggested the importance of uniform temperature distribution to long operating life.

Transient Temperature Distributions

There are two different time scales that should be distinguished when considering thermal effects in heterostructure lasers.[153] The steady-state is only reached after times of seconds or longer, while temperature gradients are formed near the active region over a much shorter time period after the application of a current pulse. Joyce has considered the magnitude and rise time of the temperature gradients.[153]

Several interesting conclusions were derived from this analysis of the transient temperature distributions.[153] The rapid local formation of temperature gradients depends almost exclusively on the thermal properties of the Al$_x$Ga$_{1-x}$As layers adjacent to the active layer. However, in the steady-state case the temperature rise is influenced by the other epitaxial layers, the metallization, and mounting structure. Also, thermal-gradient effects remain small for about 10×10^{-9} sec. Since carrier-lifetime effects were shown in Section 7.7 to have response times less than 5×10^{-9} sec, this difference in time scale can be helpful in distinguishing between electrical and thermal effects.

7.9 GAIN-COEFFICIENT MEASUREMENTS

Measurement Technique

In previous portions of this chapter, the experimental threshold current density has been compared to values derived from the calculated gain coefficient. It is also useful to consider measured values of the gain coefficient near threshold. A very straightforward and useful gain-coefficient measure-measurement technique for stripe-geometry lasers was illustrated by Hakki and Paoli.[154,155] In this part of Section 7.9, the quantitative expressions necessary for the interpretation of the experimental data will be derived. The experimental technique for measurement of the gain coefficient is based on the measurement of the ratio of the maximum to the minimum of the Fabry–Perot resonance of the spontaneous emission.[154,155] The experimental results based on this technique will be illustrated in the next part of this section.

For reflection between parallel, partially reflecting surfaces (a Fabry–Perot cavity) as illustrated in Fig. 3.8-1, the transmitted field for constructive interference $\mathscr{E}_t{}^+$ was given by Eq. (3.8-3) as

$$\mathscr{E}_t{}^+ = \mathscr{E}_i\left[\frac{t_1 t_2 \exp(-\Gamma L)}{1 - r_1 r_2 \exp(-2\Gamma L)}\right]. \tag{7.9-1}$$

For destructive interference,

$$\mathscr{E}_t{}^- = t_1 t_2 \mathscr{E}_i \exp(-\Gamma L)[1 - r_1 r^2 \exp(-2\Gamma L) + r_1{}^2 r_2{}^2 \exp(-4\Gamma L) - \cdots], \tag{7.9-2}$$

or

$$\mathscr{E}_t{}^- = \mathscr{E}_i\left[\frac{t_1 t_2 \exp(-\Gamma L)}{1 + r_1 r_2 \exp(-2\Gamma L)}\right]. \tag{7.9-3}$$

Taking the ratio of the field maxima and minima gives

$$\frac{\mathscr{E}_t{}^+ - \mathscr{E}_t{}^-}{\mathscr{E}_t{}^+ + \mathscr{E}_t{}^-} = r_1 r_2 \exp(-2\Gamma L). \tag{7.9-4}$$

From Eq. (2.2-54), the complex propagation constant $\Gamma = j(\bar{n} - j\bar{k})k_0$, with $k_0 = 2\pi/\lambda_0$, and $\bar{k} = \alpha\lambda_0/4\pi$ so that

$$\Gamma = j(2\pi\bar{n}/\lambda_0) + \alpha/2. \tag{7.9-5}$$

With Eq. (7.9-5) for Γ and by taking the magnitude of Eq. (7.9-4) gives

$$\frac{\left|\mathcal{E}_t^+\right| - \left|\mathcal{E}_t^-\right|}{\left|\mathcal{E}_t^+\right| + \left|\mathcal{E}_t^-\right|} = r_1 r_2 \exp(-\alpha L). \tag{7.9-6}$$

Since the experimental measurements give intensities $P = \left|\mathcal{E}_t\right|^2$, measurement of the adjacent interference maxima and minima intensities may be used with Eq. (7.9-6) to determine α. Replacing $\left|\mathcal{E}_t^+\right|$ by $(P_t^+)^{1/2}$ and $\left|\mathcal{E}_t^-\right|$ by $(P_t^-)^{1/2}$ and the field reflectivities r by the power reflectivities $R^{1/2}$ gives

$$-\alpha = (g - \alpha_i)\Gamma = \frac{1}{L}\left\{\frac{1}{2}\ln\left(\frac{1}{R_1 R_2}\right) + \ln\left[\frac{(P_t^+)^{1/2} - (P_t^-)^{1/2}}{(P_t^+)^{1/2} + (P_t^-)^{1/2}}\right]\right\}. \tag{7.9-7}$$

In Eq. (7.9-7), the absorption term has been written as the difference between the gain coefficient g and all of the losses α_i which were given in Eq. (7.4-4). The net gain coefficient $(g - \alpha_i)$ has been multiplied by the confinement factor Γ to take into account the portion of the propagating mode within the active layer. It should be noted that the symbol Γ was used for the complex propagation constant in Eqs. (7.9-1)–(7.9-5). Values of the confinement factor were given in Chapter 2. Equation (7.9-7) is the expression needed to obtain the gain coefficient from experimental measurements.

Experimental Results

The experimental technique requires the measurement of P_t^+ and P_t^- for the spontaneous emission as illustrated schematically in Fig. 7.9-1. The adjacent maxima P_t^+ and minima P_t^- may be measured with a grating spectrometer as a function of current. This technique is illustrated by the expanded wavelength inserts. For this example the separation of adjacent modes is 2.5 Å. Above threshold, the Fabry–Perot resonances for the spontaneous emission may still be observed at wavelengths away from the more intense stimulated emission. Lasers have to be carefully selected for uniform and stable lasing behavior along the junction plane over a substantial current range above threshold.

The gain coefficient measurements obtained by Hakki and Paoli[155] are shown in Fig. 7.9-2. The measurements were made on a GaAs–$Al_{0.36}Ga_{0.64}As$ DH laser with a 0.25-μm-thick active layer that was doped p-type with Ge to give $p_0 \approx 4 \times 10^{17}$ cm^{-3}. Lateral current confinement was provided by proton bombardmaent to give $S \approx 10 \ \mu$m. The cavity length was 380 μm. The laser was bonded on a heat sink for cw operation. A data acquisition system was used to obtain continuous measurements between 0.9 and 0.865 μm. A value of $\Gamma = 0.76$ was used in Eq. (7.9-7) so that $(g - \alpha_i)$ was plotted. Both TE and TM polarizations were measured.

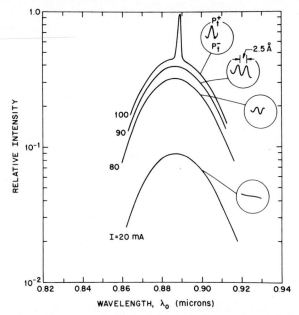

FIG. 7.9-1 Schematic representation of the emission spectra and the Fabry–Perot resonances for the spontaneous emission. The maximum P_t^+ and the minimum P_t^- are used in Eq. (7.9-7) to obtain the gain coefficient. The inserts have an expanded wavelength scale to illustrate the cavity modes.

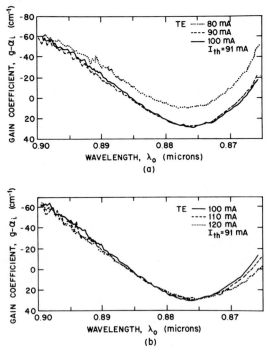

FIG. 7.9-2 Gain spectra for the TE polarization in a GaAs–$Al_{0.36}Ga_{0.64}As$ stripe-geometry DH laser between currents of 80 and 120 mA. The threshold current is 91 mA (Ref. 155).

As the current was increased, the gain coefficient at a fixed wavelength increases linearly. The wavelength for the peak gain coefficient decreases (photon energy increases) as the current is increased. The gain coefficient saturates at threshold. The variation of the gain coefficient with current at fixed wavelengths shorter than the lasing wavelength of 0.876 μm is shown in Fig. 7.9-3. Similar curves for wavelengths that are longer than the lasing wavelengths are shown in Fig. 7.9-4. These figures show that the gain coefficient above J_{th} saturates for TE polarization only at wavelengths close to the lasing wavelength, and increases slightly at shorter wavelengths. Further discussion of the gain-coefficient spectra are given in Ref. 155.

The experimental gain-coefficient dependence on current near the lasing wavelength was found to be represented by[155]

$$g = 5.45 \times 10^{-2}(J_{nom} - 4 \times 10^3) \qquad (7.9\text{-}8)$$

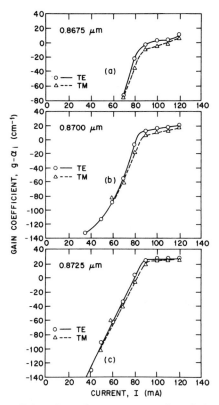

FIG. 7.9-3 Gain coefficient dependence on current in a GaAs–Al$_{0.36}$Ga$_{0.64}$As stripe-geometry DH laser for wavelengths between 0.8675 and 0.8725 μm. The lasing wavelengths in the TE mode are centered around 0.8760 μm (Ref. 155).

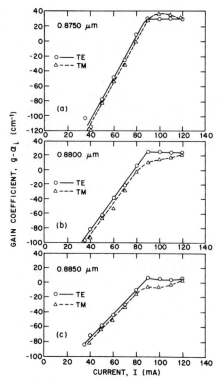

FIG. 7.9-4 Gain coefficient dependence on current in a GaAs–Al$_{0.36}$Ga$_{0.64}$As stripe-geometry DH laser for wavelengths between 0.8750 and 0.8850 μm. The TE lasing wavelengths are centered around 0.8760 μm (Ref. 155).

for $d = 1$ μm. From Stern's[60] calculated g_{max} given by Eq. (7.4-6), the prefactor was 5.0×10^{-2} and the zero current offset was 4.5×10^3. It is indeed remarkable that these experimental and calculated numerical quantities agree within $\sim 10\%$. Further comparisons are discussed in Ref. 60.

7.10 GAIN GUIDING IN STRIPE-GEOMETRY LASERS

Introductory Comments

In the early studies of the emission of stripe-geometry homostructure lasers, the Hermite–Gaussian-mode structure in the direction along the junction plane suggested the presence of a spatially varying refractive index along the junction plane.[100,156] Further measurements demonstrated the presence of nonplanar phase fronts for stripe-geometry homostructure[157] and DH lasers.[158] The nonplanar phase fronts led to the suggestion that gain provides the mode confinement along the junction plane.[159,160] As shown in Chapter 2, waveguiding is based on the spatial variation of the dielectric constant which is a complex quantity. When the real part of the dielectric constant, which is related to the refractive index, dominates the guiding both perpendicular to and along the junction plane, the phase fronts are planar.[156] If the variation of the imaginary part of the dielectric constant, which is related to the gain, is significant along the junction plane, then the phase fronts are cylindrically concave in the direction of the wave propagation. Gain guiding occurs when the gain rather than the refractive index influences the field distributions.

The wave fronts for the stripe-geometry laser in Fig. 7.10-1a are illustrated in Fig. 7.10-1b, c, d. In part (b), the phase fronts for the field determined by index guiding perpendicular to the junction plane due to the heterostructure

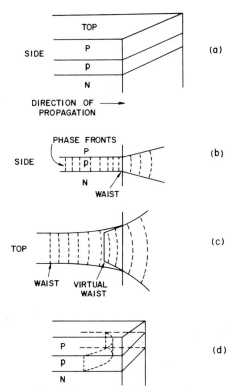

FIG. 7.10-1 Schematic representation of the phase fronts (dashed lines) for stripe-geometry lasers. (a) Geometry of waveguide. (b) Field confined by the refractive index change of the heterostructure layers perpendicular to the junction plane. (c) Field confined by gain guiding along the junction plane. (d) Cylindrical phase front.

are planar, and the waist, where the beam front is planar and beam size is a minimum, occurs at the mirror. Along the junction where the fields are influenced by gain guiding, a virtual waist is observed ~ 40 μm[158] behind the laser mirror as illustrated in part (c). These fields give the cylindrical phase front shown in part (d). This beam is astigmatic because the beam waist (source plane) is at the mirror face for the field confined perpendicular to the junction plane, while the virtual beam waist for the field confined along the junction plane is behind the mirror face. This astigmatism can be important to consider when the output is coupled into lenses.

It is necessary to consider only lasing modes that are well behaved and fill the active region rather than filamentary lasing. Hakki[127] showed that the carrier distribution along the junction plane was consistent with carrier diffusion as represented in Section 7.7. Nash[160] considered the mode guidance along the junction plane. Experimental measurements of the far-field beam divergence and beam width at the laser mirror along the junction plane permitted Cook and Nash[158] to calculate the gain distribution responsible for waveguiding. They showed that the lowest-order fundamental mode along the junction plane was approximately Gaussian, which is consistent with an approximately parabolic spatial guiding mechanism. Further measurements by Paoli[161] showed that optical confinement along the junction plane is primarily by the optical gain profile. Also, the remainder of the confinement is consistent with a refractive index profile determined by the temperature distribution in the presence of defocusing by the index change due to the injected free carriers.[161] In this section, the solution of the three-dimensional wave equation for a spatial variation of the complex dielectric constant along the junction plane is presented. Then the derived expressions will be used to explain the experimental behavior of the optical intensity along the junction plane for stripe-geometry GaAs–Al$_x$Ga$_{1-x}$As DH lasers. Although most of the analysis for waveguiding in stripe-geometry lasers has considered the proton-bombarded structure, Aiki et al.[114a] have analyzed waveguiding in the CSP structure.

Solution of the Wave Equation

For the structure given in Fig. 7.10-2, the wave equation is given by Eq. (2.4-10), and with the sinusoidal time dependence given by $\exp(j\omega t)$, the wave equation becomes

$$\nabla^2 \mathscr{E}_y + \omega^2 \mu_0 \varepsilon \mathscr{E}_y = 0. \qquad (7.10\text{-}1)$$

With Eqs. (2.2-33), (2.2-35), and (2.2-38), Eq. (7.10-1) may be written as

$$\nabla^2 \mathscr{E}_y + (k_0{}^2 \varepsilon/\varepsilon_0) \mathscr{E}_y = 0. \qquad (7.10\text{-}2)$$

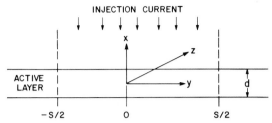

FIG. 7.10-2 Coordinate system used for the solution of the wave equation for a stripe-geometry laser with the stripe width S defined by proton bombardment.

In this equation, $\varepsilon/\varepsilon_0$ is taken as two dimensional with the form:[158,161]

$$\varepsilon(x, y)/\varepsilon_0 = [\varepsilon(0) - a^2 y^2]/\varepsilon_0 \tag{7.10-3}$$

within the active layer, and

$$\varepsilon(x, y)/\varepsilon_0 = \varepsilon_1/\varepsilon_0 \tag{7.10-4}$$

outside the active layer in the cladding layers. In Eq. (7.10-3), $\varepsilon(0)$ is the complex dielectric constant $\varepsilon_r(0) + j\varepsilon_i(0)$ at $y = 0$ in the active layer, and a is a complex constant represented as

$$a = a_r + ja_i. \tag{7.10-5}$$

A rigorous solution of Eq. (7.10-2) is not available for a dielectric constant represented by Eqs. (7.10-3) and (7.10-4). As illustrated by Paoli,[161] it is convenient to assume that a first approximation to the solutions of Eq. (7.10-2) is given by

$$\mathscr{E}_y(x, y, z) = \mathscr{E}_y(x)\mathscr{E}_y(y)\exp(-j\beta_z z). \tag{7.10-6}$$

Because $\varepsilon(x, y)$ varies slowly with y along the junction plane, it was also assumed[161] that $\mathscr{E}_y(x)$ is not significantly affected by the confinement along y, and from Eq. (7.10-2) by the separation of variables,

$$[\partial^2 \mathscr{E}_y(x)/\partial x^2] + \beta_x^2 \mathscr{E}_y(x) = 0. \tag{7.10-7}$$

Substitution of Eqs. (7.10-6) and (7.10-7) into the wave equation of Eq. (7.10-2) gives

$$\mathscr{E}_y(x)[d^2\mathscr{E}_y(y)/dy^2] + (k_0^2 \varepsilon/\varepsilon_0 - \beta_x^2 - \beta_z^2)\mathscr{E}_y(x)\mathscr{E}_y(y) = 0. \tag{7.10-8}$$

To eliminate $\mathscr{E}_y(x)$, Eq. (7.10-8) is multiplied by its complex conjugate $\mathscr{E}_y^*(x)$ and integrated over x to give

$$[d^2\mathscr{E}_y(y)/dy^2] + \{k_0^2[\varepsilon(0) - a^2 y^2]\Gamma/\varepsilon_0 + \varepsilon_1 k_0^2(1 - \Gamma)/\varepsilon_0$$
$$- \beta_x^2 - \beta_z^2\}\mathscr{E}_y(y) = 0. \tag{7.10-9}$$

In Eq. (7.10-9), the confinement factor Γ is given by

$$\Gamma = \int_{-d/2}^{d/2} |\mathcal{E}_y(x)|^2 \, dx \Big/ \int_{-\infty}^{\infty} |\mathcal{E}_y(x)|^2 \, dx. \tag{7.10-10}$$

A more standard form is

$$[d^2\mathcal{E}_y(y)/dy^2] + \{k_0^2[\Gamma\varepsilon(0)/\varepsilon_0 + (1 - \Gamma)\varepsilon_1/\varepsilon_0] - \beta_x^2 - \beta_z^2$$
$$- (\Gamma k_0^2 a^2 y^2/\varepsilon_0)\}\mathcal{E}_y(y) = 0. \tag{7.10-11}$$

The field distributions for $\mathcal{E}_y(y)$ represented by Eq. (7.10-11) are Hermite–Gaussian functions,[160] and therefore

$$\mathcal{E}_y(y) = H_p[(\Gamma^{1/2}ak_0/\varepsilon_0^{1/2})^{1/2}y]\exp[-\tfrac{1}{2}(\Gamma/\varepsilon_0)^{1/2}ak_0y^2], \tag{7.10-12}$$

where H_p is the Hermite polynomial of order p. The Hermite polynomial is given by[162]

$$H_p(\xi) = (-1)^p \exp(\xi^2)\partial^p \exp(-\xi^2)/\partial\xi^p, \tag{7.10-13}$$

and the first three Hermite polynomials are $H_0(\xi) = 1$, $H_1(\xi) = 2\xi$, and $H_2(\xi) = 4\xi^2 - 2$. Therefore, the intensity for the fundamental mode is Gaussian and is given by

$$|\mathcal{E}_y(y)|^2 = \exp[-(\Gamma/\varepsilon_0)^{1/2}a_r k_0 y^2], \tag{7.10-14}$$

which demonstrates that the intensity distribution along the junction plane is influenced by a_r.

An expression for a_r requires the assignment of the refractive index $\bar{n}$ and gain coefficient g along the junction plane. Since the dielectric constant is the complex refractive index squared (see Section 2.2), it is convenient to write Eq. (7.10-3) as

$$\bar{N} = \{[\varepsilon(0) - a^2 y^2]/\varepsilon_0\}^{1/2} = \bar{n} - j\bar{k}. \tag{7.10-15}$$

or with the complex forms of $\varepsilon(0)$ and a,

$$\bar{n} - j\bar{k} = \left[\frac{\varepsilon_r(0)}{\varepsilon_0} - \left(\frac{(a_r^2 - a_i^2)y^2 - j[\varepsilon_i(0) - 2a_r a_i y^2]}{\varepsilon_0}\right)\right]^{1/2}. \tag{7.10-16}$$

For $\varepsilon_r(0) \gg \varepsilon_i(0)$ or $\varepsilon_r(0) \gg a^2 y^2$,

$$\bar{n} - j\bar{k} = \left(\frac{\varepsilon_r(0)}{\varepsilon_0}\right)^{1/2}\left[1 - \left(\frac{(a_r^2 - a_i^2)y^2 - j[\varepsilon_i(0) - 2a_r a_i y^2]}{2\varepsilon_r(0)}\right)\right]. \tag{7.10-17}$$

Therefore, equating real and imaginary parts gives

$$\bar{n} = \left(\frac{\varepsilon_r(0)}{\varepsilon_0}\right)^{1/2} - \frac{(a_r^2 - a_i^2)y^2}{2[\varepsilon_r(0)\varepsilon_0]^{1/2}}, \tag{7.10-18}$$

and

$$\bar{k} = -\left(\frac{\varepsilon_r(0)}{\varepsilon_0}\right)^{1/2}\left[\frac{\varepsilon_i(0) - 2a_r a_i y^2}{2\varepsilon_r(0)}\right], \tag{7.10-19}$$

where $\bar{k}$ is related to the absorption coefficient α by

$$\bar{k} = \alpha\lambda_0/4\pi. \tag{2.2-61}$$

The models for the variation of the refractive index $\bar{n}(y)$ and gain coefficient $g(y) = -\alpha$, as given in Eqs. (7.10-18) and (7.10-19), are schematically represented in Fig. 7.10-3. At $y = 0$, $\bar{n}(0) = [\varepsilon_r(0)/\varepsilon_0]^{1/2}$ and at $|y| = S/2$, $\bar{n}(S/2) = \bar{n}(0) - \Delta\bar{n}$, and therefore,

$$\bar{n}(y) = \bar{n}(0) - (4\Delta\bar{n}/S^2)y^2, \tag{7.10-20}$$

and similarly,

$$g(y) = g(0) - (4\Delta g/S^2)y^2. \tag{7.10-21}$$

Equating Eqs. (7.10-18) and (7.10-20) gives

$$a_r^2 - a_i^2 = [8\bar{n}(0)\Delta\bar{n}/S^2]\varepsilon_0, \tag{7.10-22}$$

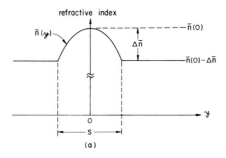

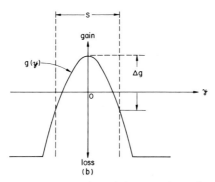

FIG. 7.10-3 Schematic representation of the complex refractive index. (a) Spatial variation of the real refractive index. (b) Spatial variation of the gain (Ref. 158).

and with Eq. (2.2-61) for $\bar{k}$, equating Eqs. (7.10-19) and (7.10-21) gives

$$a_i = \lambda_0 \Delta g \bar{n}(0) \varepsilon_0 / \pi S^2 a_r. \qquad (7.10\text{-}23)$$

With Eq. (7.10-23) in Eq. (7.10-22),

$$a_r^2 = \varepsilon_0 \left\{ \frac{4\bar{n}(0)\Delta\bar{n}}{S^2} + \left[\left(\frac{4\bar{n}(0)\Delta\bar{n}}{S^2} \right)^2 + \left(\frac{\lambda_0 \Delta g \bar{n}(0)}{\pi S^2} \right)^2 \right]^{1/2} \right\}. \qquad (7.10\text{-}24)$$

For this two-dimensional model, the refractive index $\bar{n}(0)$ by Eq. (7.10-11) is $[\Gamma\varepsilon(0)/\varepsilon_0 - (1 - \Gamma)\varepsilon_1/\varepsilon_0]^{1/2}$.[161] Equation (7.10-14) with Eq. (7.10-24) for a_r gives the intensity distribution along the junction plane.

Additional properties of the fields were derived by Cook and Nash.[158] They obtain expressions for the radius of curvature of the phase fronts, the beam width, and the location of the virtual waist. Reference 158 should be consulted for further details.

Demonstration of Gain Guiding

Studies by Nash,[160] Cook and Nash,[158] and Paoli[161] have been devoted to the demonstration of gain guiding. The basic technique has been to relate the width of the lasing region along the junction plane to the width expected for gain guiding. The results of Paoli[161] will be summarized in this part of Section 7.10.

Paoli measured the variation of the optical field by magnifying the image at the laser mirror more than 500 times.[161] The magnified image was focused onto an aperture that corresponded to a width of 0.3 μm on the laser mirror. A proton-bombarded stripe-geometry $Al_{0.36}Ga_{0.64}As|Al_{0.08}Ga_{0.92}As|$ $Al_{0.36}Ga_{0.64}As$ DH laser was used for the measurements. The active-layer thickness was 0.12 μm, and the stripe width was 12 μm. For this structure, the confinement factor Γ was 0.3.[161] The protons penetrated close to, but not into, the active layer.

The carrier distribution within the active region was shown to be determined by lateral diffusion[127,158,161] which was presented in Section 7.7. At low currents, the spontaneous optical intensity along the junction plane is taken to be proportional to the carrier concentration, and therefore the profile is given by Eqs. (7.7-15) and (7.7-16) for $I = I_e$ and $I_0 = 0$. The carrier distributions are then given for $|y| < S/2$ as[127]

$$n(y) = (I\tau_n/qSLd)[1 - \cosh(y/L_n)\exp(-S/2L_n)], \qquad (7.10\text{-}25)$$

and for $|y| > S/2$ as

$$n(y) = (I\tau_n/qSLd)\sinh(S/2L_n)\exp(-S/2L_n)\exp[-(|y| - S/2)/L_n]. \qquad (7.10\text{-}26)$$

A fit of these expressions to the experimental data shown by the solid line in Fig. 7.10-4 gives $S = 11.7 \pm 0.3$ μm and $L_n = 3.6 \pm 0.3$ μm.[161] The open

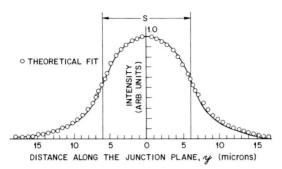

FIG. 7.10-4   Intensity of the spontaneous emission as a function of distance along the junction plane at 40 mA or less. The open circles were calculated from Eqs. (7.10-25) and (7.10-26) for $S = 11.7\ \mu$m and $L_n = 3.6\ \mu$m (Ref. 161).

circles in Fig. 7.10-4 were calculated with these parameters. Although the stripe width is 12 μm, it may be seen in Fig. 7.10-4 that the spontaneous emission extends over a considerably larger distance.

Next, the variation of the intensity distribution along the junction plane is measured as a function of current. The full width at half-power in Fig. 7.10-4 was 12.8 μm. The half-power full width is shown in Fig. 7.10-5 for the total TE emission and for the TE emission of two Fabry–Perot modes of the laser cavity. These data demonstrate the narrowing of a longitudinal mode as a function of current below threshold, and the relatively constant width at 6.5 μm above threshold. This figure also shows that the width of the total TE intensity is a measure of the width of the guided mode for $I > 1.1I_{\text{th}}$.

With the intensity represented by Eq. (7.10-14), the full width at half intensity w is given by

$$w^2 = -4\ln 0.5/(\Gamma/\varepsilon_0)^{1/2}a_r k_0. \qquad (7.10\text{-}27)$$

Therefore, the measured w^2 gives $(\Gamma/\varepsilon_0)^{1/2}a_r k_0$ and permits calculation of the optical-intensity profile. The carrier concentration and optical-intensity profile for $w = 6.5\ \mu$m are shown in Fig. 7.10-6. For gain guiding with $\Delta\bar{n}$ taken as zero, Eq. (7.10-24) gives a_r as $[\varepsilon_0\lambda_0\Delta g\bar{n}(0)/\pi S^2]^{1/2}$, so that with Eq. (7.10-27)

$$w^4 = 1.92\lambda_0 S^2/\Gamma\pi\bar{n}(0)\Delta g. \qquad (7.10\text{-}28)$$

Therefore, Eq. (7.10-28) may be used to determine whether or not the observed width w is consistent with the gain profile that is based on the carrier profile $n(y)$.

It was shown in Sections 7.4 and 7.9 that the gain-coefficient dependence on current could be represented as $g = A[J - J_0]$, and therefore the gain-coefficient profile may be related to the carrier-concentration profile by

$$g(y) = bn(y) - c. \qquad (7.10\text{-}29)$$

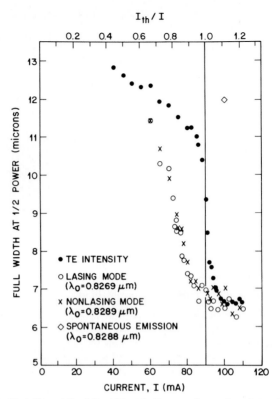

FIG. 7.10-5 Variation of the full width at half power for various intensity distributions emitted by a stripe-geometry DH laser as a function of junction current. The data represented by ○ and × are the measured half-width values for the intensity at the wavelengths of two longitudinal TE modes, while ● represents the half width of the total intensity emitted with TE polarization (Ref. 161).

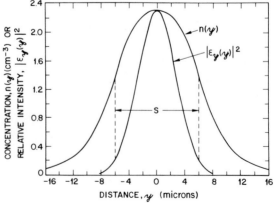

FIG. 7.10-6 Comparison of the electron concentration and optical intensity along the junction plane.

248

From Eq. (7.10-25) at $y = 0$,

$$n(0) = (I\tau_n/qSLd)[1 - \exp(-S/2L_n)], \tag{7.10-30}$$

so that Eqs. (7.10-29) and (7.10-30) give

$$g(0) = b(I\tau_n/qSLd)[1 - \exp(-S/2L_n)] - c. \tag{7.10-31}$$

With Δg defined as $g(0) - g(S/2)$ and with $n(S/2)$ given by Eqs. (7.10-25) or (7.10-26),

$$\Delta g = b(I\tau_n/qSLd)\exp(-S/2L_n)[\cosh(S/2L_n) - 1]. \tag{7.10-32}$$

Equations (7.10-31) and (7.10-32) provide expressions for $g(0)$ and Δg in Eq. (7.10-21).

Measurement of the gain-coefficient dependence on current, as described in Section 7.9, permits evaluation of the parameter b in Eq. (7.10-32), and it is Δg that determines w in Eq. (7.10-28). Measurement of the adjacent intensity maximum P_t^+ and minimum P_t^-, as described for Eq. (7.9-7), gives the variation of the gain coefficient with current as shown in Fig. 7.10-7. The slope was found to 2.22 cm^{-1}/mA and, as will be shown, it is the quantity that permits evaluation of the parameter b in Eq. (7.10-32). The gain coefficient given by Eq. (7.10-21) is the gain coefficient of an incremental volume and must be multiplied by the fraction of the propagating mode within that incremental volume to give the experimentally measured gain coefficient G_0. Therefore,

$$G_0 = \frac{\int_{-S/2}^{S/2} \int_{-d/2}^{d/2} \int_0^L \left(g(0) - \frac{4\Delta g y^2}{S^2}\right) |\mathscr{E}_y(x, y, z)|^2 \, dx \, dy \, dz}{\int_{-S/2}^{S/2} \int_{-\infty}^{\infty} \int_0^L |\mathscr{E}_y(x, y, z)|^2 \, dx \, dy \, dz}, \tag{7.10-33}$$

where $|\mathscr{E}_y(x, y, z)|^2$ is given by Eq. (7.10-6) and $|\mathscr{E}_y(y)|^2$ by Eq. (7.10-14). The gain coefficient is uniform along z so that the z-integral ratio is unity, the integral ratio over x was given in Eq. (7.10-10) as Γ, and then

$$G_0 = \frac{\Gamma \int_{-\infty}^{\infty} \left(g(0) - \frac{4\Delta g y^2}{S^2}\right) |\mathscr{E}_y(y)|^2 \, dy}{\int_{-\infty}^{\infty} |\mathscr{E}_y(y)|^2 \, dy}. \tag{7.10-34}$$

The integration limits of the upper integral have been extended to $\pm\infty$ because $\mathscr{E}_y(y)$ rapidly goes to zero for $|y| > S/2$ (see Fig. 7.10-6). This integral gives

$$G_0 = \Gamma\left[g(0) - \Delta g\left(\frac{2/k_0 a_r(\Gamma/\varepsilon_0)^{1/2}}{S^2}\right)\right], \tag{7.10-35}$$

and with Eq. (7.10-27), $2/k_0 a_r(\Gamma/\varepsilon_0)^{1/2} = 0.721w^2$.

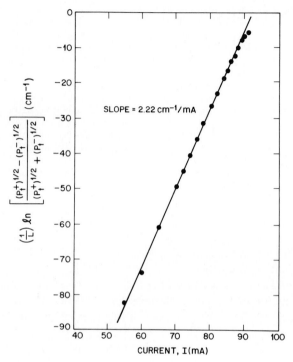

FIG. 7.10-7   Current dependence of the net gain,

$$(g - \alpha_i) - \frac{1}{L}\ln\left(\frac{1}{R}\right) = \frac{1}{L}\ln\left[\frac{(P_t^+)^{1/2} - (P_t^-)^{1/2}}{(P_t^+)^{1/2} + (P_t^-)^{1/2}}\right],$$

of a Fabry–Perot mode at 0.8269 μm (Ref. 161).

With Eq. (7.10-31) for $g(0)$ and Eq. (7.10-32) for Δg in Eq. (7.10-35), the derivative dG_0/dI times I gives

$$I\,dG_0/dI = \Gamma b(I\tau_n/qSLd)\{1 - \exp(-S/2L_n)$$
$$- (0.721w^2/S^2)\exp(-S/2L_n)[\cosh(S/2L_n) - 1]\}, \quad (7.10\text{-}36)$$

or

$$b\left(\frac{I\tau_n}{qSLd}\right)$$

$$= \frac{I(dG_0/dI)}{\Gamma\{1 - \exp(-S/2L_n) - (0.721w^2/S^2)\exp(-S/2L_n)[\cosh(S/2L_n) - 1]\}}.$$

$$(7.10\text{-}37)$$

Equation (7.10-37) in Eq. (7.10-32) gives

$$\Delta g = \frac{I(dG_0/dI)\exp(-S/2L_n)[\cosh(S/2L_n) - 1]}{\Gamma\{1 - \exp(-S/2L_n) - (0.721w^2/S^2)\exp(-S/2L_n)[\cosh(S/2L_n) - 1]\}}.$$

(7.10-38)

Equating Δg from Eq. (7.10-28) to Δg of Eq. (7.10-38) permits solving for w^2 as

$$w^2 = \frac{-1.38\lambda_0 + \{1.90\lambda_0^2 + 7.68I(dG_0/dI)\pi\bar{n}(0)\lambda_0 S^2[\exp(S/2L_n) - 1]/[\cosh(S/2L_n) - 1]\}^{1/2}}{2I(dG_0/dI)\pi\bar{n}(0)}.$$

(7.10-39)

As discussed for Eq. (7.10-24), $\bar{n}(0)$ is $[\Gamma\varepsilon(0)/\varepsilon_0 - (1 - \Gamma)\varepsilon_1/\varepsilon_0]^{1/2}$ and for this structure was 3.46 with $\Gamma = 0.3$.[161] From Fig. 7.10-7, $dG_0/dI = 2.22$ cm^{-1}/mA. With $I_{th} = 90$ mA, $\lambda_0 = 0.8269$ μm, $S = 11.7$ μm, and $L_n = 3.6$ μm, w is calculated from Eq. (7.10-39) to be 6.9 μm. This value agrees quite closely with the measured value of 6.5 μm. With $w = 6.9$ μm, Eq. (7.10-28) gives Δg as 294 cm^{-1}.

The close agreement between the measured and calculated w for the assumption of $\Delta\bar{n} = 0$ shows that the contribution from the spatial variation of the real part of the refractive index must be small. Paoli[161] has pointed out that a $\Delta\bar{n}$ of 4.6×10^{-4} in Eq. (7.10-24) would account for the 0.4 μm difference between the calculated and measured w. As discussed in Section 2.3, there will be contributions to $\Delta\bar{n}$ by both the injected electrons and the temperature variation. The change in the refractive index due to free electrons was given by Eq. (2.3-2) and gives

$$\Delta\bar{n}_{fc} = -(q^2\bar{n}/2m_n\omega^2\varepsilon)[n(0) - n(S/2)].$$

(7.10-40)

The values of the constants were given for Eq. (2.3-2), and for $\lambda_0 = 0.8269$ μm, $\Delta\bar{n}_{fc}$ becomes $-3.5 \times 10^{-22}\bar{n}[n(0) - n(S/2)]$. The electron concentrations $n(0)$ and $n(S/2)$ are given by Eq. (7.10-25). To evaluate $(I\tau_n/qSLd)$ in Eq. (7.10-25), τ_n was measured as 2.8 nsec by the time-delay method described in Section 7.7.[161] At $I_{th} = 0.09$ A, $d = 0.12$ μm, and $L = 380$ μm, Eq. (7.10-25) gives $n(0) = 2.33 \times 10^{18}$ cm^{-3} and $n(S/2) = 1.39 \times 10^{18}$ cm^{-3}. Therefore for $\bar{n} = 3.5$, the free carriers give $\Delta\bar{n}_{fc} = -1.15 \times 10^{-3}$. The negative value results in a defocusing of the optical beam. The temperature gradient along the stripe may be obtained from Eq. (7.8-1) as

$$\Delta T = \Delta\langle R\rangle IV,$$

(7.10-41)

and Ref. 145 gives the difference between the thermal resistance $\langle R\rangle$ at the center of the stripe and at the stripe edge as 9.3°K/W. With this $\Delta\langle R\rangle$ and $I_{th} = 0.09$ A and $V = 1.7$ V, ΔT is 1.4°K. Equation (2.3-1) gives $\Delta\bar{n}_T$ due to this temperature gradient as $\sim 5.6 \times 10^{-4}$.

Paoli[161] combined the effects from the free carriers and temperature as

$$\Delta \bar{n} = \Delta \bar{n}_{fc} \Gamma + \Delta \bar{n}_T \tag{7.10-42}$$

in order to account for localization of the free carriers to the active layer while the temperature is not localized. Therefore, $\Delta \bar{n}_T$ occurs in both the active layer and the adjacent $Al_x Ga_{1-x} As$ waveguiding layers. With the calculated values of $\Delta \bar{n}_{fc}$ and $\Delta \bar{n}_T$, the resulting $\Delta \bar{n}$ of $\sim 2.1 \times 10^{-4}$ is positive. Therefore, the temperature induced guiding tends to cancel the defocusing due to free carriers and is a small contribution to guiding. The example that has been considered here clearly demonstrates that the waveguiding along the junction plane is almost entirely due to gain.

7.11 EMISSION PROPERTIES OF STRIPE-GEOMETRY LASERS

Far-Field Pattern

Many of the emission properties of stripe-geometry DH lasers are identical to those that have previously been presented for broad-area lasers. Because the cross-sectional area is smaller than for broad-area lasers, lower output powers are obtained. For lasers with 15-μm-wide stripes and cavities 250 μm long, 20–30 mW of cw optical power have routinely been obtained from one mirror at a typical operating current of 200 mA.[149] Output powers up to 85 mW at 310 mA were obtained with these lasers before catastrophic mirror damage.[149] Mesa-stripe-geometry lasers have been reported with an output power of 390 mW for 80-μm-wide stripes and 300-μm-long cavities.[119] The far-field emission pattern for a stripe-geometry DH laser is illustrated in Fig. 7.11-1. For the case illustrated in this figure, the active-layer thickness

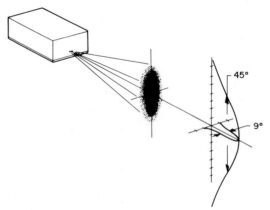

FIG. 7.11-1 Schematic representation of the far-field emission of a stripe-geometry GaAs–$Al_x Ga_{1-x} As$ DH laser. Typical values of the full angle at half power are illustrated perpendicular and along the junction plane.

and stripe width are small enough to ensure fundamental mode emission both perpendicular to and along the junction plane. Typical full beam angles between the half-power points (FAHP) are 45° in the direction perpendicular to the junction plane and 9° along the junction plane.

The variation of the relative far-field intensity with angle was illustrated for a broad-area GaAs–Al$_x$Ga$_{1-x}$As DH laser in Fig. 2.7-4.[51] The variation of the FAHP perpendicular to the junction plane $\Theta_\perp$ as a function of active layer thickness at selected values of x was given in Fig. 2.7-5. The behavior of $\Theta_\perp$ is the same for broad-area and stripe-geometry DH lasers, and the analysis of beam divergence given in Section 2.7 may be applied to stripe-geometry lasers. The coupling of stripe-geometry DH lasers to optical fibers has been considered by Brackett, and a coupling efficiency of 62% was measured.[163]

The conditions for higher-order modes perpendicular to the junction plane are the same as discussed in Chapter 2 and Section 7.4 for broad-area DH lasers [see Eq. (7.4-2)]. The far-field patterns for $m = 0$, 1, and 2 were given for GaAs–Al$_{0.43}$Ga$_{0.57}$As DH lasers in Fig. 7.4-3.

As the stripe width is increased from 12 μm, higher-order modes along the junction plane are observed. Yonezu et al.[103] illustrated the variation of mode order with stripe width for the planar-stripe laser. Their near-field and far-field patterns are shown in Fig. 7.11-2. As illustrated in Fig. 7.11-2 for $S = 20$ and 30 μm, the mode order was also found to increase as the current was increased. These modes along the junction plane are characteristic of the Hermite–Gaussian distribution represented by Eq. (7.10-12). It should be noted that well-behaved mode structure along the junction plane is not always obtained. When stripe widths exceed ~ 10–12 μm, the filamentary behavior described in Sections 7.4 and 8.2 is very commonly observed. Systematic studies of filamentary behavior in the various types of stripe-geometry lasers have not been reported, and the cause of filamentary behavior is not understood.

Longitudinal Modes

The longitudinal mode structure was given previously in Fig. 7.4-16 for a broad-area laser. It is similar to the higher-resolution lasing spectrum shown in Fig. 7.11-3 for a well-behaved cw Al$_{0.08}$Ga$_{0.92}$As–Al$_{0.36}$Ga$_{0.64}$As stripe-geometry DH laser.[164] The stripe width was 12 μm and was defined by proton bombardment. The Fabry–Perot mode spacing is given by Eq. (3.8-11). For this laser, the emission is polarized TE. It was shown in Section 2.8 that the facet reflectivity was expected to select the TE polarization. A detailed investigation of the polarization characteristics of stripe-geometry Al$_x$Ga$_{1-x}$As–Al$_y$Ga$_{1-y}$As DH lasers was made by Paoli.[164] It was found that some of these devices did not oscillate in a linearly polarized mode, but instead had elliptical or a more complex polarization.

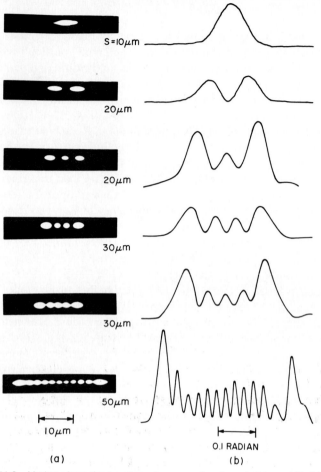

FIG. 7.11-2 Modes along the junction plane as a function of stripe width S for planar-stripe DH lasers. (a) Near-field patterns. (b) Far-field patterns (Ref. 103).

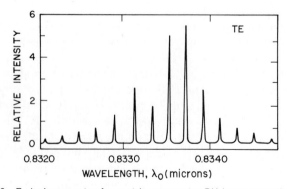

FIG. 7.11-3 Emission spectra for a stripe-geometry DH laser operating cw at 1.1 J_{th} (Ref. 164).

Ideally, the emission should be in a single longitudinal mode. Some proton-bombarded stripe-geometry GaAs–Al$_x$Ga$_{1-x}$As DH lasers do have single longitudinal-mode emission at single-mirror output powers of 3 mW, while otherwise identical lasers have many longitudinal modes.[165] The first question that arises is whether the spectral gain profile is homogeneously or inhomogeneously broadened. In the homogeneously broadened case, the carriers consumed by increased stimulated emission at one frequency are replaced by rapid thermalization within the bands. This rapid thermalization maintains the distributions determined by the quasi-Fermi levels. For the inhomogeneously broadened case, the carrier concentration at a lasing wavelength can be depleted and further excitation permits increased gain at other wavelengths and would result in longitudinal modes. Therefore, for homogeneous broadening, another mechanism is necessary to give longitudinal modes.

Some insight into this question was obtained by studies of DH lasers operated in external grating cavities. Paoli and Ripper studied cw GaAs–Al$_{0.23}$Ga$_{0.77}$As proton-bombarded stripe-geometry DH lasers at room temperature.[166] Frequency-selective optical feedback was obtained by optically coupling one cleaved facet of the laser to a diffraction grating through a microscope objective. Increased emission of the externally selected mode was accompanied by an amplitude reduction of the other longitudinal modes. This result implies that the spectral gain profile is homogeneously broadened, but it does not explain the reason for the longitudinal modes. For similar studies with pulse excitation at 77°K of Ga$_x$In$_{1-x}$P$_y$As$_{1-y}$ DH lasers, the experimental observations were interpreted in terms of both homogeneous and inhomogeneous broadening.[167,168]

With picosecond thermalization times,[169] homogeneous broadening can be assumed, and then possible explanations can be considered. Explanation of the origin of the longitudinal modes for this case has been based on the axial distribution of carriers due to the standing-wave pattern of the oscillating modes.[170–172] A single longitudinal mode gives an axial standing-wave pattern. At the intensity peaks, the stimulated emission will deplete the carriers more rapidly than at the nodes where stimulated emission will not occur. This effect will give a nonuniform carrier distribution and permits the oscillation of another longitudinal mode which has a different standing-wave pattern. Axial carrier diffusion will tend to eliminate the nonuniform carrier distribution. Streifer *et al.*[172] have evaluated an expression for the gain linewidth from Danielmeyer[171] and suggested that the more rapidly diffusing electrons can prevent longitudinal modes. If the active layer is lightly doped, then similar concentrations of holes and electrons will be injected in order to maintain electrical neutrality, and the spatial distribution will be influenced by the more slowly diffusing holes. However, an active layer doped to give $p_0 \approx 5 \times 10^{18}$ cm^{-3} will have essentially only electron injection. The stimulated emission at standing-wave peaks will only significantly affect the more rapidly diffusing electrons which would reduce axial nonuniformities in the carrier concentrations.

Scifres et al.[173] considered GaAs–Al$_x$Ga$_{1-x}$As DH lasers with active layers doped with Zn or Ge to give $p_0 > 5 \times 10^{18}$ cm^{-3}. For pulsed operation of broad-area lasers, they found single longitudinal-mode operation up to 1.4 J_{th} at room temperature. The transverse-junction-stripe laser shown in Figs. 7.6-4b and 7.7-9 has a heavily doped p-type active layer because of the Zn diffusion to form the junction. The TJS laser when operated cw has one or just a few longitudinal modes at currents up to 2J_{th}.[174] However, the CSP laser shown in Fig. 7.6-3c also gives a single longitudinal mode, but does not have a heavily doped p-type active layer. The stripe-geometry structures that spatially stabilize the lasing filament give single longitudinal mode emission. Further work is required to understand the origin of longitudinal modes.

Light–Current Nonlinearities

The observation of nonlinearities in the optical-power-output-versus-current ($L–I$) characteristic was introduced in Section 7.7 and illustrated in Fig. 7.7-6. These $L–I$ kinks are not only undesirable, but in some applications can make the device unacceptable. They can reduce the available output power and make stable operating intensities difficult to achieve. The properties and the elimination of $L–I$ kinks were a major topic of discussion at the 1976 Semiconductor Laser Conference. Fortunately, it appears that these nonlinearities can be eliminated.

The emission characteristics for the front and back mirrors of an Al$_{0.08}$Ga$_{0.92}$As–Al$_{0.36}$Ga$_{0.64}$As stripe-geometry DH laser formed by proton bombardment is shown in Fig. 7.11-4.[175] For 12-μm-wide stripes, these nonlinearities commonly occur at single-mirror output powers of less than 3 mW, and the light is not emitted symmetrically from the opposite mirrors. The light output from one mirror can be increasing while from the other mirror it is decreasing with current. The lack of symmetry hinders the use of feedback stabilization of the laser output by monitoring the emission from the opposite end.[175,176] As illustrated in Fig. 7.7-6, the loss of voltage saturation accompanies the nonlinear $L–I$ curve.

Measurement of the spatial distribution of the optical near field showed that the $L–I$ kink is accompanied by a lasing mode that shifts along the junction plane toward a stripe edge. This spatial variation of the lasing mode as the current is increased is shown in Fig. 7.11-5. The shift in position can seriously degrade the amount of light coupled into a single-mode fiber.

By reducing the stripe width to 8 μm for proton-bombarded stripe-geometry DH lasers, Dixon et al.[176] obtained linear and symmetric $L–I$ outputs below 3 mW. This reduction of stripe width to 8 μm did not always

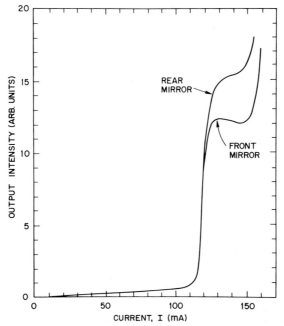

FIG. 7.11-4   Emission characteristics for the front and rear mirrors of a stripe-geometry DH laser operating cw at room temperature. Full scale corresponds to ~3 mW (Ref. 175).

eliminate the kinks, but it caused the kinks to occur at higher output powers.[176] Kinks were also eliminated for the planar-stripe lasers by Zn diffusion through the active layer as illustrated in Fig. 7.6-3b.[112] The stripe width was 15 μm and no kinks were observed for pulsed-current excitation to levels that gave 30 mW output power from one mirror. For this case, the mode patterns along the junction plane are different from the Hermite–Gaussian modes produced by gain guiding, and guiding in this case appears to be due to steps in the real part of the refractive index of about 0.1%.[112] As presented in Section 7.6, the planar-stripe laser grown on a channeled substrate that was illustrated in Fig. 7.6-3c also eliminated kinks.[114]

Chinone[177] considered the laser output power as a function of injection current by solving the carrier continuity equation and the wave equation for the optical field. This analysis showed that the gain profile obtained near threshold, as given in Section 7.10, is deformed by stimulated recombination of the carriers near the center of the stripe. Then, the optical field along the junction plane penetrates into the low-gain or lossy regions. This condition reduces the mode gain which causes power saturation and results in light–current kinks. Many of the experimental observations are explained by this model.

MIRROR   ILLUMINATION (TE)

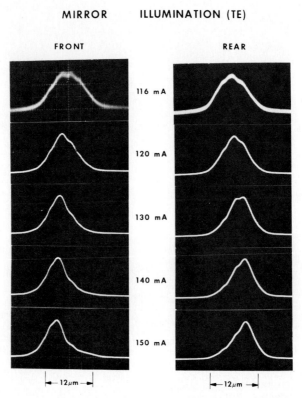

FIG. 7.11-5   Intensity distribution along the junction plane of the TE emission at the indicated currents from I_{th} into the nonlinear region of the L–I curve. The nominal stripe width is 12 μm. Note the shift of the peak of the intensity toward one edge of the stripe (Ref. 175).

Relaxation Oscillations

When a fast-rise-time current pulse is applied to a semiconductor laser, the light output power is delayed a few nanoseconds and then is characterized by a damped oscillation. This response together with the excitation current is shown in Fig. 7.11-6.[178] The ~4-nsec delay is the short time delay discussed in Section 7.7. The damped oscillation for this particular case has a frequency of ~1 GHz and a decay constant of a few nanoseconds in the light output. This behavior is called the relaxation oscillation. When the current pulse is applied, the carrier buildup is initially delayed by the carrier lifetime. The carrier concentration then builds up to concentrations that exceed the value necessary to reach threshold and the resulting high optical fields deplete the carrier concentration which reduces the optical field so

DC BIAS = O

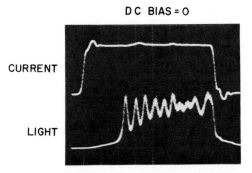

CURRENT

LIGHT

FIG. 7.11-6   Input excitation current and the resulting output light intensity for a stripe-geometry DH laser. The time scale is 2 nsec/div (Ref. 178).

that the carrier density can build up again. This process continues, but each successive cycle is diminished. This dynamic behavior of a semiconductor laser is described by the rate equations[179] for the carriers and photons. Both the relaxation oscillation and the noise resonance that is discussed in the next part of this section are related to this interaction between the carriers and photons.

Observations of relaxation oscillations began with homostructure lasers.[179,180] A first-order approximation to the relaxation or resonance frequency v_R was obtained from a linear, small-signal analysis to be approximately[181]

$$v_R = \frac{1}{2\pi}\left[\frac{1}{\tau_{ph}\tau_n}\left(\frac{I}{I_{th}} - 1\right)\right]^{1/2}, \qquad (7.11\text{-}1)$$

where τ_{ph} is the photon lifetime. The resonant frequency depends on both the material properties and current, and experimentally v_R ranges from about 0.3 to 1 GHz. There are several techniques for the reduction of the relaxation oscillations. As shown in Fig. 7.11-7, dc bias at $0.94I_{th}$ greatly

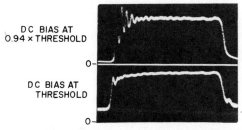

DC BIAS AT
0.94 × THRESHOLD

0—

DC BIAS AT
THRESHOLD

0—

FIG. 7.11-7   The pulsed output intensity from a stripe-geometry DH laser to illustrate suppression of the relaxation oscillations by biasing the laser at currents of $0.94I_{th}$ and I_{th}. The time scale is 2 nsec/div (Ref. 178).

reduces the relaxation oscillations, while dc bias at I_{th} eliminates these oscillations. Lang and Kobayashi[182] suppressed the relaxation oscillation with the injection of light. Reduced amplitude for the relaxation oscillations was observed for the buried-heterostructure stripe-geometry laser.[183] A more rapid damping was obtained for the planar-stripe laser with Zn diffusion through the active layer.[184,185] For the CSP lasers, the relaxation oscillations were suppressed and an almost flat response over 1 GHz was obtained.[114]

A different type of pulsation that has been observed in semiconductor lasers is characterized by a lack of damping and is called self-pulsation. These pulsations, illustrated in Fig. 8.4-5, were found by Paoli[186] to occur during device aging in devices that initially exhibited no self-pulsation. For the lasers that Paoli studied, the self-induced pulsations occur at frequencies ranging from 300 to 600 MHz, which is significantly less than the relaxation oscillation frequency of these same lasers. The mechanism by which self-induced pulsations occur is not presently understood.

Noise

A fundamental property of any signal source is the noise. The initial noise studies on broad-area homostructure lasers were by Armstrong and Smith[187–189] and on stripe-geometry homostructure lasers by Paoli and Ripper.[190] The quantum shot noise was found to be the fundamental source of the intensity fluctuations in the cw output.[190] The discrete and random spontaneous or stimulated transitions are the origin of the laser shot noise. Theoretical description of these quantum fluctuations for lasers in general was given by McCumber.[191] His calculations predicted peaks in the noise spectra at the relaxation (spiking) frequencies (resonances) discussed in the previous part of this section. Detailed calculations by Haug[192] for semiconductor lasers showed that the same general form of the noise spectrum is obtained.

Noise measurements on GaAs–Al$_x$Ga$_{1-x}$As stripe-geometry DH lasers operating cw at room temperature were made by Paoli.[193,194] The frequency spectra of the intensity fluctuations were measured from 10 MHz to 4 GHz for currents both below and above threshold. An example of the noise spectra as a function of current is shown in Fig. 7.11-8 for a laser with I_{th} of 372 mA. At currents above threshold the relaxation resonance leads to peaks in the noise spectra, and the resonant frequency ν_R varies with current approximately as $(I/I_{th} - 1)^{1/2}$. This resonant frequency just above threshold is typically 200–1000 MHz and the spectrum is flat below about 100 MHz. As shown in Fig. 7.11-9 for a lower cw threshold stripe-geometry DH laser, the noise power below the resonance frequency (50 MHz) abruptly increases near the 91-mA threshold. Further increase in current above I_{th}

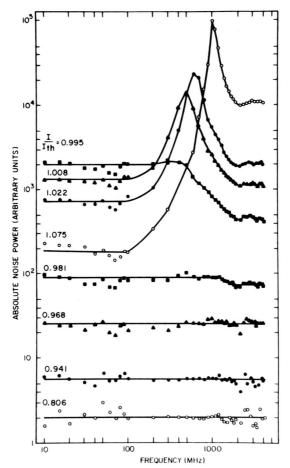

FIG. 7.11-8 Intensity noise spectra (1 MHz bandwidth) obtained for a stripe-geometry DH laser operating cw at room temperature. Laser threshold is 372 mA. The spectra have been corrected for the frequency response of the detection system (Ref. 193).

results in a rapid decrease in noise as the gain saturation stabilizes the intensity fluctuations.[194]

Ito *et al.*[195] investigated the intensity fluctuations of each longitudinal mode of a planar-stripe DH laser with 15-μm stripe widths. The frequency spectrum of the fluctuating output was measured from 1 MHz to 1.8 GHz. The noise spectrum of each longitudinal mode gave a peak near 1 GHz, as shown in Fig. 7.11-10. For currents more than 1.1 I_{th}, the lower-frequency noise of a single mode is about 30 dB larger than the noise for the total emission. The variation of the noise at 10 MHz, which is much lower than

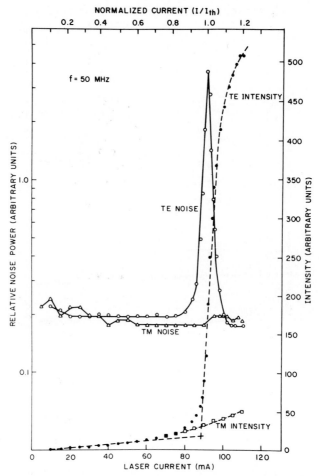

FIG. 7.11-9   Variation of the relative intensity noise for both TE and TM polarized light as a function of laser current. The noise power is measured in a 1 MHz interval centered at 50 MHz. Also shown are the intensities of the TE and TM light as a function of laser current (Ref. 194).

the resonance frequency, is shown in Fig. 7.11-11 as a function of current. These results demonstrate that the low-frequency noise for each mode increases with current, while the noise of the total emission has the same gain stabilization decrease as shown in Fig. 7.11-9. This behavior suggests the partition of the total output among the different modes, and that while one mode is increasing another is decreasing so that the total intensity fluctuation is less than for either. Recent studies of noise by Jäckel and Guekos also showed much stronger intensity fluctuations for an individual lasing mode as compared to fluctuations of the total output.[195a]

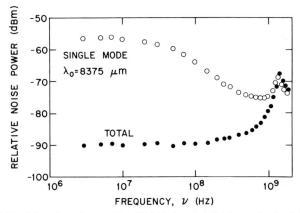

FIG. 7.11-10 Intensity noise spectra (30-kMz bandwidth) for a planar-stripe laser with I_{th} = 132 mA at I/I_{th} = 1.14 (Ref. 195).

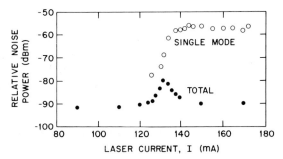

FIG. 7.11-11 Relative noise power in a 30-kMz interval centered at 10 MHz as a function of laser current for a planar-stripe laser with I_{th} = 132 mA (Ref. 195).

Modulation

Stripe-geometry DH lasers are a suitable source for fiber-optic communication systems because of their small size, low operating current and voltage (<200 mA at ~ 1.7 V), power efficiencies in excess of 5%, long operating life, and potential low cost. An additional attractive feature is the direct modulation of the emission by varying its input current. Almost all of the modulation studies of injection lasers have been devoted to pulse rather than amplitude modulation, and for that reason only pulse modulation will be considered here. There are several reasons for this choice. Most of the current communication system development, whether microwave or optical, is devoted to digital systems because of the better signal-to-noise ratio as compared to analog systems. Therefore, amplitude modulation would only be considered for short range and low performance systems where light-emitting diodes would be a more reasonable source. Summaries of the modulation characteristics of cw semiconductor lasers have been given by Paoli[178] and Kaminow and Li.[196]

Several properties of stripe-geometry DH lasers influence the performance in high-pulse rate applications. The principal problems are the initial time delay, the relaxation oscillations, and the charge storage that can affect the decay after the pulse. The time delay and relaxation oscillations were illustrated in Fig. 7.11-6. Reduction of the time delay by prebiasing to a current near threshold to reduce the initial time delay[139] was discussed in Section 7.7. Figure 7.11-7 showed that the prebias also reduces the relaxation oscillations. For pulse rates less than 50–100 Mbit/sec, the relaxation oscillations can be reduced without prebias by increasing the pulse rise time.[178] Also, equalization techniques that eliminate prebiasing have been demonstrated by Ozeki and Ito.[197] The decay after the pulse depends on the carrier lifetime[198] and can affect subsequent pulses (intersymbol interference) because residual charge can result in a lower threshold for the next pulse.

In several studies, the dynamic behavior[199–202] of semiconductor lasers and pulse modulation[203–208] have been considered. Investigation of the rate equations for carriers and photons suggested that bit rates of 3–4 Gbit/sec can be achieved.[202] Although bit rates of 1 Gbit/sec or more have been demonstrated,[203,206] it is not clear that random bit rates at frequencies this high are attainable. With a pseudorandom bit stream for a return to zero (RZ) pulse, a 200–Mbit/sec rate was demonstrated.[207] The useful pulse rates may depend on use of practical high-speed drivers and detectors.

The actual use of stripe-geometry DH lasers in pulse-modulated communication systems has begun.[209–213] Chen et al.[209] have described a 44.7-Mbit/sec experimental lightwave-communication system. In that system, the $Ga_{0.08}Al_{0.92}As$–$Ga_{0.36}Al_{0.64}As$ stripe-geometry DH laser is feedback stabilized for transmission of nonreturn to zero (NRZ) data. Experimental systems with bit rates from 50 Mbit/sec to 400 Mbit/sec have been described.[210–213] The feasibility of using pulse-modulated stripe-geometry DH lasers for lightwave communications has been demonstrated.

7.12 DISTRIBUTED-FEEDBACK LASERS

Operating Characteristics

The analysis for laser action in periodic structures was presented in Section 2.10. The feedback necessary for lasing is obtained by a periodic variation of the refractive index within the optical waveguide. The most extensive data for the lasing characteristics for a distributed-feedback (DFB) laser were reported by Aiki et al.[214] for the SCH structure illustrated in

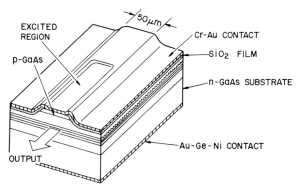

FIG. 7.12-1   Schematic representation of the DFB laser fabricated as a mesa-stripe laser (Ref. 214).

Figs. 2.10-5b and 2.10-6. The mesa-stripe SCH structure fabricated for these measurements is shown in Fig. 7.12-1. The wafer was grown by LPE, and the periodic corrugation was third order with a period of 0.3814 μm. The excited region was 500 μm long, and the contiguous unexcited waveguide was ~ 2 mm long to eliminate reflections from the back mirror. This structure is the only DFB laser that has operated cw at room temperature.[214,215]

The laser spectra for this DFB laser are shown in Fig. 7.12-2a. The lower spectrum is for 1.1 I_{th} and the upper spectrum is for 1.5I_{th}. The spectra for a cleaved Fabry–Perot (FP) laser fabricated from the same material are shown in Fig. 7.12-2b for comparison. This comparison illustrates the

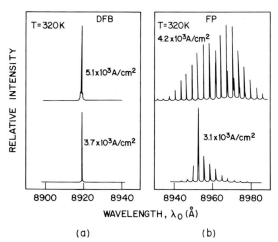

FIG. 7.12-2   Laser spectra of devices prepared from the same wafer. (a) DFB laser. (b) Fabry–Perot laser (Ref. 214).

wave length selectivity of the DFB laser and also shows that the emission wavelength is stable as the excitation is varied. The emission properties of this DFB laser and the Fabry–Perot laser are summarized in Fig. 7.12-3 for operation between 150° and 400°K. Both the lasing wavelength and threshold current density are shown as a function of temperature. Over this temperature range, two transverse TE modes and one TM mode were observed. The diode lased in the TE $m = 0$ (fundamental transverse) mode between 300° and 360°K, and J_{th} was about 20% higher than for the cleaved mirror laser. The lowest J_{th} was 3.4×10^3 A/cm^2 at 320°K. The mismatch between the Bragg frequency and the gain spectrum resulted in a rapid increase in J_{th} below 300°K and above 360°K. Figure 7.12-3 clearly illustrates the more rapid shift of the lasing wavelength with temperature for the Fabry–Perot structure as compared to the DFB laser. The laser emission of the Fabry–Perot laser follows the temperature dependence of the energy gap, while the lasing wavelength of the DFB laser follows the smaller temperature dependence of the refractive index. High-resolution spectral measurements showed that the spectral width of the single longitudinal TE $m = 0$ mode was ≈ 0.5 Å at $1.5\ J_{th}$ at room temperature.

The output power for the DFB laser as a function of current for several temperatures is shown in Fig. 7.12-4. The maximum cw output power of

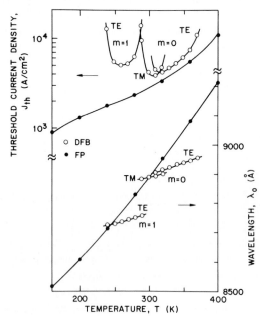

FIG. 7.12-3 Threshold current density and lasing wavelength as a function of the junction temperature (Ref. 214).

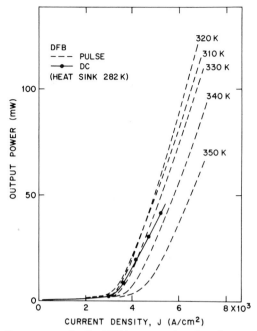

FIG. 7.12-4   Output power for the DFB laser as a function of current (Ref. 214).

40 mW was obtained at $282°K$. Previously, 10 mW was obtained for cw operation at $300°K$.[215] The pulsed output powers are shown in Fig. 7.12-4 to be greater than 100 mW. These results demonstrate that adequate power and good spectral performance can be obtained with DFB lasers.

This SCH–DFB laser was extended to the waveguide-coupled structure shown in Fig. 7.12-5.[216] The laser emission is coupled into the $Al_{0.1}Ga_{0.9}As$

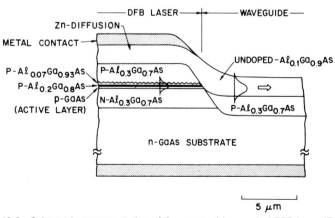

FIG. 7.12-5   Schematic representation of the waveguide coupled DFB laser (Ref. 216).

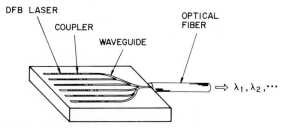

FIG. 7.12-6   Schematic representation of the frequency-multiplexing light source. Six DFB lasers with emission wavelengths separated by ~20 Å are monolithically integrated with passive waveguides (Ref. 217).

layer through the stepped coupling region shown in the figure. As illustrated schematically in Fig. 7.12-6,[217] six of these lasers were fabricated on a single LPE wafer and coupled into the single waveguide. The grating period of each laser was individually exposed with a different period to give an emission wavelength separation of ~20 Å. At room temperature, J_{th} of each DFB laser varied from 3 to 6 × 10^3 A/cm². The lasing wavelengths were separated by 20 ± 5 Å, with a spectral width of ~0.3 Å. This structure illustrates a technique for frequency multiplexing light sources.

Other Periodic Waveguide Structures

Much of the initial work with DFB lasers was limited to temperatures near or at 77°K. Preparation of the periodic corrugation directly on the active layer of a DH laser reduced the recombination efficiency due to interface nonradiative recombination and prevented lasing at room temperature. The SCH laser was used to separate the periodic corrugation from the active layer to achieve room-temperature DFB operation.[214–216,218] Separation of the Bragg grating from the active layer was also achieved by Reinhart et al.[219] They used a taper-coupled laser[220] with the corrguation on the passive waveguide to give room-temperature operation of a distributed Bragg reflection laser. The taper-coupled laser with a distributed Bragg reflector (DBR) is represented schematically in Fig. 7.12-7. The

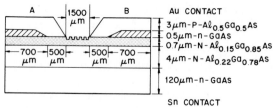

FIG. 7.12-7   Schematic representation of the taper-coupled distributed Bragg reflector (DBR) laser (Ref. 219).

active layer is the cross-hatched n-type GaAs layer. The window in the P–$Al_{0.5}Ga_{0.5}As$ layer was formed by selective etching or the taper layer was grown in segments in a manner similar to that used to grow the tapered-active regions. A third-order grating was formed on the N–$Al_{0.15}Ga_{0.85}As$ layer. Pulsed current was applied to section A of the structure and section B served as an unexcited termination for the laser radiation. Threshold at room temperature was 5×10^3 A/cm^2 and the spectral width of the dominant mode was ≈ 0.2 Å. Bragg reflectors were used on both ends of a DH laser as illustrated in Fig. 7.12-8. Third-order gratings were used, and at room temperature the threshold current density was between 6 and 7×10^3 A/cm^2.[221]

Distributed feedback has also been used with the buried heterostructure[222] (see Fig. 7.6-6). For these lasers, the layer sequence was $N_{0.5}$–$P_{0.04}$–$P_{0.3}$–$P_{0.1}$–$P_{0.4}$ with the $p_{0.04}$ layer as the active layer. The periodic corrugation was between the $P_{0.1}$ and $P_{0.4}$ layers so that this structure also provided separate confinement. The room-temperature threshold was higher than for the usual buried heterostructure. Laser operation with DFB was also demonstrated in a stripe-geometry $Pb_{1-x}Sn_xTe$ DH laser grown by molecular-beam epitaxy.[223] Pulsed operation near a wavelength of 13 μm was obtained at 58°K.

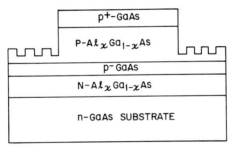

FIG. 7.12-8   Schematic representation of the DH distributed Bragg reflector (DBR) laser (Ref. 221).

7.13   CONCLUDING COMMENTS

The fabrication procedures for the preparation of broad-area and stripe-geometry GaAs (or $Al_yGa_{1-y}As$)–$Al_xGa_{1-x}As$ DH lasers and their operating properties were presented in this chapter. The fabrication procedures showed how the heteroepitaxial wafers whose growth was presented in Chapter 6 are made into discrete lasers with cleaved mirrors. The discussion of the fabrication procedures also permitted illustration of various stripe-geometry configurations. Numerous operating properties were presented and the calculated current dependence of the gain coefficient was compared to the experimental values for uncompensated active layers.

The question of the current dependence of the gain coefficient g_{max} was considered. The theoretical results from Chapter 3 showed that for $g_{max} \lesssim$ 100 cm^{-1} the gain coefficient varies superlinearly with current, while for $g_{max} \gtrsim$ 100 cm^{-1} the gain coefficient varies linearly with current. In both cases, it is necessary to include the offset current J_0 where g_{max} goes to zero. Low threshold lasers have small active-layer thicknesses d, which means that g_{max} at threshold is generally greater than ~ 100 cm^{-1}. Therefore, these lasers are most conveniently represented by a linear gain-coefficient–current dependence. Close agreement between the calculated and experimental g_{max} dependence on current as well as the variation of the room-temperature threshold current density $J_{th}(300°K)$ with d was demonstrated.

For stripe-geometry lasers, it was shown that $J_{th}(300°K)$ approximately doubles as the stripe width is reduced from ~ 25 μm to ~ 10 μm. This increased $J_{th}(300°K)$ is largely due to the lateral diffusion along the junction plane of the carriers injected into the active layer. The temperature of the active region was shown to increase by $\sim 5°–10°C$ near threshold. Light confinement along the junction plane for proton-bombarded stripe-geometry DH lasers was demonstrated to be due to gain guiding. The emission properties such as transverse modes, longitudinal modes, modes along the junction plane, and the beam divergence were described. The relaxation oscillations and noise were also discussed. As demonstrated in this chapter, the concepts that were presented in the previous chapters represent the experimental behavior very well.

REFERENCES

1. N. E. Schumaker, Private communication.
2. B. Schwartz, F. Ermanis, and M. H. Brastad, *J. Electrochem. Soc.* **123**, 1089 (1976).
3. B. Schwartz, J. C. Dyment, and S. E. Haszko, "Gallium Arsenide and Related Compounds," 1972, p. 187. Inst. of Phys. London, 1973.
4. R. A. Logan and F. K. Reinhart, *J. Appl. Phys.* **44**, 4172 (1973).
5. W. D. Johnston, Jr. and B. I. Miller, *Appl. Phys. Lett.* **23**, 192 (1973).
6. R. Ito, H. Nakashima, and O. Nakada, *Jpn. J. Appl. Phys.* **12**, 1272 (1973).
7. F. R. Nash, R. W. Dixon, P. A. Barnes, and N. E. Schumaker, *Appl. Phys. Lett.* **27**, 234 (1975).
8. C. H. Henry and R. A. Logan, *J. Appl. Phys.* **48**, 3962 (1977).
9. V. L. Rideout, *Solid-State Electron.* **18**, 541 (1975).
10. H. C. Casey, Jr. and M. B. Panish, *Trans. Metall. Soc. AIME* **242**, 406 (1968).
11. J. S. Harris, Y. Nannichi, G. L. Pearson, and G. F. Day, *J. Appl. Phys.* **40**, 4575 (1969).
12. A. M. Andrews and N. Holonyak, Jr., *Solid-State Electron.* **15**, 601 (1972).
13. W. D. Edwards, W. A. Hartman, and A. B. Torrens, *Solid-State Electron.* **15**, 387 (1972).
14. K. K. Shih and J. M. Blum, *Solid-State Electron.* **15**, 1177 (1972).
15. N. Yokoyama, S. Ohkawa, H. Ishikawa, *Jpn. J. Appl. Phys.* **14**, 1071 (1975).
16. W. L. Bond, B. G. Cohen, R. C. C. Leite, and A. Yariv, *Appl. Phys. Lett.* **2**, 57 (1963).

17. M. Ettenberg, H. F. Lockwood, and H. S. Sommers, Jr., *J. Appl. Phys.* **43**, 5047 (1972).
18. R. L. Hartman and A. R. Hartman, *Appl. Phys. Lett.* **23**, 147 (1973).
19. Y. Shima, N. Chinone, and R. Ito, *Appl. Phys. Lett.* **31**, 625 (1977).
20. M. H. Pilkuhn and H. Rupprecht, *J. Appl. Phys.* **38**, 5 (1967).
21. M. B. Panish, I. Hayashi, and S. Sumski, *IEEE J. Quantum Electron.* **QE-5**, 210 (1969).
22. I. Hayashi, M. B. Panish, and P. W. Foy, *IEEE J. Quantum Electron.* **QE-5**, 211 (1969).
23. H. Kressel and H. Nelson, *RCA Rev.* **30**, 106 (1969).
24. I. Hayashi and M. B. Panish, *J. Appl. Phys.* **41**, 150 (1970).
25. H. T. Minden and R. Premo, *J. Appl. Phys.* **45**, 4520 (1974).
26. R. B. Gill, *Proc. IEEE* **58**, 949 (1970).
27. A. R. Goodwin and P. R. Selway, *IEEE J. Quantum Electron.* **QE-6**, 285 (1970).
28. H. Yonezu, I. Sakuma, and Y. Nannichi, *Jpn. J. Appl. Phys.* **9**, 231 (1970).
29. E. A. Ulmer, Jr. and I. Hayashi, *J. Quantum Electron.* **QE-6**, 297 (1970).
30. H. Nelson and H. Kressel, *Appl. Phys. Lett.* **15**, 7 (1969).
31. H. C. Casey, Jr., B. I. Miller, and E. Pinkas, *J. Appl. Phys.* **44**, 1281 (1973).
32. C. J. Hwang, *J. Appl. Phys.* **42**, 4408 (1971).
33. W. Shockley, "Electrons and Holes in Semiconductors," p. 242. Van Nostrand–Reinhold, Princeton, New Jersey, 1950.
34. H. K. Gummel, *Solid-State Electron.* **10**, 209 (1967).
35. H. Kressel, H. Nelson, and F. Z. Hawrylo, *J. Appl. Phys.* **41**, 2019 (1970).
36. H. Kressel, H. Nelson, and F. Z. Hawrylo, *IEEE J. Quantum Electron.* **QE-6**, 290 (1970).
37. N. E. Byer and J. K. Butler, *IEEE J. Quantum Electron.* **QE-6**, 291 (1970).
38. G. D. Henshall and J. E. A. Whiteaway, *Electron. Lett.* **10**, 326 (1974).
39. J. A. Rossi, H. Heckscher, and S. R. Chinn, *Appl. Phys. Lett.* **23**, 257 (1973).
40. J. E. Ripper and J. A. Rossi, *IEEE J. Quantum Electron.* **QE-10**, 435 (1974).
41. K. Konnerth and C. Lanza, *Appl. Phys. Lett.* **4**, 120 (1964).
42. J. E. Ripper and J. C. Dyment, *Appl. Phys. Lett.* **12**, 365 (1968).
43. S. Gründorfer, M. J. Adams, and B. Thomas, *IEEE J. Quantum Electron.* **QE-11**, 532 (1975).
44. F. D. Nunes, N. B. Patel, and J. E. Ripper, *Electron. Lett.* **12**, 574 (1976).
45. I. Hayashi, M. B. Panish, P. W. Foy, and S. Sumski, *Appl. Phys. Lett.* **17**, 109 (1970).
46. Zh. I. Alferov, V. M. Andreev, D. Z. Garbuzov, Yu. V. Zhilyaev, E. P. Morozov, E. L. Portnoi, and V. G. Triofim, *Sov. Phys.–Semicond.* **4**, 1573 (1971) [*Translated from*: *Fiz. Tekh. Poluprovodn.* **4**, 1826 (1970)].
47. J. C. Dyment, L. A. D'Asaro, J. C. North, B. I. Miller, and J. E. Ripper, *Proc. IEEE* **60**, 726 (1972).
48. R. L. Hartman, N. E. Schumaker, and R. W. Dixon, *Appl. Phys. Lett.* **31**, 756 (1977).
49. E. Pinkas, B. I. Miller, I. Hayashi, and P. W. Foy, *J. Appl. Phys.* **43**, 2827 (1972).
49a. G. D. Henshall, *Appl. Phys. Lett.* **31**, 205 (1977).
50. H. Yonezu, K. Kobayashi, and I. Sakuma, *Jpn. J. Appl. Phys.* **12**, 1593 (1973).
51. H. C. Casey, Jr., M. B. Panish, and J. L. Merz, *J. Appl. Phys.* **44**, 5470 (1973).
52. J. C. Dyment, F. R. Nash, C. J. Hwang, G. A. Rozgonyi, R. L. Hartman, H. M. Marcos, and S. E. Haszko, *Appl. Phys. Lett.* **24**, 481 (1974).
53. M. Ettenberg, *Appl. Phys. Lett.* **27**, 652 (1975).
54. H. Kressel and M. Ettenberg, *J. Appl. Phys.* **47**, 3533 (1976).
55. H. C. Casey, Jr., M. B. Panish, W. O. Schlosser, and T. L. Paoli, *J. Appl. Phys.* **45**, 322 (1974).
56. F. R. Nash, W. R. Wagner, and R. L. Brown, *J. Appl. Phys.* **47**, 3992 (1976).
57. D. L. Rode, *J. Appl. Phys.* **45**, 3887 (1974).
58. P. R. Selway and A. R. Goodwin, *J. Phys. D: Appl. Phys.* **5**, 904 (1972).

59. I. Hayashi, M. B. Panish, and F. K. Reinhart, *J. Appl. Phys.* **42**, 1929 (1971).
60. F. Stern, *J. Appl. Phys.* **47**, 5382 (1976).
60a. R. D. Dupuis, P. D. Dapkus, and L. A. Moudy, *Techn. Digest 1977 Int. Electron Devices Meeting*, p. 575 (1977).
60b. H. C. Casey, Jr., *J. Appl. Phys.* (May 1978).
60c. G. H. B. Thompson, P. A. Kirby, and J. E. A. Whiteaway, *IEEE J. Quantum Electron.* **QE-11**, 481 (1975).
61. M. B. Panish, I. Hayashi, and S. Sumski, *Appl. Phys. Lett.* **16**, 326 (1970).
62. A. R. Goodwin, J. R. Peters, M. Pion, G. H. B. Thompson, and J. E. A. Whiteaway, *J. Appl. Phys.* **46**, 3126 (1975).
63. H. C. Casey, Jr. and M. B. Panish, *J. Appl. Phys.* **46**, 1393 (1975).
64. J. K. Butler, H. Kressel, and I. Ladany, *IEEE J. Quantum Electron.* **QE-11**, 402 (1975).
65. W. Streifer, R. D. Burham, and D. R. Scifres, *IEEE J. Quantum Electron.* **QE-12**, 177 (1976).
66. D. R. Scifres, W. Streifer, and R. D. Burham, *Appl. Phys. Lett.* **29**, 23 (1976).
67. W. G. French, J. B. MacChesney, P. B. O'Connor, and G. W. Tasker, *Bell Syst. Tech. J.* **53**, 951 (1974).
68. B. I. Miller, J. E. Ripper, J. C. Dyment, E. Pinkas, and M. B. Panish, *Appl. Phys. Lett.* **18**, 403 (1971).
69. K. Itoh, M. Inoue, and I. Teramoto, *IEEE J. Quantum Electron.* **QE-11**, 421. (1975).
70. H. Kressel and F. Z. Hawrylo, *Appl. Phys. Lett.* **28**, 598 (1976).
71. Zh. I. Alferov, V. M. Andreev, T. Ya. Belousova, V. I. Borodulin, V. A. Gorbylev, G. T. Pak, A. I. Petrov, E. L. Portnoi, N. P. Chernousov, V. I. Shveikin, and I. V. Yashchumov, *Sov. Phys.–Semicond.* **6**, 495 (1972) [*Translated from: Fiz. Tekh. Poluprovodn.* **6**, 568 (1972)].
72. H. Kressel, H. F. Lockwood, F. H. Nicoll, and M. Ettenberg, *IEEE J. Quantum Electron.* **QE-9**, 383 (1973).
73. H. Kressel and H. F. Lockwood, *Appl. Phys. Lett.* **20**, 175 (1972).
74. G. H. B. Thompson, *Opto-Electronics* **4**, 257 (1972).
75. M. Cross, *Phys. Status Solidi (a)* **16**, 167 (1973).
76. P. A. Kirby and G. H. B. Thompson, *Appl. Phys. Lett.* **22**, 638 (1973).
76a. J. E. A. Whiteaway and G. H. B. Thompson, *Solid-State and Electron Dev.* **1**, 81 (1977).
76b. C. H. Henry, R. A. Logan, and F. R. Merritt, *Appl. Phys. Lett.* **31**, 454 (1977).
77. H. S. Sommers, Jr. and D. O. North, *Solid-State Electron.* **19**, 675 (1976).
78. D. O. North, *IEEE J. Quantum Electron.* **QE-12**, 616 (1976).
79. R. Keller, C. Voumard, and H. Weber, *Appl. Phys. Lett.* **26**, 50 (1975).
80. H. F. Lockwood, K.-F. Etzold, T. E. Stockton, and D. P. Marinelli, *IEEE J. Quantum Electron.* **QE-10**, 567 (1974).
81. Zh. I. Alferov, V. M. Andreev, V. I. Korol'kov, V. G. Nikitin, E. L. Portnoi, and A. A. Yakovenko, *Sov. Phys.–Semicond.* **6**, 637 (1972) [*Translated from: Fiz. Tekh. Poluprovodn.* **6**, 739 (1972)].
82. F. K. Reinhart and B. I. Miller, *Appl. Phys. Lett.* **20**, 36 (1972).
83. F. K. Reinhart, *Appl. Phys. Lett.* **22**, 372 (1973).
84. T. P. Lee, C. A. Burrus, Jr., and B. I. Miller, *IEEE J. Quantum Electron.* **QE-9**, 820 (1973).
85. H. F. Lockwood, H. Kressel, H. S. Sommers, Jr., and F. Z. Hawrylo, *Appl. Phys. Lett.* **17**, 499 (1970).
86. H. Kressel, H. F. Lockwood, and F. Z. Hawrylo, *Appl. Phys. Lett.* **18**, 43 (1971).
87. H. Kressel, H. F. Lockwood, and F. Z. Hawrylo, J. Appl. Phys. **43**, 561 (1972).
88. J. K. Butler and H. Kressel, *J. Appl. Phys.* **43**, 3403 (1972).

89. T. L. Paoli, B. W. Hakki, and B. I. Miller, *J. Appl. Phys.* **44**, 1276 (1973).
90. B. W. Hakki, *J. Appl. Phys.* **45**, 288 (1974).
91. B. W. Hakki and C. J. Hwang, *J. Appl. Phys.* **45**, 2168 (1974).
92. B. W. Hakki, *IEEE J. Quantum Electron.* **QE-11**, 149 (1975).
93. D. C. Krupka, *IEEE J. Quantum Electron.* **QE-11**, 390 (1975).
94. M. B. Panish, H. C. Casey, Jr., S. Sumski, and P. W. Foy, *Appl. Phys. Lett.* **22**, 590 (1973).
95. G. H. B. Thompson and P. A. Kirkby, *Electron. Lett.* **9**, 295 (1973).
96. I. Hayashi, U.S. Patent No. 3,691,476 (1972).
97. G. H. B. Thompson and P. A. Kirkby, *IEEE J. Quantum Electron.* **QE-9**, 311 (1973).
98. G. H. B. Thompson, G. D. Henshall, J. E. A. Whiteaway, and P. A. Kirkby, *J. Appl. Phys.* **47**, 1501 (1976).
99. R. A. Furnanage and D. K. Wilson, U.S. Patent No. 3,363,195 (January 1968).
100. J. C. Dyment, *Appl. Phys. Lett.* **10**, 84 (1967).
101. J. C. Dyment and L. A. D'Asaro, *Appl. Phys. Lett.* **11**, 292 (1967).
102. J. C. Dyment and T. H. Zachos, *J. Appl. Phys.* **39**, 2923 (1968).
103. H. Yonezu, I. Sakuma, K. Kobayashi, T. Kamejima, M. Ueno, and Y. Nannichi, *Jpn. J. Appl. Phys.* **12**, 1585 (1973).
104. L. A. D'Asaro, *J. Lumin.* **7**, 310 (1973).
105. H. Kan, H. Namizaki, M. Ishii, and A. Ito, *Appl. Phys. Lett.* **27**, 138 (1975).
106. K. Wohlleben and W. Beck, *Z. Naturforsch.* **A21**, 1057 (1966).
107. A. G. Foyt, W. T. Lindley, C. M. Wolfe, and J. P. Donnelly, *Solid-State Electron.* **12**, 209 (1969).
108. J. C. Dyment, J. C. North, and L. A. D'Asaro, *J. Appl. Phys.* **44**, 207 (1973).
109. P. N. Favennec and D. Diguet, *Appl. Phys. Lett.* **23**, 546 (1973).
110. J. M. Blum, J. C. McGroddy, P. G. McMullin, K. K. Shih, A. W. Smith, and J. F. Ziegler, *IEEE J. Quantum Electron.* **QE-11**, 413 (1975).
111. P. N. Favennec, *J. Appl. Phys.* **47**, 2532 (1976).
112. H. Yonezu, Y. Matsumoto, T. Shinohara, I. Sakuma, T. Suzuki, K. Kobayashi, R. Lang, Y. Nannichi, and I. Hayashi, *Jpn. J. Appl. Phys.* **16**, 209 (1977).
113. M. Takusagawa, S. Ohsaka, N. Takagi, H. Ishikawa, and H. Takanashi, *Proc. IEEE Lett.* **61**, 758 (1973).
114. K. Aiki, M. Nakamura, T. Kuroda, and J. Umeda, *Appl. Phys. Lett.* **30**, 649 (1977).
114a. K. Aiki M. Nakamura, T. Kuroda, J. Umeda, R. Ito, N. Chinone, and M. Maeda, *IEEE J. Quantum Electron.*, **QE-14**, 89 (1978).
115. W. Susaki, H. Namizaki, H. Kan, and A. Ito, *J. Appl. Phys.* **44**, 2893 (1973).
116. H. Namizaki, H. Kan, M. Ishii, and A. Ito, *J. Appl. Phys.* **45**, 2785 (1974).
117. H. Namizaki. *IEEE J. Quantum Electron.* **QE-11**, 427 (1975).
118. T. Tsukada, H. Nakashima, J. Umeda, S. Nakamura, N. Chinone, R. Ito, and O. Nakada, *Appl. Phys. Lett.* **20**, 344 (1972).
119. N. Chinone, R. Ito, and O. Nakada, *J. Appl. Phys.* **47**, 785 (1976).
120. T. Tsukada, *J. Appl. Phys.* **45**, 4899 (1974).
120a. W. T. Tsang, R. A. Logan, and M. Ilegems, *Appl. Phys. Lett.* **32**, 311 (1978).
120b. W. T. Tsang, Private communication.
121. R. D. Burnham, D. R. Scifres, J. C. Tramontana, and A. S. Alimonda, *IEEE J. Quantum Electron.* **QE-11**, 418 (1975).
122. K. Itoh, M. Inoue, and I. Teramoto, *IEEE J. Quantum Electron.* **QE-11**, 421 (1975).
123. W. T. Tsang and R. A. Logan, *Appl. Phys. Lett.* **30**, 538 (1977).
124. R. D. Burnham and D. R. Scifres, *Appl. Phys. Lett.* **27**, 510 (1975).
125. P. A. Kirkby and G. H. B. Thompson, *J. Appl. Phys.* **47**, 4578 (1976).
126. T. P. Lee and A. Y. Cho, *Appl. Phys. Lett.* **29**, 164 (1976).

127. B. W. Hakki, *J. Appl. Phys.* **44**, 5021 (1973).
128. W. T. Tsang, *J. Appl. Phys.* (March 1978).
129. W. B. Joyce and S. H. Wemple, *J. Appl. Phys.* **41**, 3818 (1970).
130. W. P. Dumke, *Solid–State Electron.* **16**, 1279 (1973).
130a. I. Ladany, *J. Appl. Phys.* **48**, 1935 (1977).
130b. J. J. Hseih and C. C. Shen, *Appl. Phys. Lett.* **30**, 429 (1977).
131. R. W. Dixon, *Bell Syst. Tech. J.* **55**, 973 (1976).
132. T. L. Paoli and P. A. Barnes, *Appl. Phys. Lett.* **28**, 714 (1976).
133. P. A. Barnes and T. L. Paoli, *IEEE J. Quantum Electron.* **QE-12**, 633 (1976).
134. W. B. Joyce and R. W. Dixon, *J. Appl. Phys.* **47**, 3510 (1976).
135. T. L. Paoli, *Appl. Phys. Lett.* **29**, 673 (1976).
136. P. G. Eliseev, A. I. Krasil'nikov, M. A. Man'ko, and V. P. Strakhov, "Physics of p-n Junctions and Semiconductor Devices" (S. M. Ryvkin and Yu. V. Shmartsev, eds.), p. 150. Plenum Press, New York, 1971.
137. T. L. Paoli, *IEEE J. Quantum Electron.* **QE-9**, 267 (1973).
138. H. S. Sommers, Jr., *Appl. Phys. Lett.* **19**, 424 (1971).
139. J. C. Dyment, J. E. Ripper, and T. P. Lee, *J. Appl. Phys.* **43**, 452 (1972).
140. J. E. Ripper, *J. Appl. Phys.* **43**, 1762 (1972).
141. C. J. Hwang and J. C. Dyment, *J. Appl. Phys.* **44**, 3240 (1973).
142. H. Namizaki, H. Kan, M. Ishii, and A. Ito, *Appl. Phys. Lett.* **24**, 486 (1974).
143. H. Namizaki, H. Kan, M. Ishii, A. Ito, and W. Susaki, *Jpn. J. Appl. Phys.* **13**, 1618 (1974).
144. W. Susaki, T. Tanaka, H. Kan, and M. Ishii, *IEEE J. Quantum Electron.* **QE-13**, 587 (1977).
145. W. B. Joyce and R. W. Dixon, *J. Appl. Phys.* **46**, 855 (1975).
146. M. A. Afromowitz, *J. Appl. Phys.* **44**, 1292 (1973).
147. P. D. Maycock, *Solid-State Electron.* **10**, 161 (1967).
148. H. S. Carslaw and J. C. Jaeger, "Conduction of Heat in Solids," 2nd ed., Chapter 5. Oxford Univ. Press, London and New York, 1959.
149. H. Yonezu, T. Yuasa, T. Shinohara, T. Kamejima, and I. Sakuma, *Jpn. J. Appl. Phys.* **15**, 2393 (1976).
150. R. Berman, "Physical Properties of Diamond," p. 387. Oxford Univ. Press, London and New York, 1965.
151. D. E. Gray (ed.), "American Institute of Physics Handbook," Table 4g-8. McGraw-Hill, New York, 1972.
152. T. L. Paoli, *IEEE J. Quantum Electron.* **QE-11**, 498 (1975).
152a. T. Kobayashi and G. Iwane, *Jpn. J. Appl. Phys.* **16**, 1403 (1977).
153. W. B. Joyce, unpublished.
154. B. W. Hakki and T. L. Paoli, *J. Appl. Phys.* **44**, 4113 (1973).
155. B. W. Hakki and T. L. Paoli, *J. Appl. Phys.* **46**, 1299 (1975).
156. T. H. Zachos and J. E. Ripper, *IEEE J. Quantum Electron.* **QE-5**, 29 (1969).
157. T. H. Zachos and J. C. Dyment, *IEEE J. Quantum Electron.* **QE-6**, 317 (1970).
158. D. D. Cook and F. R. Nash, *J. Appl. Phys.* **46**, 1660 (1975).
159. W. O. Schlosser, *Bell Syst. Tech. J.* **52**, 887 (1973).
160. F. R. Nash, *J. Appl. Phys.* **44**, 4696 (1973).
161. T. L. Paoli, *IEEE J. Quantum Electron.* **QE-13**, 662 (1977).
162. A. E. Siegman, "An Introduction to Lasers and Masers," p. 329. McGraw–Hill, New York, 1971.
163. C. A. Brackett, *J. Appl. Phys.* **45**, 2636 (1974).
164. T. L. Paoli, *IEEE J. Quantum Electron.* **QE-11**, 489 (1975).
165. R. L. Hartman, Private communication.

166. T. L. Paoli and J. E. Ripper, *Appl. Phys. Lett.* **25**, 744 (1974).
167. P. D. Wright, J. J. Coleman, N. Holonyak, Jr., M. J. Ludowise, and G. E. Stillman, *Appl. Phys. Lett.* **29**, 18 (1976).
168. P. D. Wright, J. J. Coleman, N. Holonyak, Jr., M. J. Ludowise, and G. E. Stillman, *J. Appl. Phys.* **47**, 3580 (1976).
169. Y. Nishimura, *Jpn. J. Appl. Phys.* **13**, 109 (1974).
170. H. Statz, C. L. Tang, and J. M. Lavine, *J. Appl. Phys.* **35**, 2581 (1964).
171. H. G. Danielmeyer, *J. Appl. Phys.* **42**, 3125 (1971).
172. W. Streifer, R. D. Burnham, and D. R. Scifres, *IEEE J. Quantum Electron.* **QE-13**, 403 (1977).
173. D. R. Scifres, R. D. Burnham, and W. Streifer, *Appl. Phys. Lett.* **31**, 112 (1977).
174. H. Namizaki, *Trans. IECE Jpn.* **E59**, 8 (1976).
175. T. L. Paoli, *IEEE J. Quantum Electron.* **QE-12**, 770 (1976).
176. R. W. Dixon, F. R. Nash, R. L. Hartman, and R. T. Hepplewhite, *Appl. Phys. Lett.* **29**, 372 (1976).
177. N. Chinone, *J. Appl. Phys.* **48**, 3237 (1977).
178. T. L. Paoli, *Techn. Digest 1976 Int. Electron Devices Meeting* p. 136 (1976).
179. V. D. Kurnosov, V. I. Magalyas, A. A. Pleshkov, L. A. Rivlin, V. G. Trukhan, and V. V. Tsvetkov, *JETP Lett.* **4**, 303 (1966) [*Translated from*: *ZhETF Pis'ma* **4**, 449 (1966)].
180. R. Roldan, *Appl. Phys. Lett.* **11**, 346 (1967).
181. M. J. Adams, *Opto-Electronics* **5**, 201 (1973).
182. R. Lang and K. Kobayashi, *IEEE J. Quantum Electron.* **QE-12**, 194 (1976).
183. T. Kobayashi and S. Takahashi, *Jpn. J. Appl. Phys.* **15**, 2025 (1976).
184. R. Lang, *Jpn. J. Appl. Phys.* **16**, 205 (1977).
185. K. Kobayashi, R. Lang, H. Yonezu, I. Sakuma, and I. Hayashi, *Jpn. J. Appl. Phys.* **16**, 207 (1977).
186. T. L. Paoli, *IEEE J. Quantum Electron.* **QE-13**, 351 (1977).
187. J. A. Armstrong and A. W. Smith, *Phys. Rev.* **140**, A155 (1965).
188. A. W. Smith and J. A. Armstrong, *IBM J. Res. Develop.* **10**, 225 (1966).
189. J. A. Armstrong and A. W. Smith, *Progress in Optics*, Vol. VI, ed. by E. Wolf (Wiley, New York, 1967), p. 211.
190. T. L. Paoli and J. E. Ripper, *Phys. Rev. A* **2**, 2551 (1970).
191. D. E. McCumber, *Phys. Rev.* **141**, 306 (1966).
192. H. Haug, *Phys. Rev.* **184**, 338 (1969).
193. T. L. Paoli, *Appl. Phys. Lett.* **24**, 187 (1974).
194. T. L. Paoli, *IEEE J. Quantum Electron.* **QE-11**, 276 (1975).
195. T. Ito, S. Machida, K. Nawata, and T. Ikegami, *IEEE J. Quantum Electron.* **QE-13**, 574 (1977).
195a. J. Jäckel and G. Guekos, *Opt. and Quantum Electron.* **9**, 233 (1977).
196. I. P. Kaminow and T. Li, "Optical Fiber Telecommunications" (A. G. Chynoweth and S. E. Miller, eds.) Chapter 17 Academic Press (in press).
197. T. Ozeki and T. Ito, *IEEE J. Quantum Electron.* **QE-9**, 1098 (1973).
198. T. P. Lee and R. M. Derosier, *Proc. IEEE* **62**, 1176 (1974).
199. P. M. Boers and M. T. Vlaardingerbroek, *Electron. Lett.* **11**, 206 (1975).
200. W. Harth, *AEU* **29**, 149 (1975).
201. P. Russer, *AEU* **29**, 231 (1975).
202. M. Danielsen, *IEEE J. Quantum Electron.* **QE-12**, 657 (1976).
203. M. Chown, A. R. Goodwin, D. F. Lovelace, G. H. B. Thompson, and P. R. Selway, *Electron. Lett.* **9**, 34 (1973).
204. T. Ozeki and T. Ito, *IEEE J. Quantum Electron.* **QE-9**, 388 (1973).

205. J. E. Carroll and J. G. Farrington, *Electron. Lett.* **9**, 166 (1973).
206. P. Russer, *AEU* **27**, 193 (1973).
207. V. Ostoich and P. Jeppesen, *Electron. Lett.* **11**, 515 (1975).
208. P. R. Selway and A. R. Goodwin, *Electron. Lett.* **12**, 25 (1976).
209. F. S. Chen, P. W. Dorman, and M. A. Karr, *Bell Syst. Tech. J.* (July–August 1978).
210. P. K. Runge, *IEEE Trans. Commun.* **COM-24**, 413 (1976).
211. K. Nawata, K. Takano, T. Ikegami, and S. Ohara, *Electron. Lett.* **11**, 583 (1975).
212. J. E. Goell, *Proc. IEEE* **61**, 1504 (1973).
213. T. Ito, S. Machida, T. Ikegami, and S. Ohara, *Electron. Lett.* **11**, 375 (1975).
214. K. Aiki, M. Nakamura, and J. Umeda, *IEEE J. Quantum Electron.* **QE-12**, 597 (1976).
215. M. Nakamura, K. Aiki, J. Umeda, and A. Yariv, *Appl. Phys. Lett.* **27**, 403 (1975).
216. K. Aiki, M. Nakamura, and J. Umeda, *Appl. Phys. Lett.* **29**, 506 (1976).
217. M. Nakamura, Private communication.
218. H. C. Casey, Jr., S. Somekh, and M. Ilegems, *Appl. Phys. Lett.* **27**, 142 (1975).
219. F. K. Reinhart, R. A. Logan, and C. V. Shank, *Appl. Phys. Lett.* **27**, 45 (1975).
220. J. L. Merz, R. A. Logan, W. Wiegmann, and A. C. Gossard, *Appl. Phys. Lett.* **26**, 337 (1975).
221. W. Ng, H. W. Yen, A. Katzir, I. Samid, and A. Yariv, *Appl. Phys. Lett.* **29**, 684 (1976).
222. R. D. Burnham, D. R. Scrifres, and W. Streifer, *Appl. Phys. Lett.* **29**, 287 (1976).
223. J. N. Walpole, A. R. Calawa, S. R. Chinn, S. H. Groves, and T. C. Harman, *Appl. Phys. Lett.* **29**, 307 (1976).

8.1 INTRODUCTION

Injection lasers degrade by a variety of mechanisms that occur only during the passage of current. Which mechanism is dominant depends upon factors that include heteroepitaxial wafer growth procedures, wafer quality, device fabrication and mounting procedures, and operating conditions. While many of the fundamental details of the degradation mechanisms are not known, extensive empirical observations of GaAs–Al$_x$Ga$_{1-x}$As DH heterostructure laser degradation have been made. From these observations, the laser degradation may be conveniently separated into three categories:

(1) catastrophic mirror damage at high power densities,
(2) "dark-line defect" formation, and
(3) gradual degradation.

In this chapter, the experimental behavior that characterizes each of these categories is described and, where possible, reasonable models are discussed.

Catastrophic degradation due to mirror damage is observed for every type of injection laser. It usually occurs during pulsed high-power-density operation when the optical intensity per unit area at the laser facet exceeds a critical value of $\sim 6 \pm 2 \times 10^6$ W/cm^2. The experimental observations for this degradation mechanism are presented in Section 8.2. Catastrophic degradation is characterized by gross damage to the mirror and the generation of gross crystal faults in the interior of the laser near the mirror. Damage occurs where the optical intensity is the greatest. Mirror damage can be the most rapid form of laser degradation, and whenever the critical optical field intensity is exceeded, the destruction of the laser mirror can be virtually instantaneous.

The second mechanism of laser degradation to be considered is the dark-line defect (DLD) described in Section 8.3. The DLD is a network of dislocations that can form during laser operation, and it intrudes upon the optical cavity. Once started, it can grow extensively in a few hours. The DLD is also a localized region of high nonradiative recombination and relatively high absorption, and its growth is accompanied by an increase in J_{th}. Although the DLD usually starts within minutes to hours after the start of cw laser operation, its initiation may occasionally take much longer. There have been elegant observations of the DLD dislocation network, of its growth, and of the recombination enhanced motion of native point defects that may be required for its growth. Although the source and exact nature of those point defects and the detailed way that they interact with the growing DLD or initiate its growth has not been definitively established, a plausible model is described.

The empirical observations of relatively slow laser degradation, which exclude the instantaneous catastrophic failure or the fairly rapid degradation by DLD formation, are presented in Section 8.4 on gradual degradation. This category includes, therefore, lasers that may degrade by one or more undefined mechanisms.

In spite of the empirical nature of the study of heterostructure laser degradation, the practical aim of long laser operating life has been achieved. For low-power (~ 3 mW) cw lasers needed for optical communications, the DLD formation may be thwarted by growth and processing procedures that reduce the concentration of inclined dislocations that appear to be necessary to initiate its growth. Gradual degradation, although not well understood, can be slow enough for low-power applications to give extrapolated laser operating lifetimes considerably greater than 10^5 hr at 300°K. A fundamental limit to laser operating life has not been identified.

8.2 CATASTROPHIC FAILURE

Catastrophic Failure of Homostructure Lasers

In 1966, Cooper et al.[1] and Dobson and Keeble[2] reported that attempts to operate GaAs homostructure injection lasers at high pulse power resulted in gross damage to the emitting region. The visible evidence of this damage was the formation of pits, grooves, and "spherical mounds" at the mirror surface where the optical-flux density was the greatest. A detailed examination of catastrophic damage in GaAs homostructure lasers by Shaw and Thornton[3] utilized scanning-electron microscopy, cathodoluminescence, and x-ray microanalysis and showed that the damaged regions had fractured areas coexisting with melted and fissured regions. An example is shown in Fig. 8.2-1. In addition, there were solidified droplets over the length of the damaged region. The cathodoluminescence studies revealed that the fissured regions with low luminescence extended from the melted–fractured region on the p-side into the n-side of the p–n junction. Successive etching showed that the damage, as revealed by etch-pit studies, extended as far as 400 μm into the device in an irregular manner.

Simultaneous with the damage to the mirror was a decrease in the emitted light.[1,2] Several such decreases could be observed with a single laser, and each was apparently associated with damage occurring at the location of the end of a lasing filament at the mirror.[1] Similar damage for homostructure

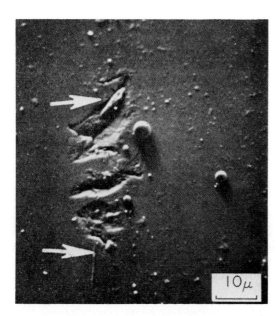

FIG. 8.2-1   A scanning-electron photomicrograph of a catastrophically damaged homo-structure laser mirror showing fractures and droplets. The arrows show the location of the p–n junction (Ref. 3).

lasers was reported by Kressel and Mierop[4] in 1967. In the temperature range between 77° and 300°K, they observed that the optical power level required for damage is lower at low temperature than at high temperature. A further pertinent observation[1,2] was that for a given current density the damage only occurred if the unit was lasing. Kressel and Mierop[4] assumed a uniform distribution of optical flux for a recombination region $1–1.5$ μm wide so that the critical-flux density ranged from 1.8 to 2.5 MW/cm² at 77°K and 5.8 to 8 MW/cm² at 300°K. These numbers are, of course, very approximate. The flux distribution is certainly not uniform, and the recombination-region thickness must increase with temperature because the minority-carrier diffusion length in GaAs increases by a factor of about five between 77° and 300°K.[5]

All of these early observations suggested that catastrophic failure of injection lasers is associated with the optical-power density at the mirror which results in an abrupt and large temperature increase that is sufficient to cause localized melting. The literature on degradation has described the damage limit in several ways: the optical power at the damage limit for a given laser P^c, the optical-power density at the damage limit over the cross-sectional area of the waveguide P^c_{AV}, the peak optical power at the damage limit P_{peak}, and the optical power emitted per unit width W of the waveguide at the damage limit $P_W{}^c$. Unfortunately, catastrophic degradation for homostructure and heterostructure lasers has most often been reported as $P_W{}^c$ obtained from P^c/W without regard to filaments and other emission nonuniformities. Primarily for that reason, data on catastrophic degradation are badly scattered.

Catastrophic Failure of Heterostructure Lasers

In spite of the emission nonuniformities due to the filamentary behavior of broad-area lasers, useful results have been obtained.[6–13] Kressel et al.[6] noted that with SH lasers catastrophic failure occurs at lower $P_W{}^c$ than with homostructure lasers. Also, for the SH laser, there is essentially no temperature dependence of $P_W{}^c$ between 77° and 300°K.[7] These observations are consistent with the fact that in the SH laser, electrons are usually injected into a GaAs active region 1–2 μm thick (Section 7.3). Except at quite low temperatures, the injected electrons have a longer diffusion length than the active-region thickness. Therefore, if the damage limit is determined by the optical-field density, the critical value will be less temperature sensitive in an SH laser than in a homostructure laser. Kressel et al.[7,8] also showed that the critical value for catastropic damage in the SH laser decreases markedly as the pulse length becomes shorter, just as it does in the homostructure laser.[2] Therefore, for all injection lasers, care must be taken to compare damage limits measured under the same pulse conditions.

An indication of the relation of the optical field to the catastrophic mirror damage was illustrated by Ettenberg et al.[13] They compared the catastrophic mirror damage for otherwise identical GaAs–Al$_x$Ga$_{1-x}$As SH lasers with and without an antireflection coating on one mirror. The coated mirror reflectivity was determined by considering the reflection at the partially reflecting mirrors illustrated in Fig. 3.8-1. At surface 2 after a round trip of $2L$, the field $t_1 r_1 r_2 \mathscr{E}_i \exp(-3\Gamma L)$ must equal the field $t_1 \mathscr{E}_i \exp(-\Gamma L)$ which requires that

$$\exp(-2\Gamma L) = 1/r_1 r_2, \qquad (8.2\text{-}1)$$

where the field reflectivity r is related to the power reflectivity R as $r = R^{1/2}$. Since the emitted power is the incident power less the reflected power, the emitted power at surface 1 is

$$P_1 = (1 - R_1)[t_1 r_2 \mathscr{E}_i \exp(-2\Gamma L)]^2, \qquad (8.2\text{-}2)$$

and the emitted power at surface 2 is

$$P_2 = (1 - R_2)[t_1 \mathscr{E}_i \exp(-\Gamma L)]^2. \qquad (8.2\text{-}3)$$

The ratio P_1 to P_2 with Eq. (8.2-1) for $\exp(-2\Gamma L)$ is

$$P_1/P_2 = (R_2^{1/2}/R_1^{1/2})(1 - R_1)/(1 - R_2). \qquad (8.2\text{-}4)$$

With the reflectivity of the uncoated mirror taken as 0.3, the reflectivity of the coated mirror was obtained from Eq. (8.2-4) by measuring the emission power for each mirror of a laser with one coated mirror.

Ettenberg et al.[13] compared the emission power for catastrophic mirror damage for SH lasers with one mirror coated to similar devices with uncoated mirrors. The mirror reflectivity was obtained from Eq. (8.2-4) as described above. The experimental ratio of the emission power for a laser with coated mirror P_{t_1} to a laser with an uncoated mirror P_{t_0} is given in Fig. 8.2-2. The effect of mirror reflectivity on the emitted power was described by Hakki and Nash[9] and may be derived from the relationships given in Chapter 2. From Eqs. (2.4-46) to (2.4-48) and with the definitions of β and ω from Section 2.2,

$$P = \tfrac{1}{2}\mathscr{E} \times \mathscr{H} = (\beta/2\omega\,\mu_0)\mathscr{E}^2 = (\bar{n}/2)(\varepsilon_0/\mu_0)^{1/2}\mathscr{E}^2. \qquad (8.2\text{-}5)$$

The electric field is continuous at the mirror so that the field of the transmitted wave is

$$\mathscr{E}_t = \mathscr{E}_i + \mathscr{E}_r = (1 + R^{1/2})\mathscr{E}_i, \qquad (8.2\text{-}6)$$

where $\mathscr{E}_i$ and $\mathscr{E}_r$ are the electric fields for the incident and reflected wave on the inside of the mirror. Since the transmitted power P_t is the incident power less the reflected power, Eq. (8.2-5) gives

$$P_t = (\bar{n}/2)(\varepsilon_0/\mu_0)^{1/2}(1 - R)\mathscr{E}_i^2, \qquad (8.2\text{-}7)$$

which can be rewritten with Eq. (8.2-6) as

$$P_t = \bar{n}(\varepsilon_0/\mu_0)^{1/2}(1 - R)\mathscr{E}_t^2/2(1 + R^{1/2})^2. \qquad (8.2\text{-}8)$$

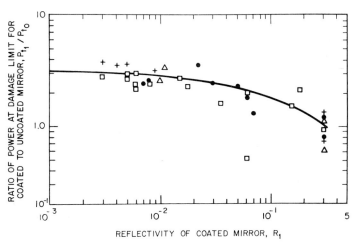

FIG. 8.2-2 Ratio of the catastrophic damage limit with and without antireflective coating as a function of reflectivity of the coated mirror. The data are from Ref. 13. The theoretical curve is calculated from Eq. 8.2-11 (Ref. 9).

If $\mathscr{E}_t$ of two similar lasers with and without antireflective coatings is the same, then the ratio of the transmitted power from the two lasers is [9]

$$P_{t_1}/P_{t_0} = (1 - R_1)(1 + R_0^{1/2})^2/(1 - R_0)(1 + R_1^{1/2})^2, \qquad (8.2\text{-}9)$$

where P_{t_1} is the transmitted power with an antireflective coating and P_{t_0} the transmitted power without a coating. From Eq. (2.6-19), the reflectance of a wave at normal incidence on a dielectric interface with refractive index $\bar{n}$ and unity is related to R by

$$\bar{n} = (1 + R_0^{1/2})^2/(1 - R_0). \qquad (8.2\text{-}10)$$

With Eq. (8.2-10), Eq. (8.2-9) becomes

$$P_{t_1}/P_{t_0} = \bar{n}(1 - R_1)/(1 + R_1^{1/2})^2. \qquad (8.2\text{-}11)$$

Then, if $\mathscr{E}_{t_1}$ and $\mathscr{E}_{t_0}$ are the same at the catastrophic damange limit, the ratio P_{t_1}/P_{t_0} should increase by the factor $\bar{n}$ as R_1 approaches zero. The curve drawn through the data of Fig. 8.2-2 was obtained by Hakki and Nash[9] by fitting Eq. (8.2-11) at one point. Within the scatter of the data, the power ratio does increase by about $\bar{n}$ as R_1 approaches zero.

Hakki and Nash[9] observed with stripe-geometry DH and PpnN lasers that, as with the homostructure, damage starts at the mirror and moves into the semiconductor bulk. This damage is, however, confined primarily to the region of the optical cavity. Electroluminescence studies reveal the damage as a dark line of internal crystal damage extending into the active region by as much as 250 μm. It grows at an average velocity of 10–20 μm/sec along the $\langle 110 \rangle$-axis of the cavity. They obtained an emission power of 4–8×10^6 W/cm^2 for catastrophic mirror damage of DH lasers for 100-nsec pulse lengths.[9] This emission power may be converted to an electric field with Eq. (8.2-8). With $\mu_0 = 1.26 \times 10^{-8}$ H/cm, $\varepsilon_0 = 8.86 \times 10^{-14}$ F/cm, and $R = 0.3$, the critical optical field intensity becomes 5.4×10^4 to 7.6×10^4 V/cm. Since these field strengths are at least a factor of four lower than the dc avalanche field strength in GaAs, it does not appear reasonable to consider heating due to large currents caused by avalanche breakdown as the reason for the catastrophic damage.

Effect of Emission Uniformity on Catastrophic Failure Limits of the Heterostructure Lasers

A particularly interesting study of catastrophic failure was reported by Henshall.[14] He studied the near-field uniformity, differential efficiency, and catastrophic damage limit of SH, DH, and asymmetric SCH lasers for an excitation pulse width of 200 nsec. The uniformity U is taken to be the ratio of the average emission intensity parallel to the junction plane to the maximum intensity of the brightest filament. The variation of the near-field optical

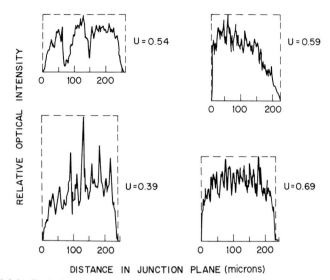

FIG. 8.2-3   Typical optical intensity distribution along the junction plane for heterostructure laser. The asymmetric SCH lasers described in Section 7.5 were used for these studies (Ref. 14).

intensity for several representative asymmetric SCH lasers is shown in Fig. 8.2-3. Similar behavior for DH lasers was presented in Section 7.4. Qualitatively the emission may be considered to result from a number of filaments, each with its own threshold and current density. At threshold the filament with the lowest J_{th} starts to lase. As current is increased, other filaments lase and the optical distribution ceases to change markedly after the last filament is above its threshold. As shown in Fig. 8.2-4, Henshall[14] observed that U generally remains approximately constant with increasing current I for a given laser when $I/I_{th} > 3$, where I_{th} is the threshold current.

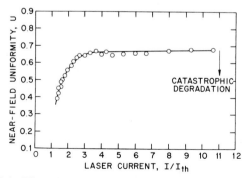

FIG. 8.2-4   Effect of injection level on near field uniformity (Ref. 14).

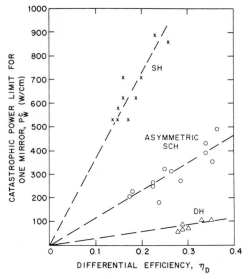

FIG. 8.2-5   Catastrophic damage limits for various heterostructure lasers as a function of differential efficiency (Ref. 14).

Henshall[14] showed experimentally that both the differential efficiency η_D and $P_W{}^c$ vary linearly with U for $I > 3I_{th}$, and therefore $P_W{}^c$ varies linearly with η_D. A plot of $P_W{}^c$ versus η_D is given in Fig. 8.2-5 for SH, DH, and asymmetric SCH lasers. The significant features of this plot are the range of $P_W{}^c$ for a given structure and the differences in slope and absolute magnitude for the different types of lasers. Figure 8.2-5 shows that the asymmetric SCH laser of Fig. 7.5-5 is a compromise between a lower $P_W{}^c$ than the SH laser and a higher $P_W{}^c$ than the DH laser. Its advantage is a J_{th} of $0.5-1.5 \times 10^3$ A/cm² which is similar to that of low-J_{th} DH lasers and much lower than the $J_{th} > 10^4$ A/cm² for SH lasers. Although the SH laser has a higher $P_W{}^c$, the asymmetric SCH laser has the advantage of a much higher power conversion efficiency near threshold as well as a smaller temperature dependence of J_{th}.

The results[14] of a study of the variation of $P_W{}^c$ with the effective waveguide thickness S_{eff} and beam divergence perpendicular to the junction plane $\Theta_\perp$ are given in Fig. 8.2-6 for a group of asymmetric SCH lasers very similar to those in Table 7.5-1. These lasers were selected to have uniform emission and for the absence of internally circulating modes. The latter are modes that result from reflection at the sawn side walls. They produce no emission in the near-field but contribute to the local electric field at the mirror and thus to scatter in $P_W{}^c$. The linear relation between $P_W{}^c$ and S_{eff} suggests that a

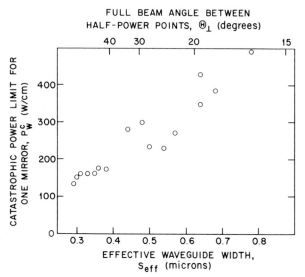

FIG. 8.2-6 $P_W{}^c$ versus S_{eff} and $\Theta_\perp$ for a uniform set of asymmetric SCH lasers (Ref. 14).

useful quantity for predicting the catastrophic damage limit of uniform lasers may be the effective average optical power density $P_e{}^c = P_W{}^c$ (W/cm)/ S_{eff}(cm). As defined in Section 7.5, $S_{eff} \approx d/\Gamma$, and therefore S_{eff} represents spreading of the optical intensity in the direction perpendicular to the junction plane. In Fig. 8.2-5, $P_W{}^c$ is larger for SH lasers than the SCH or DH lasers because of the larger S_{eff}. This difference emphasizes that it is the spatial peak intensity of the emission that causes catastrophic mirror damage. From Fig. 8.2-6, $P_e{}^c$ for an uncoated GaAs laser mirror is approximately 5.5 ± 0.5 MW/cm² for a 200-nsec pulse width. Figure 7.5-6, which gives S_{eff} versus $\Theta_\perp$ for various structures, may be used with $P_e{}^c$ to predict $P_W{}^c$ for other uniform lasers. For example, curve 1 of Fig. 7.5-6 is for large d and may be taken to approximate the SH laser case. For SH lasers, $\Theta_\perp$ is normally about 15°–20° (Ref. 14) and $S_{eff} \approx 1.7$ μm from Fig. 7.5-6. The expected value of $P_W{}^c$ is then 5.5 (MW/cm²) × S(cm) $\approx$ 900 W/cm, which is approximately the value given in Fig. 8.2-5 for the best SH lasers.

Unfortunately, there is very little information on catastrophic degradation limits and $\Theta_\perp$ for DH lasers. Kirkby and Thompson[10] have reported values of $P_W{}^c$, $\Theta_\perp$, η_D, and S_{eff} for several groups of slightly asymmetric DH lasers with thin active layers. The excitation pulse width was 200 nsec. The parameters for these lasers are given in Table 8.2-1. Although the lasers of Table 8.2-1 were apparently not selected for high uniformity, the measured differential efficiency for lasers from slices 1 and 2 were as high or higher than η_D of the

TABLE 8.2-1 Properties of Narrow-Active-Region DH Lasers[a]

Slice number	d (μm)	Mole fraction AlAs, x N-layer	Mole fraction AlAs, x P-layer	η_D (%)	$J_{th}(300°\text{K})$ (A/cm²)	$\Theta_\perp$ (deg)	Effective optical width, S_{eff} (μm)	$P_W°$(W/cm) measured	$P_W°$(W/cm) predicted
1	0.14	0.24	0.20	25–40	1150	30	0.36	80–110	200
2	0.12	0.23	0.17	25–52	1300	~20	0.44	230–320	240
3	0.11	0.24	0.17	14–31	1450	16	0.60	340–410	330

[a] Ref. 10.

"best," and thus most uniform, DH and SCH lasers of Fig. 8.2-5. The lower differential efficiencies of lasers from slice 3 suggest that they are less uniform. The predicted and measured values of $P_W{}^c$ in Table 8.2-1 are in reasonable agreement, but the trend with efficiency is not entirely consistent with Henshall's SCH laser data. This inconsistency may arise because the critical parameter is probably the peak power and not $P_W{}^c$. Nevertheless, this approach permits an approximate empirical prediction of $P_W{}^c$ that can be useful.

The mechanism by which catastrophic damage occurs is not known. Several have been suggested. It was proposed that optical absorption at inhomogeneities resulted in heating and melting of the facet.[2,3] Ettenberg et al.[13] rejected this mechanism on the basis of a simple model that considers the power absorbed near the facet by an inhomogeneity to be proportional to the optical power inside the crystal. Their estimate of the maximum change in damage limit as a function of mirror reflectivity with this model is, however, only about 30% lower than the observed change. The rather small scatter of the data plotted in Figs. 8.2-5 and 8.2-6 suggests that chance occurrences of inhomogeneities is not required. However, it seems reasonable to point out that the surface space-charge region of the cleaved laser immediately adjacent to the mirror must be absorbing. The GaAs or $Al_xGa_{1-x}As$ surface provides rapid nonradiative recombination, and therefore there will be a thin region adjacent to the surface in which the absorption rate exceeds the stimulated emission rate. It is possible that catastrophic failure near the mirror occurs when and where the surface recombination optical power absorption are great enough to cause runaway heating. In studies by Henry et al.,[15] catastrophic damage was induced by exciting superradiance in a $GaAs–Al_xGa_{1-x}As$ DH wafer by photo-excitation with a cavity dumped Ar laser. Local melting due to intense nonradiative recombination of minority carriers at a cleaved surface or on a defect was observed. This recent work suggests a cause of catastrophic degradation and a technique for its study.

8.3 THE DARK-LINE DEFECT (DLD)

Experimental Observation

Perhaps the single most important observation leading to the achievement of cw operation of injection lasers for long periods of time at or above room temperature was reported by De Loach et al.[16] They demonstrated a major degradation mechanism in $GaAs–Al_xGa_{1-x}As$ stripe-geometry DH lasers that involved nonuniform changes in the optical cavity. Previously, degradation studies had involved measurement of light output and current characteristics,[17–19] frequently for pulsed operation of homostructure lasers. From the earlier studies, it appeared that degradation involved the formation of nonradiative centers and that it was more rapid in structures made from material with, than without, high concentrations of dislocations and precipitates.[19]

To observe the degree of uniformity of the active region of a stripe-geometry DH laser, De Loach et al.[16] used devices that were fabricated with a window in the n-side contact directly above the stripe, as shown in Fig. 8.3-1. Thus the spontaneous emission from the active region was observed and photographed through the substrate during cw-lasing operation. A dominant set of features that developed during minutes to hours of operation were thin dark regions that started at one edge or within the stripe and crossed it in a $\langle 100 \rangle$ direction while gradually thickening. The development of these dark regions with operating time is illustrated in Fig. 8.3-2. As the dark lines formed and increased in width, J_{th} increased while the external differential quantum efficiency decreased. Because of these observations, it has become common practice to refer to such a defect as a dark-line defect (DLD).

The observation of the DLD is consistent with studies of spectral emission from both ends of degraded lasers[20] and with changes in the gain[21] that suggested the presence of nonuniform optical absorption. De Loach et al.[16] also noted the similarity of the DLD to features observed by Biard et al.[22] in GaAs light-emitting diodes. Biard et al. attributed this degradation to strain introduced during bonding. Similar features at dislocations were reported by Zschauer[23] for alloyed GaAs p–n junctions. The features they[22,23] observed were qualitatively different from each other, and from the DLD usually observed in lasers. It was important at this stage, however, for the association between a severe localized reduction in radiative efficiency

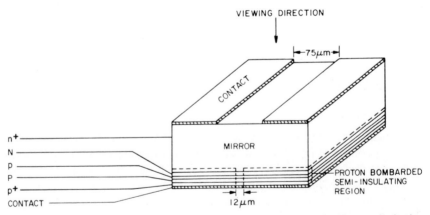

FIG. 8.3-1 A stripe-geometry DH laser with a partial n-type contact to permit viewing of the electroluminescence of the active region during lasing (Ref. 16).

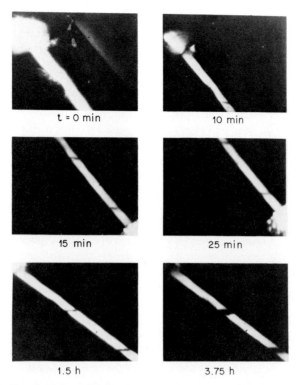

FIG. 8.3-2 Development of dark-line defects during room-temperature cw operation of a stripe-geometry DH laser as viewed with electroluminescence through the window in the partial n^+-contact of Fig. 8.3-1 (Ref. 16).

and the presence of strain and dislocations to be made. In a laser, such localized regions will have reduced gain and even become lossy. The small active-region volume and the necessity of maintaining a high gain region render the presence of a DLD far more deleterious to lasers than to light-emitting diodes. In fact, it had already been demonstrated that short-term cw laser degradation, occurring during times similar to those involved in the DLD formation, was dramatically reduced when bonding strain was reduced.[24]

Yonezu et al.[25] observed what is apparently the same DLD feature in GaAs–$Al_xGa_{1-x}As$ stripe-geometry and broad-area DH lasers. Their devices were forward biased at current densities comparable to those used by De Loach et al.,[16] however, because of poor thermal heat sinking the devices were nonlasing.[25] In addition, Johnston et al.,[26] Petroff et al.,[27] and Ito et al.[28] observed that DLD features could be produced by optical excitation in some areas of a DH wafer that contained dislocations or stacking faults.

These optical excitation results are significant observations because they establish that the DLD formation is not dependent upon the current flow, but rather upon carrier recombination and some defect feature that can sometimes be related to strain.

Detailed studies have been made of the DLD in DH lasers by utilizing the transmission-electron microscope (TEM).[29–33] The DLD's formed during injection lasing and optical excitation are apparently identical in nature. The TEM studies revealed that each DLD is a three-dimensional network of dislocations. In stripe-geometry lasers, the DLD networks are confined to the stripe area. In the early work by Petroff and Hartman,[29,30] relatively short-lived lasers that operated for 5–500 hr at ~300°K were studied. The networks were only observed to have nucleated at dislocations (see Section 5.6) that passed through the multilayer structure.[29,30] Presumably these dislocations that served as nucleating sites for the DLD in such short-lived lasers originated in the substrate or by plastic flow during processing. It is important to note, however, that dislocations may also result from the presence of precipitates or other foreign particles that are either incorporated during growth of the structure or form during laser operation.[33] Such dislocations may reasonably be expected to also act as nucleating sites for growth of the DLD.

An electron micrograph of the dislocation network that forms the DLD is shown in Fig. 8.3-3. On the basis of stereoelectron micrographs, Petroff and Hartman[30] claimed that the DLD originated at a point usually located in the P–$Al_xGa_{1-x}As$ layer. It is somewhat surprising that the DLD origin would be outside the active layer, and confirmation by cross-section TEM would be helpful. Hutchinson et al.[31,32] have observed with TEM that the

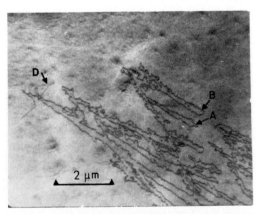

FIG. 8.3-3   Bright-field transmission-electron micrograph of part of a dislocation network associated with a DLD. Note that the DLD originates from the dislocation at D (Ref. 29).

networks lie in a region approximately as thick as the active region and suggest that they are probably confined to the active region. In addition, they observe that some of the dislocation networks do not appear to originate at threading dislocations. This may be consistent with other observations by Petroff and Hartman,[34] that occasionally, in longer-lived lasers, DLD features are associated with faulted loops associated with precipitates or possibly even with precipitates alone.

The dislocations that form the networks are primarily observed to be ragged helices, and usually these helices are roughly parallel to a {100} plane. They are elongated in the ⟨100⟩ and ⟨210⟩ directions and only occasionally in the ⟨110⟩ direction.[29,30] Such continuous elongated dislocation structures are designated by A and B in Fig. 8.3-3 and are usually called dipoles. In addition to the dipole helices, the network structure is associated with dislocation loops. These are dislocation structures in which the dislocation closes upon itself so as to enclose a region with an extra pair of planes of group III and group V atoms (an extrinsic or interstitial loop) or a region with a missing pair of planes of atoms (an intrinsic or vacancy type loop). Since the region away from the immediate vicinity of the dislocation is perfect, only the loop boundary, consisting of the dislocation itself, is seen in the TEM. An analysis of the TEM image contrast reveals whether a given loop is intrinsic or extrinsic.

Petroff's image-contrast analysis of the dipoles and loops revealed that pure edge and mixed dislocations are present in the network,[29] and that the dislocations are not impurity decorated.[30] The contrast analysis in the early work indicated that all of the loops were of the intrinsic type. It was thought that these loops resulted from the interaction or pinching off of portions of the helical dipoles, so that the dipoles and loops were *both* thought to be intrinsic. Hutchinson *et al.*[32] showed, however, that at least some of the dislocation loops are boundaries within an extrinsic dipole so that they would appear to have been intrinsic relative to the surrounding medium. The question of the intrinsic or extrinsic nature and the origin of the loops bears closely on the mechanism of DLD formation. Subsequent studies by Petroff and Kimerling[35] confirm the Hutchinson *et al.*[32] observation that some of the loops are within the large dipole which is extrinsic. Those loops are small (<200 Å diameter) and intrinsic.[35] Other larger extrinsic loops are outside the boundaries of the dipole and probably those result from pinching off of portions of the dipole.

In addition to the detailed observations described above, the DLD growth can be extremely erratic.[36] Usually the DLD, if it is to form at all, will be observed within hours after the start of cw operation. In some cases, however, the start of DLD formation has been observed to be delayed for hundreds of hours. In addition, DLD growth rate has also been observed to vary greatly without apparent reason and to sometimes cease abruptly after a period of rapid growth.

DLD Growth by Climb or Glide

The detailed mechanism of DLD growth is not yet known. Discussion of DLD growth requires considering whether the dislocation is extended primarily by climb as is claimed by Petroff and Hartman[29,30] and Petroff and Kimerling[35] or primarily by glide as claimed by Matsui et al.[37] and Nannichi et al.[38] This distinction is important because climb requires the presence of fairly high concentrations of point defects while glide does not.

Petroff and Hartman[30] have, for example, estimated that a typical DLD has 40 dipoles with an average length and width of 10 μm and 0.2 μm, respectively. If the dipoles result entirely from climb and are formed by pure edge dislocations, the number of point defects (equivalent vacancies or interstitials), N_V, required for its formation is the total dipole volume divided by the atomic volume. The atomic radius was taken to be 1.41 Å so that $N_V \approx 5 \times 10^{18}$. If these point defects were evenly distributed in the volume of the active region of a typical stripe-geometry laser (400 μm $\times$ 10 μm $\times$ 0.2 μm), their concentration would be $\sim 6 \times 10^{17}$ cm^{-3}, and if the surrounding Al$_x$Ga$_{1-x}$As regions were included, this concentration would decrease by more than a factor of 10. Although DLD formation can usually be thwarted by the elimination of the inclined dislocation upon which it nucleates, the implied presence of high point defect concentrations suggests their potential involvement in subsequent more gradual degradation. The point defect that contributes to climb has not been identified. However, the donor level in Al$_x$Ga$_{1-x}$As that controls the resistivity appears to be a donor-vacancy complex.[39] This point defect is present in concentrations that approach the donor impurity concentration. The direct relationship between this defect and degradation has not been established.

It is useful at this point to consider briefly the dislocation climb mechanism proposed by Petroff and Kimerling.[35] The 60° dislocation described in Section 5.6 and illustrated in Fig. 5.6-4 is shown projected on the (1$\bar{1}$0) plane in Fig. 8.3-4a. A supersaturation of one type of defect is postulated. For their example, Petroff and Kimerling chose Ga interstitials Ga$_i$. These defects migrate to the vicinity of the dislocation and occupy the dangling bond site at the dislocation core as shown in Fig. 8.3-4b. An As vacancy V_{As} is thus created at the core. An As atom from an adjacent site occupies the core site vacancy as illustrated in Figs. 8.3-4b,c. In part (d) the resulting V_{As} moves into a location where it tends to compensate local stresses, and another Ga$_i$ has diffused near to the dislocation. The process may then be repeated. Thus, climb by the effective addition of a Ga and As atom at the dislocation has been effected. Supersaturation with only one kind of point defect, Ga$_i$, was needed, but a trail of point defects V_{As} remains.

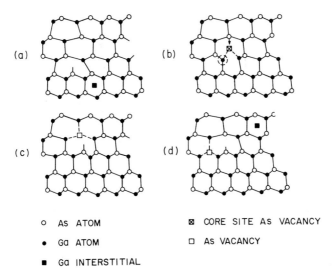

○ AS ATOM	⊠ CORE SITE AS VACANCY
● Ga ATOM	□ AS VACANCY
■ Ga INTERSTITIAL	

FIG. 8.3-4 (a) The zinc-blende lattice with a 60° dislocation projected normal to the $(1\bar{1}0)$ plane. (b), (c), (d) Schematic representations of the point defect diffusion required for the dislocation climb (Ref. 35).

Qualitative thermodynamic justification for such a model results[35,40] if it is assumed that Ga_i and V_{As} are the dominant defects at equilibrium at the growth temperature. The driving force for the climb reaction was postulated[35] to be the lower chemical potential of V_{As} relative to Ga_i at temperatures below the growth temperature as the result of the larger volume of Ga_i as compared to V_{As}.[41] Petroff and Kimerling[35] further postulate that the As vacancies cluster and then collapse to form the intrinsic loops observed inside the DLD dipoles with the emission of an antisite defect Ga_{As}. Although this latter suggestion is certainly speculative, it is consistent with Petroff and Kimerling's TEM studies[35] of injection-stimulated climb that are described in the next part of this section on recombination-enhanced defect motion. It is also interesting to note that Van Vechten[42] has suggested that the vacancy–antisite defect complex $V_{As}Ga_{As}V_{As}$ may be relatively stable compared to V_{As} and may also be a nonradiative recombination center. The complex would also be effective in using up V_{As} while aiding in the formation of intrinsic loops.

It is quite possible to start with essentially the same experimental facts and obtain a different model for DLD climb. Intrinsic climb in the model by Petroff and Kimmerling[35] results from the absorption of interstitial point defects whose reaction has been enhanced by nonradiative recombination. O'Hara et al.[43] suggested that intrinsic climb results from the emission of vacancy pairs at the dislocation as the result of a reaction enhanced by nonradiative recombination. As these two models demonstrate, considerable controversy exists in the description of dark-line defects.

Matsui *et al.*[37] and Nannichi *et al.*[38] have suggested that the DLD dipoles extend themselves primarily by a glide mechanism. They suggest that a screw segment of a threading dislocation cross slips alternately in the $[1\bar{1}0]$ direction on the $(1\bar{1}1)$ plane and then in the $[\bar{1}\bar{1}0]$ direction on the $(\bar{1}\bar{1}1)$ plane so as to give an overall dipole direction of $[\bar{1}00]$ as illustrated in Fig. 8.3-5. Matsui *et al.*[37] also postulated a very similar glide mechanism for propagation of a branch of the dislocation in the ⟨210⟩ direction. A clear advantage of this model is that it predicts the usual preferential directions for dipole extension in the DLD. It does not explain the width of the dipoles nor their very ragged nature that was illustrated in Fig. 8.3-3. Therefore, Matsui *et al.*[37] proposed additionally that after the formation of long narrow dipoles by slip, these dipoles widen by climb, and in the process form the other features such as the raggedness and loops that are associated with the DLD.

Since the suggested DLD growth mechanisms require that important features result from climb, the major point of contention is whether glide contributes to DLD growth in a major or a minor way. Matsui *et al.*[37] have noted and Nannichi *et al.*[38] have discussed more fully the requirement of a localized stress, probably due to local heating, for DLD growth by glide. Nannichi *et al.*[38] contend that a ∼200°C localized temperature increase is sufficient, but Kobayashi *et al.*[44,45] measured the localized temperature rise at a DLD to be between ∼25° and 70°C. The localized stress resulting from heating during laser operation is presumed to be superimposed upon a preexisting stress field that determines the direction of the glide motion. The initiation of DLD growth by glide at localized hot-spots suggests that the initial dislocation from which the DLD grows should be a site for nonradiative recombination.

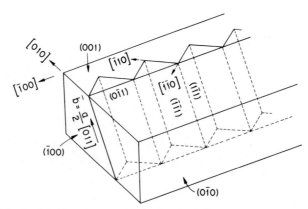

FIG. 8.3-5 Propagation of a screw segment in the $[\bar{1}00]$ direction by alternate glide on $(1\bar{1}1)$ and $(\bar{1}11)$ planes (Ref. 37).

A correlation between DLD behavior during laser degradation and the nature of the available nucleating sites does not appear to have been demonstrated. The TEM studies[29–32] show the DLD grown from an inclined dislocation (Fig. 8.3-3) that is presumed to be grown-in and not from the typically very straight slip dislocations. However, this observation may occur because virtually all lasers studied by TEM were fabricated by techniques that do not induce slip. In the early work, there certainly was a strong correlation between fabrication induced strain and rapid degradation that presumably resulted from DLD formation. In that case, the fabrication introduced strain probably caused slip dislocations that were the nuclei for the DLD's. In a more recent study, Kamejima et al.[46] appear to have modified the arguments concerning the glide growth of DLD's and show that ⟨110⟩ DLD's can be produced by glide and require both stress and carrier injection for growth. Once the ⟨110⟩ DLD's are present, ⟨100⟩ DLD's propagate, apparently as the result of climb and injection.

The observations and speculations described above suggest that climb certainly does play an important part in DLD growth, but leave considerable uncertainty about the role of glide. Long smooth dipoles such as would be expected if the initial step in dipole extension were from slip have never been seen in stress-free degraded lasers. In addition, it is difficult to understand how the delayed start or abrupt ending of DLD growth could happen with a glide and local heating mechanism. These events are, however, expected with climb if the interstitial point defects are needed. Delayed DLD initiation is expected if climb requires nucleating sites, presumably jogs, that are relatively unavailable on the starting dislocation. Once DLD growth starts, the ragged dipole is rich in such sites and growth continues as long as there is recombination and until the needed point defects are depleted. (See the discussion of recombination-enhanced defect motion below.) It does not seem unreasonable to expect that dipole extension by climb will have a preferred orientation because preferred climb sites probably are jogs along the dislocation. Presumably, it is the jogs that provide the source of the preferred dipole orientation.

Recombination-Enhanced Defect Motion

In support of the climb mechanism, Kimerling et al.[47] have shown that climb can be induced on localized regions of misfit dislocations when radiation induced point defects and carrier recombination are simultaneously present. In addition, Petroff and Kimerling[35] have shown experimentally that the freshly formed parts of a dislocation network can be stimulated to grow by carrier injection from the electron beam of a transmission electron microscope. This experimental behavior is illustrated in the circled area of Fig. 8.3-6. Loop and point-defect clusters were observed to occur only in

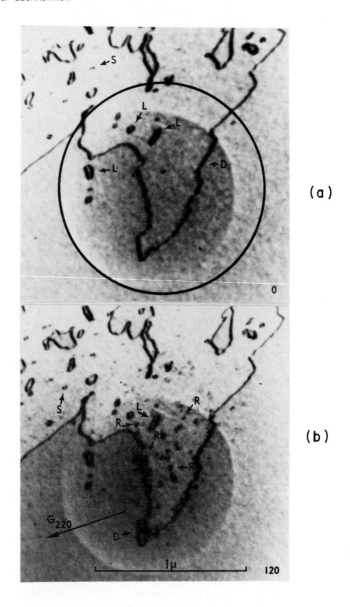

FIG. 8.3-6 (a) Bright-field transmission-electron micrograph of part of a dislocation dipole D and of large and small dislocation loops L and S formed by climb during the degradation of a GaAs–Al$_x$Ga$_{1-x}$As DH laser. New small loops and point-defect clusters R were produced in (b) by stimulating the defect motion with an electron beam in the indicated circular area (Ref. 35).

the vicinity of the dislocation line, and the entire process was observed to saturate. Thus many of the major features suggested by a climb model are accounted for, including symptoms that suggest the initial presence of a limited source (supersaturation) of point defects. One further requirement of the climb mechanism is that it be operative, as observed, only with carrier recombination. It seems reasonable to suggest that this feature of DLD formation results partly because the point defects responsible for climb do not diffuse rapidly enough to give DLD growth when only thermally excited at or near room temperature. Because of this role of recombination-enhanced defect motion, the studies of deep traps using the deep-level transient spectroscopy (DLTS) technique developed by Lang[48] are of particular interest.

The DLTS technique employs high-frequency capacitance transient thermal scanning for observing a variety of deep traps in semiconductors. With it, a trap spectrum is obtained from which the energy level and concentration of each trap, among other properties, can be determined. With DLTS studies, particularly of GaAs and GaP, Lang et al.[49-51], and Kimerling and Lang[52] have directly observed recombination-enhanced annealing of point defects. The 20°C annealing behavior, as observed by DLTS,[52a] of the defect-state concentrations induced in a GaAs p–n junction by 1-MeV electron irradiation is shown in Fig. 8.3-7. Without a diode forward current, no recovery was observed at this temperature, while for a forward current density of 20 A/cm², the defects annealed with time as shown in the figure.

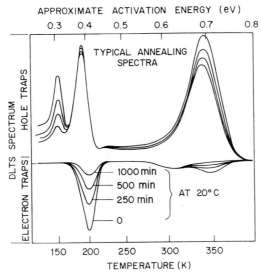

FIG. 8.3-7   Recombination activated annealing of electron and hole traps in GaAs at 300°K. Diode current is 10 mA. No 300°K annealing is seen without current flow (Ref. 52a).

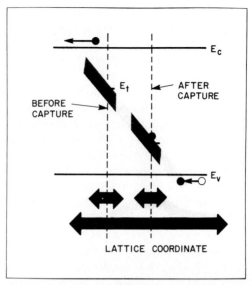

FIG. 8.3-8 Illustration of nonradiative capture of an electron. The equilibrium energies and lattice coordinates before and after capture are illustrated with dashed lines. The shaded regions within the energy gap suggest how the energy of the defect level changes relative to the band edges as the lattice vibrates. The smaller arrows represent the amplitude of the thermal vibrations before and after electron capture. The large arrow represents the amplitude of the lattice vibrations about the new equilibrium position immediately after electron capture (Ref. 54).

As described by Lang and Henry,[53,54] nonradiative capture of minority carriers can sometimes occur as the result of the variation in the energy of a deep trap as the crystal lattice vibrates. Thus, as illustrated in Fig. 8.3-8, the energy of the trap E_t extends over a range that can overlap the conduction band edge and nonradiatively capture an injected electron.[54] Subsequently the lattice relaxes so as to lower the energy of the level. Immediately upon electron capture the lattice is considerably distorted from its equilibrium configuration so that there is a violent lattice vibration localized near the trap. The vibration will rapidly damp down to the amplitude of the thermal vibrations by the emission of multiple phonons. The configuration coordinate diagram is given in Fig. 8.3-9. It shows the model in which the trap is a potential well U_t that can bind an electron. The energies of the conduction and valence band edges U_c and U_v also vary as the lattice vibrates.

The capture of the minority electron (or hole) in this manner can give rise to the low-temperature defect motion that is usually called recombination-enhanced defect motion. Weeks et al.[55] have analyzed the introduction of the recombination energy into the lattice in terms of unimolecular reaction

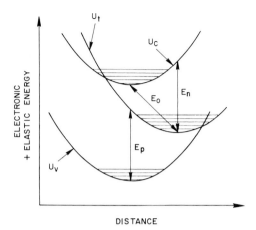

FIG. 8.3-9   The configuration coordinate diagram for energy versus distance. E_p and E_n are the optical excitation thresholds at equilibrium before and after recombination. The energies of the conduction and valance band edges are U_c and U_v, and the trap energy is U_t (Ref. 53).

rate theory and find that the annealing behavior of defects in GaAs is consistent with a reasonable theoretical interpretation. A direct connection between the frequently observed phenomenon of recombination-enhanced defect motion and the recombination requirement for DLD growth has not been established. Nevertheless, it seems obvious that if climb is important for DLD growth, the required point defects probably do have their motion enhanced by carrier recombination.

It is useful to note the more recent work of Shen et al.[56,57] with $InP|Ga_xIn_{1-x}P_yAs_{1-y}|InP$ DH lasers. The lattice match at the $InP-Ga_xIn_{1-x}P_yAs_{1-y}$ heterojunction must be achieved by precise compositional control during the epitaxial growth. It seems reasonable to expect that, with such lasers, difficulties due to DLD growth as the result of the presence of mismatch dislocations and strain would be encountered. However, cw operation without observable degradation for more than 5000 hr has been obtained.[57] These tests were still underway at the time of this writing. This result suggests that because the narrower-energy-gap material provides less nonradiative recombination energy for defect motion than does $Al_xGa_{1-x}As$, degradation in the $InP-Ga_xIn_{1-x}P_yAs_{1-y}$ lasers is appreciably slower.

Reduction of Dark-Line Defects

Whatever the mechanism of DLD growth, it is clear that to increase the cw life of injection lasers beyond minutes to hours, the DLD had to be eliminated. Most of the initial progress that was made in increasing laser life resulted from elimination of the DLD that starts to grow almost immediately upon initial operation of the devices. Elimination of the DLD is achieved primarily by the prevention of the source dislocations by careful bonding of the laser to the heat sink, usually with In in order to minimize strain. Therefore, if the dislocation density in the substrate is relatively low ($\lesssim 1 \times 10^3/\text{cm}^2$), then each ($\sim 400$ μm $\times$ 10 μm) stripe-geometry laser has a fairly small ($\lesssim 4\%$) chance of incorporating a dislocation if new defects have not been introduced during crystal growth or device fabrication. A burn-in test period can be used to eliminate most devices that fail rapidly due to DLD's.

The most obvious source of defects, particulate matter, has been shown to generate stacking faults and dislocations in GaAs–Al$_x$Ga$_{1-x}$As layers,[33] and Ishii et al.[58] have demonstrated that oxygen contamination during LPE can have a profound effect upon defect concentration. The use of small amounts of Al in the laser active region to slightly increase the lasing photon energy (Chapter 5) also improves reliability because the added Al getters oxygen. The success that has been achieved in drastically reducing the probability of DLD formation in fabricated lasers has resulted from the care paid to cleanliness and gas purity during heteroepitaxial wafer growth, and the use of fabrication techniques that eliminate bonding strain. The careful inspection, such as that reported by Goodwin et al.[59] for defects in the grown wafer, has also been beneficial.

8.4 GRADUAL DEGRADATION OF GaAs–Al$_x$Ga$_{1-x}$As STRIPE-GEOMETRY LASERS

The achievement of "useful operating life" has permitted many potential applications of heterostructure lasers. However, there is no uniform definition of laser operating life and each worker tends to use his own. To circumvent this difficulty, the appropriate time and the reported operating conditions will be given for each case that is considered. Hartman et al.[60] first produced stripe-geometry GaAs–Al$_x$Ga$_{1-x}$As DH lasers with operating life exceeding 1000 hr in a 30°C nitrogen ambient atmosphere by paying particular attention to processing cleanliness and reduction of bonding strain. The 13-μm-wide stripes were produced by proton bombardment. They were operated at constant current starting at $I = 1.3I_{th}$, and at least one degraded only 10% from its initial 10-mW output from one mirror after several thousand hours of operation. Nakada et al.[61] obtained several thousand hours of cw operation at high output power of 40–50 mW from one mirror with an increase in J_{th} of about 20%. Their devices were carefully selected and mounted 40-μm-wide mesa-stripe lasers. Nakada et al.[61] periodically readjusted the diode current to maintain 40-mW operation. An additional feature of their lasers was the inclusion of Al ($x = 0.05$) in the active region. There have been indications by other workers[62,63] that a small Al addition to the active region improved crystal growth and degradation behavior. The results of Ishii et al.[58] suggest that this improvement results from gettering of oxygen and thus the removal of gross defects and the resulting DLD's. Kan et al.[64] have shown that the use of procedures to eliminate oxygen permits long operating life of over 1×10^4 hr for lasers with GaAs active regions. Double-heterostructure lasers that can operate continuously for thousands of hours apparently require the elimination of the early forming DLD by the use of substrates with low dislocation densities, ultraclean processing, and low-strain bonding.

The achievement of lasers that did not degrade by the formation of a DLD and therefore operated for thousands of hours at room temperature made it desirable to use a testing procedure that would permit studies in a shorter time. Hartman and Dixon[65] described studies of proton-bombardment-defined stripe-geometry DH lasers operated cw in dry-nitrogen ambient atmosphere at temperatures of 30°, 50°, 70°, and 90°C. Two groups of lasers were used, one with GaAs active regions and $Al_{0.36}Ga_{0.64}As$ waveguide layers, while the second had a small amount of phosphorus added to the ternary solutions before growth. In the latter case, the proper amount of phosphorus reduces grown in lattice stress[66,67] that results from the slight mismatch between GaAs and $Al_xGa_{1-x}As$.

Hartman and Dixon[65] studied laser life by operating the lasers cw at 30% above the threshold current (corresponding to 5–10 mW of optical output per mirror). The current was adjusted to restore the same power when the output had decayed by about 50%. The experiments were terminated when a "useful" output of 1 mW could no longer be maintained. When the operating life as defined above is plotted at the junction temperature for a number of lasers, an activation energy E_A for the operating life τ is obtained by assuming that

$$\tau(T) = K \exp(E_A/kT). \tag{8.4-1}$$

This representation may be oversimplified, but the data for the best of these lasers were consistent with $E_A \approx 0.7$ eV, and extrapolated τ of 10^5 hr at room temperature appeared feasible.[65]

Statistical studies by Joyce et al.[68] and Hartman et al.[69] of the distribution of the time-to-failure for several groups of lasers that were temperature stress tested in a manner very similar to the lasers of Ref. 65 are particularly interesting. The lasers for those studies were proton-bombarded stripe-geometry $Al_{0.36}Ga_{0.64}As|Al_{0.08}Ga_{0.92}As|Al_{0.36}Ga_{0.64}As$ DH lasers intended for optical fiber communication systems. The lasers for the earlier study by Joyce et al.[68] were fabricated from twelve consecutively grown LPE wafers that were not preselected. Twenty-five percent of those lasers were initially rejected for failure to meet voltage and current requirements. Of the remaining lasers, 104 were randomly selected for testing by cw operation at 70°C in a dry-nitrogen ambient atmosphere. An additional selection was made by rejecting from the statistical distribution, fourteen lasers that failed during the first 10 hr of operation. The emission was about 5 mW output per mirror with a drive current less than 30% above $J_{th}(70°C)$. The initial light output at 70°C was maintained by periodic increases in the drive current. When the laser would no longer emit 0.5 mW per face of predominantly coherent radiation at 70°C it was taken to have failed. As with the work of Ref. 65, the operating conditions and failure criteria for the studies of Ref. 68 are arbitrary. They do, however, provide very useful insight into the gradual degradation behavior of DH lasers. The set of data labeled A in Fig. 8.4-1 shows the time to failure of each of the lasers. The lognormal plot of Fig. 8.4-1 is linear for lasers that lived more than 100 hr.

The more recent studies by Hartman et al.[69] were done with selected wafers. Randomly chosen lasers from those wafers had been observed to have longer lives, on the average, than lasers from the wafers used for data set A of

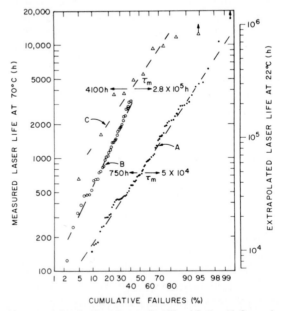

FIG. 8.4-1   Measured distribution of operating life of GaAs–Al$_x$Ga$_{1-x}$As DH lasers aged in a 70°C dry nitrogen ambient. The median operating life is τ_m. Extrapolated room temperature operating lives are 67 times longer assuming an activation energy $E_A = 0.7$ eV. ● Unselected wafers (Ref. 68). ○ Selected wafers (Ref. 69). △ One selected wafer (Ref. 69a). The symbols ● and △ indicate that these lasers were still operating.

Fig. 8.4-1. No other selection was done, and additional lasers from those wafers were chosen randomly for life testing using an identical testing procedure to that described above. The 70°C life tests for the lasers from selected wafers were still underway at the time the data were plotted and about 60% of the lasers were still operating. The data set labeled B in Fig. 8.4-1 represents the failure distribution for most of the 40% that had failed. The data set labeled C in Fig. 8.4-1 is for one of the selected wafers for which tests had begun earlier and for which nine out of the ten lasers studied had failed at the time the data were plotted. These plots suggest, but do not prove, that failure results from a single dominant failure mechanism over the range of times covered by the lasers included in the linear plot. Also, it suggests that an order-of-magnitude or greater increase in lifetime would result from elimination of the unknown failure mechanism.

Joyce et al.[68] and Hartman et al.[69] have chosen to additionally character-ize the distribution of Fig. 8.4-1 by the median life of 750 hr at 70°C. As with the work of Ref. 65, the further assumption was made that a temperature change is equivalent to a constant factor change in the rate of passage of time. This assumption is now rendered more plausible by the absence of evidence of more than one failure mechanism in the groups of lasers studied. From Ref. 65, E_A in Eq. (8.4-1) was conservatively taken as 0.7 eV to yield the extrapolated laser life at 22°C given on the right side of Fig. 8.4-1. The temperatures given are ambient heat sink temperatures. The corresponding junction temperature at 70° and 22°C ambient temperature under the condi-tions of the experiment are 95° and 29°C, respectively. For the set of lasers represented by plots A and C, the predicted median lifetimes τ_m at 22°C are 5×10^4 hr and 2.8×10^5 hr, respectively, at the time the data were plotted. The data set labeled B gave a median 70°C life of 4500 hr for the 100 lasers randomly selected from the 10 wafers. This 70°C median lifetime is thought to correspond to 3×10^5 hr (34 yrs) of continuous operation at 22°C and a mean-time-to-failure of 1×10^6 hr.[69] Although the speculative nature of this treatment must be kept in mind, it suggests that very long laser lifetimes are already at hand. Furthermore, the scatter in the data suggest that much further improvement will result from improvement in processing procedures.

The definition of laser life described here is expected to be useful for lasers intended for fiber-optic communications systems. Definitions of laser life that differ from those used in the studies of Ref. 65, 68, and 69 may be expected to be for higher power output and for operation without increasing the current to maintain light output. In either of those instances, the redefined laser life will be shorter than for the conditions described above.

The normalized light output at constant current versus operating time for a long-lived laser that was aged at 70°C is shown in Fig. 8.4-2.[69] This figure also illustrates that the lasing emission spectrum broadens and

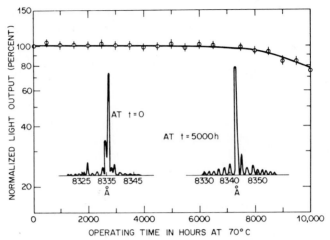

FIG. 8.4-2   Constant-current light output versus time for a typical long-lived laser operated at 70°C ambient. The spectra are typical for those observed in the long-lived proton-bombarded stripe-geometry DH lasers (Ref. 69.).

shifts to slightly longer wavelengths. For lasers that have been aged sufficiently to require a current increase to maintain an emission power per mirror face greater than 1 mW, the spectrum broadening may be quite pronounced with many new longitudinal modes appearing. When long-lived lasers are aged to the point where they no longer can maintain the required minimum output power at 70°C, their spontaneous emission has decreased by about 50% at a given current, and failure is preceded by a significant decrease in differential quantum efficiency.[70] These observations are consistent with a uniform decrease in quantum efficiency in the active region such as would be caused by nonradiative defects that are uniformly distributed. Optical output nonlinearities (kinks) show no systematic change with degradation and dark-line defects are generally not observed.

Unfortunately, there is presently very little information available that would permit a much deeper understanding of the failure mechanism for these long-lived lasers. Joyce *et al.*[68] point out that the lognormal distribution would not be expected if the lasers were initially all equivalent and then died from random nucleation of DLD's. The distribution can be interpreted in terms of a single mechanism that kills each laser at a rate that is fixed by growth and/or processing variations that result in initially inequivalent lasers. This is consistent with earlier observations[68] that similar relatively long-lived lasers exhibited uniform degradation without DLD's. However, it tells very little about what that uniform degradation mechanism might be.

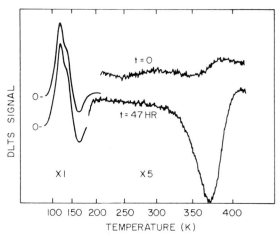

FIG. 8.4-3 DLTS spectra of a typical laser before ($t = 0$) and after ($t = 47$ hr) accelerated aging at 70°C. Note the large increase in the negative peak at 370°K (0.89-eV trap) (Ref. 71).

A clue may be provided by DLTS studies of degraded DH $Al_xGa_{1-x}As|Al_yGa_{1-y}As|Al_xGa_{1-x}As$ proton-bombarded stripe-geometry lasers by Lang et al.[71] These lasers, in which x was varied from 0.2 to 0.4 and y from 0 to 0.1, were aged at 70°C under conditions identical to those studied by Joyce et al.[68] The DLTS spectra shown in Fig. 8.4-3 consisted of three dominant peaks: two comparatively shallow peaks, one positive and one negative, near 125° and 175°K, and a very deep peak near 370°K. The very deep peak is a majority carrier trap with an activation energy of 0.89 eV. The original studies[71] suggested that the comparatively shallow peaks were a minority carrier trap and a majority carrier trap with activation energies of 0.21 and 0.31 eV, respectively. More recently, Lang and Logan[72] have speculated that the shallow peaks may result from a single trap with the 0.21-eV peak due to electron capture and the 0.31-eV peak due to electron emission. All of the peaks increase during aging of the laser although the change for the 0.89-eV peak is most obvious.

Figure 8.4-4 shows the magnitude of the 0.89-eV trap signal as a function of aging time at 70°C for a dozen lasers from four different wafers. Wafers 1–3 produced lasers that lived from several hundred to several thousand hours. These lasers seem to be typical of the range of lasers shown in set A of Fig. 8.4-1. They presumably die by the same unknown mechanism. For all of them, the 0.89 eV trap increases very rapidly during the first 100 hr of operation and more slowly thereafter for lasers that lived longer. While this correlation is probably significant, it is important to note that during the

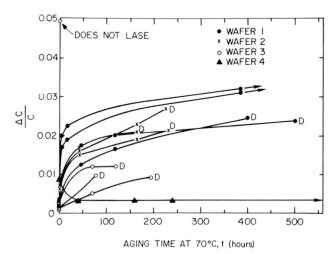

AGING TIME AT 70°C, t (hours)

FIG. 8.4-4 Normalized DLTS signal of the 0.89-eV trap in lasers from four wafers as a function of cw operating time at 70°C. The DLTS signal is ΔC, and the laser capacitance is C. The point at which a laser ceases to operate is denoted by the letter D. Lasers which operated longer than 500 hr at 70°C are denoted by an arrow at the end of the curve (Ref. 71).

rapid increase in the trap concentration a simple and consistent relationship to threshold current density behavior is not observed. Perhaps more significant is the observation for wafer 4. For that wafer the deep-trap signal actually decreased with time and when aged by the procedures used for the lasers of Ref. 68, these lasers lasted for very long times, some longer than 1.5×10^4 hr at $70°C$.[36] This extrapolates to about 10^6 hr at room temperature.

Deep-level transient spectroscopy studies of structures with varying degrees of proton bombardment damage showed that the 0.89-eV trap is associated with proton damage and is not seen in unbombarded devices. Related studies showed that it is present at the damage–undamaged interface in the $N-Al_xGa_{1-x}As$ layer and that it is very likely the so-called E3 radiation-damage electron trap observed in 1-MeV-irradiated GaAs.[73] Recent studies by Lang et al.[74] suggest that it is a Ga vacancy. These observations seem to show that the E3 defect moves from the high-concentration proton-bombarded region to the undamaged waveguide region during laser operation. However, since only the $N-Al_xGa_{1-x}As$ region can be studied in these lasers with p-type active regions, the connection to what happens in the active region has not been directly made. Nevertheless the DLTS studies suggest that mobile point defects are closely associated with gradual degradation and that their influence can potentially be minimized to yield very long lived lasers.

A form of gradual degradation that has been observed in GaAs–$Al_xGa_{1-x}As$ lasers by many workers is mirror damage characterized by roughening or discoloration of the laser mirror surface. Kressel and Ladany[11] have observed mirror damage to occur in stripe-geometry lasers run cw at relatively high powers of 25–100 mW per mirror. The extent of such damage after a given operating time depends upon the power. For unprotected mirrors on lasers run in dry air, the mirror damage was observed to significantly affect the emitted power after several thousand hours of operation. Mirror damage may reasonably be expected to be a source of gradual degradation for lasers run cw at lower power. Shima et al.[75] and Chinone et al.[76] observed facet damage to be a major cause of gradual degradation in their lasers, and Dixon and Hartman[70] have observed very shallow damage to the mirror surfaces in lasers run cw at low power for long periods of time ($> 10^4$ hr) in dry nitrogen.

Studies of the mechanism of facet damage during cw operation have been done by Yuasa et al.[77] Using Auger electron spectroscopy, they found that an oxide layer formed on the mirror surface during lasing. Both the initial rapid laser degradation during the first hundred hours of operation and the subsequent slow degradation were attributed to the buildup of this oxide layer. These observations are consistent with measurements by Suzuki and Ogawa[78] on the optical enhanced oxidation of GaAs surfaces.

Dixon and Hartman[70] found that mirror damage under the conditions of their experiments, including the 70°C studies already described, occurs reproducibly and is always present. However, in their lasers it has no observable effect on the threshold current density. This result is clearly established from the work of Ref. 70, in which gradual degradation of lasers similar to those of Refs. 68 and 69 were studied. In that work, half of the lasers were studied as LED's in which there was no mirror damage and half as lasers and showed characteristic noncatastrophic mirror damage. By using the same failure criteria as in Refs. 68 and 69, the statistical failure distribution was the same for both groups when corrected for active region temperature.

Obviously much more experimentation is required. In particular, it is not established whether the differences in the extent of mirror damage observed by different workers results from differences in the lasers, differences in the testing procedures, or both. In any case, Kressel and Ladany,[11] Yuasa et al.,[77] and Ladany et al.[79] claim that mirror damage may be prevented by protection of the mirror surfaces with dielectric coatings. Shima et al.[75] find that CVD Al_2O_3 coatings are superior to SiO_2 for this purpose.

Recently, Paoli[80] has observed that changes in the optical properties of cw lasers may occur during the early stage of operation, without any corresponding change in J_{th}. He studied proton-bombarded stripe-geometry

$Al_{0.36}Ga_{0.64}As|Al_{0.08}Ga_{0.92}As|Al_{0.36}Ga_{0.64}As$ DH lasers during cw operation at 70°C for 50–60 hr. During these studies no statistically important changes in $J_{th}(70°C)$ occurred and the light output, both TE (lasing) and TM (spontaneous), was not the same from opposite mirrors in about 60% of the lasers. The emission asymmetry increased with accelerated aging, but appeared to be uncorrelated to changes in $J_{th}(70°C)$. The most striking change that was observed was the development of regular self-induced laser intensity pulsations at room temperature in about half of the lasers studied. These pulsations are possibly similar to pulses observed by Yang et al.[81] and are illustrated in Fig. 8.4-5. The frequency of these pulsations was as low as 200 MHz but typically is much higher. This behavior occurred even in lasers

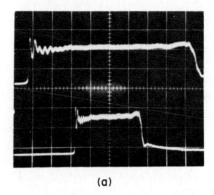

(a)

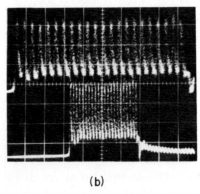

(b)

FIG. 8.4-5   Time variation of the output intensity from a DH laser operated pulsed with a dc bias current. Part (a) shows the stable behavior of the device prior to aging, and part (b) shows the sustained pulsations occurring after continuous operation at 70°C for 50 hr. For both (a) and (b) the current is 13% above the threshold and the horizontal scale is 2 nsec/div for the top trace and 5 nsec/div for the bottom trace (Ref. 80).

that initially exhibited no intensity modulation. These pulsations appeared to be uncorrelated to initial asymmetry, changes in threshold current density, axial nonuniformities in pumping current, or the formation of DLD's. Nevertheless, their appearance at the initial stage of aging demonstrates that changes occurred that were not initially revealed by changes in threshold or efficiency.

8.5 CONCLUDING COMMENTS

In this chapter, a number of empirical observations of the ways in which injection lasers fail have been described. Although a detailed mechanism has not been elucidated for it, catastrophic degradation of GaAs–$Al_xGa_{1-x}As$ lasers appears to represent a fundamental limitation of the peak optical power permissible at the laser cavity and air interface. If, as has been suggested here, this limitation results from surface recombination and absorption in the surface-space charge region near the cleaved mirror, modifications to the structure that reduce surface recombination and absorption will increase the power possible at the damage limit.

Fundamental studies of deep traps and radiation-enhanced defect motion have provided insight into the mechanism by which the DLD grows. It seems reasonable to expect that continued work will eventually lead to a detailed understanding of the DLD. However, it has already been determined empirically that this cause of rapid degradation can be largely eliminated by care in substrate selection, strain-free fabrication and ultraclean processing.

An understanding of the mechanisms of gradual degradation of GaAs–$Al_xGa_{1-x}As$ stripe-geometry DH lasers has not been achieved. The development of new experimental techniques that will permit studies leading to an understanding of the way in which point defects are generated, move, and are eliminated is of vital importance. In addition, the long tedious process of life testing of a variety of laser structures under a variety of operating conditions, and the subsequent detailed examination of degraded devices is still underway. However, much progress has been made toward extending laser operating life and no intrinsic failure mechanism has been uncovered.

This progress is illustrated with data from a program at Bell Laboratories in Fig. 8.5-1.[82] Two plots of extrapolated laser life at room temperature that were obtained during the period 1970 through 1976 are shown. The lasers studied are stripe-geometry DH lasers with proton-bombardment-defined stripes that were usually temperature stress tested at low power in a manner identical to that described in Ref. 68. The upper curve shows the expected useful life of the best lasers encountered at a given time, and the lower curve shows the corresponding expected life for lasers that could be obtained reproducibly in the laboratory. There are at least existence proofs[36]

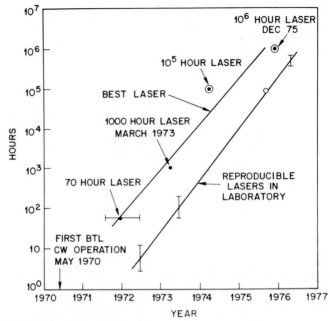

FIG. 8.5-1   Laser life at 22°C under low-power operation (<10 mW) for proton-bombarded stripe-geometry GaAs–Al$_x$Ga$_{1-x}$As DH lasers studied from 1970 through 1976 during a program at Bell Laboratories. The data were obtained from extrapolation of experimental data at elevated temperature. The upper curve shows the estimated 22°C life of the best lasers obtained at a given time. The lower curve shows the estimated life of lasers that could be obtained reproducibly in the laboratory at the time (Ref. 82).

for real-time, low-power (<10 mW per mirror) cw operation longer than 2.6×10^4 hr (3 yr) at 30°C. If the simple extrapolations of Ref. 65 are used for the data of Refs. 68 and 69, there are, as shown in Fig. 8.5-1, also existence proofs for similar operation of a few lasers for more than 10^6 hr at a 22°C heat sink temperature. Such long life at low power may meet the requirements for large scale lightwave communications systems. Most other applications will be less demanding of long life but will require higher power. The studies of Nakada[61] and of Kressel and Ladany[11] suggest that for output powers in the 20–40 mW range per mirror, it is reasonable to expect almost 1×10^4 hr of operation at the present state-of-the-art without very drastic reduction in light output or increase in lasing threshold. Initial correlation by Lang et al.[71] of point defects with gradual degradation and the observations by Paoli[80] of early changes in emission symmetry and aging dependent self pulsations show the need for more study and basic understanding of the degradation processes. It is possible that the early monitoring of such changes will provide a tool for the prediction of the behavior of lasers over longer periods of time of operation.

REFERENCES

1. D. P. Cooper, C. H. Gooch, and R. J. Sherwell, *IEEE J. Quantum Electron.* **QE-2**, 329 (1966).
2. C. D. Dobson and F. S. Keeble, "Gallium Arsenide: 1966 Symposium Proceedings," p. 68. Inst. of Phys. and Phys. Soc., London, 1967.
3. D. A. Shaw and P. R. Thornton, *Solid-State Electron.* **13**, 919 (1970).
4. H. Kressel and H. Mierop, *J. Appl. Phys.* **38**, 5419 (1967).
5. C. J. Hwang, *J. Appl. Phys.* **42**, 4408 (1971).
6. H. Kressel, H. Nelson, and F. Z. Hawrylo, *J. Appl. Phys.* **41**, 2019 (1970).
7. H. Kressel, H. S. Sommers, Jr., H. F. Lockwood, and M. Ettenberg, Tech. Rep. AFAL-TR-71-83 (April 1971).
8. H. Kressel, "Lasers" (A. K. Levine and A. J. DeMaria, eds.), Vol. 3, pp. 1–110. Dekker, New York, 1971.
9. B. W. Hakki and F. R. Nash, *J. Appl. Phys.* **45**, 3907 (1974).
10. P. A. Kirkby and G. H. B. Thompson, *Appl. Phys. Lett.* **22**, 638 (1973).
11. H. Kressel and I. Ladany, *RCA Rev.* **36**, 230 (1975).
12. H. F. Lockwood, H. Kressel, H. S. Sommers, Jr., and F. Z. Hawrylo, *Appl. Phys. Lett.* **17**, 499 (1970).
13. M. Ettenberg, H. S. Sommer, Jr., H. Kressel, and H. F. Lockwood, *Appl. Phys. Lett.* **18**, 571 (1971).
14. G. P. Henshall, *Solid-State Electron.* **20**, 595 (1977).
15. C. H. Henry, P. M. Petroff, and R. A. Logan, to be published.
16. B. C. De Loach, Jr., B. W. Hakki, R. L. Hartman, and L. A. D'Asaro, *Proc. IEEE* **61**, 1042 (1973).
17. H. Kressel and N. E. Byer, *Proc. IEEE* **57**, 25 (1969).
18. D. H. Newman and S. Ritchie, *IEEE J. Quantum Electron.* **QE-9**, 300 (1973).
19. H. Kressel, N. E. Byer, H. F. Lockwood, F. Z. Hawrylo, H. Nelson, M. S. Abrahams, and S. H. McFarlane, *Metall. Trans.* **1**, 635 (1970).
20. T. L. Paoli and B. W. Hakki, *J. Appl. Phys.* **44**, 4108 (1973).
21. B. W. Hakki and T. L. Paoli, *J. Appl. Phys.* **44**, 4113 (1973).
22. J. R. Biard, G. E. Pittman, and J. F. Leezer, "Gallium Arsenide: 1966 Symposium Proceedings," p. 113. Inst. of Phys. and the Phys. Soc., London, 1967.
23. K. H. Zschauer, *Solid State Commun.* **7**, 335 (1969).
24. R. L. Hartman and A. R. Hartman, *Appl. Phys. Lett.* **23**, 147 (1973).
25. H. Yonezu, I. Sakuma, T. Kamejima, M. Ueno, K. Nishida, Y. Nannichi, and I. Hayashi, *Appl. Phys. Lett.* **24**, 18 (1974).
26. D. W. Johnston, Jr., W. M. Callahan, and B. I. Miller, *J. Appl. Phys.* **45**, 505 (1974).
27. P. M. Petroff, W. D. Johnston, Jr., and R. L. Hartman, *Appl. Phys. Lett.* **25**, 226 (1974).
28. R. Ito, H. Nakashima, and O. Nakada, *Jpn. J. Appl. Phys.* **13**, 1321 (1974).
29. P. M. Petroff and R. L. Hartman, *Appl. Phys. Lett.* **23**, 469 (1973).
30. P. M. Petroff and R. L. Hartman, *J. Appl. Phys.* **45**, 3899 (1974).
31. P. W. Hutchinson and P. S. Dobson, *Phil. Mag.* **32**, 745 (1975).

32. P. W. Hutchinson, P. S. Dobson, S. O'Hara, and D. H. Newman, *Appl. Phys. Lett.* **26**, 250 (1975).
33. G. R. Woolhouse, A. E. Blakeslee, and K. K. Shih, *J. Appl. Phys.* **47**, 4349 (1976).
34. P. M. Petroff and R. L. Hartman, Private communication.
35. P. M. Petroff and L. C. Kimerling, *Appl. Phys. Lett.* **29**, 461 (1976).
36. R. L. Hartman, Private communication.
37. J. Matsui, K. Ishida, and Y. Nannichi, *Jpn. J. Appl. Phys.* **14**, 1555 (1975).
38. Y. Nannichi, J. Matsui, and K. Ishida, *Jpn. J. Appl. Phys.* **14**, 1561 (1975).
39. D. V. Lang, R. A. Logan, and M. Jaros, Phys. Rev., to be published.
40. P. M. Petroff and L. C. Kimerling, unpublished.
41. J. Friedel, "Dislocations," p. 105. Addison-Wesley, Reading Massachusetts, 1964.
42. J. A. Van Vechten, *J. Electrochem Soc.* **122**, 1556 (1975).
43. S. O'Hara, P. W. Hutchinson, and P. S. Dobson, *Appl. Phys. Lett.* **30**, 368 (1977).
44. T. Kobayashi, T. Kawakami, and Y. Furukawa, *Jpn. J. Appl. Phys.* **14**, 508 (1975).
45. T. Kobayashi and Y. Furukawa, *Jpn. J. Appl. Phys.* **14**, 1175 (1975).
46. T. Kamejima, K. Ishida, and J. Matsui, *Jpn. J. Appl. Phys.* **16**, 233 (1977).
47. L. C. Kimerling, P. M. Petroff, and H. J. Leamy, *Appl. Phys. Lett.* **28**, 297 (1976).
48. D. V. Lang, *J. Appl. Phys.* **45**, 3023 (1974).
49. D. V. Lang and L. C. Kimerling, *Phys. Rev. Lett.* **33**, 489 (1974).
50. D. V. Lang and L. C. Kimerling, *Appl. Phys. Lett.* **28**, 248 (1976).
51. D. V. Lang, L. C. Kimerling, and S. Y. Leung, *J. Appl. Phys.* **47**, 3587 (1976).
52. L. C. Kimerling and D. V. Lang, "Lattice Defects in Semiconductors 1974," Inst. Phys. Conf. Ser. No. 23, p. 589, Inst. Phys., London, 1975.
52a. D. V. Lang, Private communication.
53. D. V. Lang and C. H. Henry, *Phys. Rev. Lett.* **35**, 1525 (1975).
54. C. H. Henry and D. V. Lang, *Phys. Rev. B* **15**, 989 (1977).
55. J. D. Weeks, J. C. Tully, and L. C. Kimerling, *Phys. Rev. B* **12**, 3286 (1975).
56. C. C. Shen, J. J. Hsieh, and T. A. Lind, *Appl. Phys. Lett.* **30**, 353 (1977).
57. C. C. Shen, Private communication.
58. M. Ishii, H. Kan, W. Susaki, and Y. Ogata, *Appl. Phys. Lett.* **29**, 375 (1976).
59. A. R. Goodwin, P. A. Kirkby, J. R. Peters, and M. Pion, *IEEE Semicond. Laser Conf., Nemu-No-Sato, Japan* (September 1976).
60. R. L. Hartman, J. C. Dyment, C. J. Hwang, and M. Kuhn, *Appl. Phys. Lett.* **23**, 181 (1973).
61. O. Nakada, N. Chinone, S. Nakamura, H. Nakashima, and R. Ito, *Jpn. J. Appl. Phys.* **13**, 485 (1974).
62. Y. Nannichi and I. Hayashi, *J. Cryst. Growth* **27**, 126 (1974).
63. M. Ettenberg, H. Kressel, and H. F. Lockwood, *Appl. Phys. Lett.* **25**, 82 (1974).
64. H. Kan, H. Namizaki M. Ishii, and A. Ito, *Appl. Phys. Lett.* **27**, 138 (1975).
65. R. L. Hartman and R. W. Dixon, *Appl. Phys. Lett.* **26**, 239 (1975).
66. G. A. Rozgonyi and M. B. Panish, *Appl. Phys. Lett.* **23**, 533 (1973).
67. G. A. Rozgonyi, P. M. Petroff, and M. B. Panish, *J. Cryst. Growth* **27**, 106 (1974).
68. W. B. Joyce, R. W. Dixon, and R. L. Hartman, *Appl. Phys. Lett.* **28**, 684 (1976).
69. R. L. Hartman, N. E. Schumaker, and R. W. Dixon, *Appl. Phys. Lett.* **31**, 756 (1977).
69a. R. L. Hartman, N. E. Schumaker, and R. W. Dixon, Private communication.
70. R. W. Dixon and R. L. Hartman, *J. Appl. Phys.* **48**, 3225 (1977).
71. D. V. Lang, R. L. Hartman, and N. E. Schumaker, *J. Appl. Phys.* **47**, 4986 (1976).
72. D. V. Lang and R. A. Logan, Private communication.
73. D. V. Lang and L. C. Kimerling, "Lattice Defects in Semiconductors 1974," Inst. Phys. Conf. Ser. No. 23, p. 581. Inst. Phys., London, 1975.

74. D. V. Lang, R. A. Logan, and L. C. Kimerling, *Phys. Rev. B* **15**, 4874 (1977).
75. Y. Shima, N. Chinone, and R. Ito, *IEEE Semicond. Laser Conf.*, *Nemu-No-Sato, Japan* (September 1976).
76. N. Chinone, H. Nakashima, and R. Ito, *J. Appl. Phys.* **48**, 1160 (1977).
77. T. Yuasa, M. Ogawa, K. Endo, and H. Yonezu, *Digest of Late Papers, 1977 Intern. Conf. Integrated Optics and Optical Fiber Communication*, July 18–20, Tokyo, p. 13.
78. T. Suzuki and M. Ogawa, *Appl. Phys. Lett.* **31**, 473 (1977).
79. I. Ladany, M. Ettenberg, H. F. Lockwood, and H. Kressel, *Appl. Phys. Lett.* **30**, 87 (1977).
80. T. L. Paoli, Techn. Digest 1976 Int. Electron. Devices meeting p. 136 (1976).
81. E. S. Yang, P. G. McMullin, A. W. Smith, J. Blum, and K. K. Shih, *Appl. Phys. Lett.* **24**, 324 (1974).
82. B. C. De Loach Jr., Private communication.

INDEX FOR PART A